Infections and Inequalities

"A strangely uplifting read. . . . One starts this book with a sense of help-lessness . . . reading on, though, Farmer's lived example gradually engen-ders hope. As a founder member of the non-governmental organisation Partners in Health he is, through direct action and a genuinely humble al-truism, making a difference. His work is burnished by a heartening moral-ity and a demonstration of high ideals made reality. There is a painful awareness that these are drops in an ocean, but rather than overwhelm, the result is to inspire." *The Guardian* (London)

"In *Infections and Inequalities*, Paul Farmer, who was trained in both infec-tious diseases and anthropology, uses these disciplines and his medical experience in Haiti to provide a trenchant analysis of the biologic and so-cial realities of chronic infectious disease." *New England Journal of Medicine*

"Farmer's meticulous description of the stories of some patients, and of the circumstances in which they live, reminds us of the enormous suffering of a large part of humanity that has practically no access to the most basic medical care. Even today, entire family groups unacceptably succumb to tuberculosis, the world's leading infectious cause of death, despite the fact that effective treatment has been available for many decades."
British Medical Journal

"Farmer's ability to integrate poignant case studies with epidemiological data and structural analysis are very effective in highlighting the barriers to appropriate care—either primary or tertiary care—and countering the shibboleths about infectious disease being a result of poor compliance."
Social Science and Medicine

"In every speech and in all his books, Farmer is at pains to assert the inter-connectedness of the rich and poor parts of the world. . . . Most modern descriptions of human behavior give selfishness great explanatory power, even over what look like selfless acts. But after I'd spent a month with Farmer altruism had begun to seem plausible, even normal."
Tracy Kidder, *The New Yorker*

"Bolstered by thorough knowledge of the countries in which he practiced, relevant and cogent case histories, and a caring but disciplined attitude, Farmer powerfully argues for substantial changes in epidemiological the-ory and practice. He raises thought-provoking and necessary questions, and he provides answers that, if often unsettling, are pertinent and capa-ble of being put to use by individuals and governments truly interested in solving, not sidestepping, life-threatening situations."
William Beatty, *Booklist*

"In his moving and angry book [Farmer] gives a real-time account of contemporary plagues—AIDS and tuberculosis in Haiti and Peru. It is a truly *fin de siécle* story of unfinished business with an old plague, the fight against a new one, and immorality—immorality because effective remedies are there but are being unreasonably and unfairly denied. Technical incompetents, stiff-necked bureaucrats, hard-hearted capitalists, altruistic priests and starving peasants are all there as well. The only things that distinguish Farmer's account from a Dostoevskian novel is a meed of hard, effective science and a depressingly familiar story of the powerfully malignant effects of racism. . . . It is hard to think of more compelling examples to underpin his arguments. It makes the book and its message accessible to the general reader and forcefully reminds doctors, nurses, scientists, sociologists, economists and aid workers of their unfinished business. . . . But the main lessons he draws are for us all. We must do all we can to diminish social inequality."

Hugh Pennington, *The Times Higher Education Supplement*

"Farmer's work diverges strikingly from the current 'emerging infectious disease' literature, much of which misses essential points about causation that Farmer brings out very well. . . . It is sure to appeal to those general readers attracted to books like Garrett's *The Coming Plague*, as well as to readers in medicine, public health, and the sociomedical sciences."

Frederick L. Dunn, M.D.

"Farmer argues against those who would insist that the health problems of the poor require and must await structural changes, that underdevelopment negates the efforts of physicians. He believes there is much that doctors can do, not simply as activists but as physicians."

Randall Packard, author of *White Plague, Black Labor*

"The physician Paul Farmer has written a lucid, solid, well-documented book that shows that the epidemiological demon is a social demon. . . . It is no longer adequate to make this case to the rich or for the advocates of the least well off to address the rich on their behalf. It would presage far better things for the improvement of international public health if the poor were to call on Paul Farmer to become the lynchpin of a new Tricontinental movement. . . . Called by a priest to work among peasant farmers, as the densest chapter of his book explains, this physician has genuinely listened to the poor, and he expresses the collective thinking of a people confronting AIDS. This book is a call to action."   *Le Monde Diplomatique*

Infections and Inequalities

Infections and Inequalities

THE MODERN PLAGUES

PAUL FARMER

UNIVERSITY OF CALIFORNIA PRESS
Berkeley   Los Angeles   London

Material included in Chapters 2, 3, 4, 6, and 9 has been adapted from earlier work by the author, which appeared in the following publications: "Social Inequalities and Emerging Infectious Diseases," *Emerging Infectious Diseases* 2, no. 4 (1996): 259–69; "Women, Poverty, and AIDS— An Introduction," in *Women, Poverty, and AIDS: Sex, Drugs, and Structural Violence*, edited by P. E. Farmer, M. Connors, and J. Simmons (Monroe, Maine: Common Courage Press, 1996); "The Exotic and the Mundane: Human Immunodeficiency Virus in Haiti," *Human Nature* 1, no. 4 (1990): 415–46; "Sending Sickness: Sorcery, Politics, and Changing Concepts of AIDS in Rural Haiti," *Medical Anthropology Quarterly* 4, no. 1 (1990): 6–27; and "Social Scientists and the New Tuberculosis," *Social Science and Medicine* 44, no. 3 (1997): 347–58.

University of California Press
Berkeley and Los Angeles, California

University of California Press, Ltd.
London, England

First paperback printing 2001

Library of Congress Cataloging-in-Publication Data
Farmer, Paul, 1959–.
   Infections and inequalities : the modern plagues / Paul Farmer.
     p. cm.
   Includes bibliographic references (p.   ) and index.
   ISBN 0-520-22913-4 (pbk. : alk. paper)
   1. Poor— Health and hygiene.   2. Socially handicapped—Health and hygiene.   3. Communicable diseases—Social aspects.   I. Title.
  RA418.5.P6F37   1998
   306.4'61—DC21   98-23807

Printed in the United States of America
09 08 07 06 05 04 03 02 01
9 8 7 6 5 4 3 2 1

The paper used in this publication meets the minimum requirements of ANSI/NISO Z39.48-1992 (R 1997) (*Permanence of Paper*). ∞

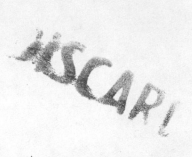

For Haun Saussy,
in celebration of two decades of friendship

The loss of equality was succeeded by the most
appalling disorder. . . . It was at last impossible
for men not to devote some thought to this awful
situation and the calamities that had befallen them.
JEAN-JACQUES ROUSSEAU, *1755*

The health effects of inequality have shown us
how deeply people are affected by these structural
features of our society. But even more important
than the few extra years which great equity would
add to the average length of life is the improvement
in the social quality of life which it would also give
us. Not only is the cost of inequality a cost we incur
for no economic benefit, but all the indications are
that it imposes a substantial economic burden which
reduces the competitiveness of the whole society.
RICHARD WILKINSON, *1996*

Contents

Preface to the Paperback Edition

Anthrax.[1] The word conjures images of germ warfare, which is pretty ridiculous when you discover that we're not really sure anthrax has ever been used in this fashion.[2] Germ warfare is certainly not what came to mind in June of this year, when a six-year-old girl showed up in our clinic with half her face puffed up like a balloon, her right eye swollen shut. We were in rural Haiti, where a very different sort of germ warfare is the rule. So what came to mind that day was the word *epidemic*, and sure enough a young woman from the same village was also diagnosed with cutaneous anthrax—called *charbon* in Haiti, "malignant pustule" in the older textbooks—on her right chest wall. Soon after their arrival, both were receiving intravenous penicillin; they would recover completely.

Later that night, the clinic's medical staff held a meeting. Another anthrax case had been diagnosed a few days earlier, and the patient was from the same area. It seemed increasingly likely that we were dealing with an epidemic. By morning, we learned that a young man from the village had just died of *charbon*. "Why?" I asked the woman who told me the news. "Because he didn't have enough money to get here." It costs no more than four dollars to take a truck from their village to our clinic. It was an epidemic, all right, and it had already taken a life.

In the United States, this conclusion might have provoked little short of calling up the National Guard. But in Haiti we had not triggered much in the way of government response in announcing previous epidemics of communicable disease. Just five months previously, we'd seen several cases of meningococcal meningitis, first diagnosed when a baby presented with what is called purpura fulminans—his skin was covered with distinctive patches of purple hemorrhage. He was in shock. Although he received antibiotics within minutes of reaching the clinic, the infant died while I was trying to get intravenous fluids into a vein, any vein, as his mother stood by wailing.

The baby's death was the harbinger of three more cases of meningococcal disease; the other patients survived. Since the bacterium, *Neisseria meningiditis*, is contagious, we gave family members rifampin, an antibiotic that can kill the organisms before they cause invasive disease. Rifampin, usually reserved for the treatment of tuberculosis, has few serious side effects. But it does cause one rather curious transformation: it turns urine, tears, and other body fluids reddish orange. The doctors and nurses who cared for these meningitis patients also took rifampin prophylaxis. We had so many cases that my urine ran red for a month; I don't recall ever seeing orange tears.

Epidemics of communicable and potentially lethal infections evoke very different official responses in different settings. In Haiti, very *real* epidemics of anthrax and meningococcal meningitis did not even result in an investigation. When I recently asked the beleaguered public-health officer why he did not come to investigate, he responded that, although he did have access to a jeep, he did not have money for gasoline. Meanwhile, in the United States, even the *theoretical possibility* of bioterrorism has moved hundreds of millions of dollars into research and conferences on a subject of dubious public-health significance.[3] The U.S. government has certainly poured substantial resources into preventing and responding to bioterrorism. In January 1999, President Clinton presented to Congress a budget that included $10 billion for antiterrorism efforts, $1.4 billion of which was allocated to biological- and chemical-attack preparedness, a twofold increase from 1997. In his almost incomprehensible remarks announcing the initiative, Clinton allowed that "there is no market for the kind of things we need to develop; and if we are successful there will never be a market for them. But we have got to do our best to develop them."[4] In contrast to these hypothetical epidemics, very real epidemics are being ignored. In a recent editorial, Cohen and colleagues remark, "The proponents of antibioterrorism programmes have it backwards. Instead of pumping more resources into ill advised and risky bioterrorism programmes, we should build national and international public health systems that can adequately reduce, detect, and respond to natural disease outbreaks and industrial chemical spills. Then, in the unlikely event of a bioterrorist attack, these systems will be available to manage the challenge."[5]

Infections and inequalities: in a wealthy country, the specter of biological warfare, for which there is exceedingly slender evidence, triggers a sort of officially blessed paranoia. In a poor country tightly bound to the rich one, real infections continue to kill off the poor, and we are told sternly to look harder for cheaper, more "cost-effective" interventions. At best, those of us working in places like Haiti can hope for trickle-down funds if the plagues of the poor are classed as "U.S. security interests."[6]

I cannot look back at the predictions made in the first edition of this book with the slightest satisfaction. Oh, they've all come true: if you want to feel like a prophet these days, predict that the poor will continue to do poorly, even in boom times. Take tuberculosis. *Infections and Inequalities* made the bold prediction that the poor would continue to die of readily treated tuberculosis and that newer multidrug-resistant strains would continue to spread. On the former score, take the example of Dominique, a twenty-six-year-old man from a town far from the clinic. In chapter 8 of this book's first edition, I noted that TB deaths were exceedingly rare in the area of central Haiti served by a comprehensive, community-based TB project. But for those beyond the boundaries of our project, TB remains the scourge it has been for centuries. Just a month or so ago, Dominique reached the clinic in terrible shape, gaunt and pale and bearded. I remarked that he looked somehow Christlike. Dominique could scarcely breathe. His chest film showed complete destruction of his left lung, even though he said he'd been sick "for only five months." He died shortly after starting therapy—collapsing in mid-sentence, as he spoke to his mother. The pain of starting therapy too late does not diminish with experience, I've learned. Nor did knowing that Dominique will be one of millions to die of tuberculosis lessen the pain. Had I still been on rifampin prophylaxis, I might have seen, just then, what orange tears look like.

Turning to the second prediction—that strains of TB resistant to rifampin and isoniazid, the most powerful antituberculous drugs, would spread—we do not need to turn to Russia or northern Lima, the "MDR-TB hot spots" mentioned in this book. Nor do we have to look to the latest global surveillance updates, which paint a grim picture of rising rates of drug resistance in these and other sites.[7] We see that this prediction has come true even in Haiti, a country with supposedly little in the way of MDR-TB, because rifampin was not routinely used there until recently. Since *Infections and Inequalities* was published, we built a TB referral hospital in central Haiti, and it is already full to bursting with young people with MDR-TB. They have been referred from all over the country, because other hospitals, including a few far better funded than our own, have decided that MDR-TB, like HIV disease, is too costly to treat. But MDR-TB, unlike HIV or Ebola, is airborne. So it does not take prophetic powers to predict that, if untreated, the disease will spread from family member to family member.

Take the Josephs, who might be termed a typical lower-middle-class Haitian family, if not for MDR-TB. They were a large family crowded into a small house in Carrefour Feuilles, a poor neighborhood in the sprawling city. Mme. Joseph sells wares in the streets of Port-au-Prince, the capital city; her husband is an irregularly employed construction worker. Although they live in poverty by any standard, theirs was a household in which it might be expected that all eight children would attend school; one or two of them might even be expected to find jobs.

One of their most talented children is Jean, in 1997 a twenty-one-year-old student. The way Jean recalls it, his family's problems began when he started to cough. At first he sought to treat his persistent hack with herbal teas. But when his cough worsened, he began to think he might have something other than a banal cold. In the second month of his illness, with new back pain and a fever, Jean took himself to a TB hospital in Port-au-Prince. "It's not that I thought I had tuberculosis," he recalled recently, as we sat on a ledge in front of the new hospital. "Not at all. It's rather that I knew they could take a chest x-ray." But Jean did indeed have TB, and he was started that day on a four-drug regimen that included not only rifampin, but also streptomycin, a drug that is injected intramuscularly. "I took all my medications," he recalled anxiously, "but I kept coughing."

Toward the end of the year, Jean's fears were heightened by an episode of hemoptysis. Coughing up bright red blood terrified the young man, as it did his entire family. "I knew I was getting worse, so I went to a pulmonologist." The specialist wondered why streptomycin had been included in the initial regimen, since most rifampin-containing regimens do not include the injectable drug. He referred Jean to the national TB sanatorium in January 1998. There Jean was found to be floridly smear-positive—which means that there were many TB bacilli in his sputum—and admitted for further therapy.

Jean was an inpatient for almost three months, during which he received directly observed therapy with the same drugs he had received previously. He remained smear-positive throughout his time there. "I was discouraged; I wanted to stop [taking the medications]. I was sure these medicines wouldn't do anything for me, since I had taken them for over a year and been positive the whole time. I stopped taking them and went to an herbalist (*doktè fey*) for a few weeks." At the herbalist's, Jean was treated with various concoctions containing the bark and leaves of trees held, he said, to cure "tuberculosis and other lung disease." But Jean's symptoms persisted, and when he again began to cough up blood, he returned to the sanatorium. Again he was prescribed the same first-line drugs, including rifampin and isoniazid. During that time, he recalls, he was placed in an open ward with other patients, many of them, he knew, with drug-resistant disease. "None of them were getting better," Jean recounted. "They started talking about other medicines that were better, but they said that the government either didn't have the medicines or wasn't going to distribute them."

Those drugs—kanamycin, cycloserine, ethionamide, and ciprofloxacin—are far more expensive, more toxic, and less effective than are rifampin and isoniazid. Little reason, then, to take them—unless you have the misfortune to have MDR-TB. In that case, such "second-line" drugs often hold the only real hope of cure. Once Jean's parents had the names of the drugs and a prescription from one of the pulmonologists, they started selling off assets—furniture, livestock, a small parcel of land—to buy the medications. "I started taking [second-line] medicines inside the sanatorium, and I was soon [smear-]negative. In July, I went home. But after five months of treatment, my parents couldn't buy any more medicines, and so I had to stop. I became positive again."

Jean soon had fevers every night, and drenching sweats. He coughed incessantly, and lived in fear of hemoptysis (he'd learned during his sanatorium stay that this symptom could prove rapidly fatal). But the situation, Jean reports, was to become even worse. "Even though I had stopped coughing blood, my sister Maryse began coughing in about October, and then she started coughing up blood." One after another, the Joseph children became ill: after Maryse, the oldest, came Myrlene, who had for years suffered with sickle-cell anemia. Then came Kenol, the youngest. Finally, Shella started coughing.

And one by one the Joseph siblings began treatment with first-line drugs. None of them improved. "I felt terrible," Jean recalled wistfully. "I was getting sicker, but I mostly felt guilty. I just knew they had drug-resistant TB, and that's why they weren't getting better. I knew it was my fault."

Because the Joseph children did not get better on first-line drugs, the nurse who was administering their streptomycin injections referred them back to the nongovernmental organization that had originally diagnosed Jean with TB. "She knew we were failing therapy," recalled Jean, "and she knew it was MDR-TB. But she said the government could not buy the drugs for patients with MDR-TB, it could only buy first-line drugs. So she referred us to [the nongovernmental organization]." There, Jean was asked to submit a sputum sample for culture and drug-susceptibility testing. "I never got the results. I kept going back every couple of weeks, and they kept telling me to come back again in a couple of weeks."

Jean worsened. Recurrent hemoptysis and cough kept him sleepless and on edge. He woke up before dawn on those mornings he'd been lucky enough to sleep. He became wasted, gaunt. His sisters knew that Jean was deeply depressed. "He blamed himself for making us all sick," said Myrlene. "We tried to reason with him, but he didn't listen. He still blames himself."

But Jean didn't give up. "I had heard that there was one place in the country where we could be treated, and couldn't believe it. It seemed even more strange that it would be out in the middle of nowhere when the big hospitals in Port-au-Prince didn't have the medicines for anyone but people who could pay for them. So I came to see for myself."

In October 1999, Jean left for central Haiti in a crowded truck—what the Haitians call "public transport." He was coughing and short of breath, drawing the attention of the people among whom he was sandwiched. Once at the clinic, he did not speak to any of us involved in treating MDR-TB. "I just spent the morning looking around," he later recounted. He liked what he saw, evidently, because in November all of the Joseph siblings came to the Clinique Bon Sauveur and, following the requisite laboratory work, began therapy for MDR-TB. All became smear-negative within two months, and remain so after eight months of therapy.

I should add that the TB clinic does not charge for its services. What happens if diseases such as that afflicting the Joseph family are declared too expensive to treat? More honestly, since MDR-TB treatment is mandated by law in most affluent nations, what happens when people are declared too poor to treat? The cost to families of doing nothing—or, more commonly, of doing something ineffective or noxious, such as repeated courses of the wrong drugs—becomes painfully obvious from the case studies in the following chapters. It is clear that a single infectious family member can rapidly transform a cramped dwelling—or a prison cell—into a setting of daily bombardment with viable, drug-resistant bacilli. Universal infection can be expected in such households.[8]

But there are other costs to such double standards. One is the costs to caregivers: in settings throughout the world, we've met doctors and nurses who are highly uncomfortable—at times, distraught—about lowering standards of care on the grounds of "cost-effectiveness." For example, the administration of ineffective first-line drugs or "isoniazid for life" to patients with documented MDR-TB is regarded by many as a violation of the social contract between patient and healer.[9] In the eyes of many within and without the medical profession, patients with MDR-TB have moral claims on all of those charged with treating the sick.

These patients also have claims on those charged with protecting the public health. Failure to treat patients with infectious MDR-TB means that drug-resistant strains will continue to spread. A number of positions regarding transmission of MDR-TB have emerged, but they are more ideological than evidence-based. Scarce resources and vested interests have led, as predicted in this book, to unrealistically confident claims regarding the spread of drug-resistant organisms. Slender evidence of "variable fitness" or "decreased infectiousness," inflated to suit the needs of the argument, has already engendered projections in which MDR-TB epidemics "burn themselves out" even if active cases are left untreated. When we ask to examine the data suggesting that drug-resistant strains are less readily transmitted than are drug-susceptible strains, we are steered to a small study from *rural* Mexico.[10] Meanwhile, ample evidence of MDR-TB's epidemic spread within slums and hospitals and prisons, reviewed in this book and elsewhere,[11] is discounted because so many of its victims were co-infected with HIV—as if the virus added wings to the bacterium. Such exercises would be merely wishful thinking if they did not lull us into complacency and lead to ill-conceived policies.

Failure to intervene effectively—to bring necessary resources to bear on the plagues of the poor—also undermines support for TB control and for public health in general. In setting after setting, patients like the Joseph children have remained untreated or have received regimens that could not cure them. In Peru, it has taken years to alter ineffective treatment policies—ineffective but formulated by international experts reluctant to reverse their position. In Russia, the situation—hinted at in this volume's footnotes—has gone from bad to worse. Again, substandard care—endorsed by international authorities—led to the use of the wrong drugs for the substantial fraction of patients with drug-

resistant disease. The result has been cure rates about half those registered in dirt-poor central Haiti.[12] But it doesn't much matter, it seems, if
we got it wrong. Who's shedding tears over Russian prisoners? When
the irrationality of improper recommendations was brought to public
attention, it engendered mostly irritation, even anger. Humility has
been in short supply among the experts; tears, of any color, absent. One
suspects that some of the tears shed by the prisoners were orange for
no good reason, since many of them were sick with strains of tuberculosis resistant to rifampin.

What, then, is to be done about MDR-TB in settings in which resources are scarce? Since *Infections and Inequalities* was written, this
question has emerged as one of the new century's more important public-health dilemmas. Commentaries to date have been long on rhetoric
and short on data. As predicted in chapter 2, vested interests have at
times prevented clear analysis of the dynamics of emerging drug resistance. Indeed, ideological positions have at times led to confident claims
unencumbered by evidence. At the same time, it has been possible to
advance evidence-informed and novel strategies that promise to stop
MDR-TB by bringing patients to cure. We have done so in an urban
slum in Peru and in a squatter settlement in rural Haiti.[13] Successful ex-
pansion of these strategies will require global leadership from the
World Health Organization and other bodies charged with formulating
health policy.[14]

The justifications for such ambitious initiatives are many: the needs
of those already sick, the prevention of ongoing transmission, and the
rectification of previous clinical and policy errors. But perhaps the most
compelling justification is to be found in considering the impact of differential standards of care for the poor. While the global era makes it
increasingly difficult to live in ignorance of the suffering of others, it
has not led to a more just partition of the fruits of science and technology. If we are to stay the ongoing spread of MDR-TB, global health equity must become a central component of TB-control policy in the
coming years.

A similar message emerges as regards AIDS, as *Infections and Inequalities* tries to show. Forecasts were also made, in its first edition, regarding HIV. The spread of this novel pathogen has been at least as rapid as

predicted, and so has its concentration among the poor—at this writing, HIV incidence is declining in wealthy countries, and more than 95 percent of new infections occur in the developing world.[15] Close to 80 percent of cumulative AIDS deaths to date have occurred in Africa, the world's poorest continent.[16] I also predicted, in the last chapter of this book, that patients in rural Haiti would soon ask for the new antiviral "cocktails." Adeline Merçon did not ask for the medications, even though more than a decade of battle with HIV had worn her down to less than 80 pounds. Her father asked, instead, for money for a coffin: he could see, by November 1999, that Adeline wasn't going to last much longer. Instead of a coffin, however, we gave Adeline a three-drug cocktail of anti-HIV drugs. And between November 29, when she began therapy, and January 2000, she gained twenty-six pounds. Adeline is aware of the debates surrounding the use of these agents in what are euphemistically termed "resource-poor settings." She is now devoting her time to the HIV Equity Initiative based in our clinic, not far from her home village.[17] "If the drugs cost a lot, there must be a reason," she commented in a recent meeting. "Science made them, so science will have to find a way to get them to poor people, since we're the ones who have AIDS."

Attending international AIDS conferences might not bolster Adeline's optimism, since the logic of limited resources holds sway here. It is fitting, perhaps, that I am finishing this preface not in rural Haiti, but in Durban, South Africa. Outside, the XIII International Conference on AIDS is in full swing. The air in this lovely seaside city, which is prosperous compared to many, is rife with tension. And no wonder: globally, billions of dollars have been invested in AIDS prevention and treatment, but the epidemic marches on. AIDS-prevention efforts have failed in precisely those areas where they are needed most. No genuinely interested party could in all honesty deny this fact and others that bring us together in Durban:

- The increasing concentration of HIV among the poor and marginalized, most of them in the so-called developing countries.[18]
- The increasing concentration of wealth in the hands of the powerful, most of them in the industrialized nations.[19]
- The development, since the Vancouver AIDS conference ambi-

tiously titled "One World, One Hope," of new therapies that have transformed HIV from an inevitably lethal annihilation of cell-mediated immunity to a chronic illness.[20] But the benefits of these therapies are reserved for those in industrialized countries, where far fewer than 10 percent of those infected live.

- The failure of primary and, indeed, of secondary prevention, especially on this continent of Africa. In other words, not only have we failed to prevent HIV transmission, we have failed to prevent HIV progression in those already infected.[21]

As these trends become further entrenched, there has been a marked tendency to regard therapy as the province of the first world; in developing countries, we are encouraged to restrict our "AIDS-related activities" to prevention alone. Take, as an example, the world's largest pot of AIDS funding targeted to the developing world. The hundreds of millions of dollars disbursed by the U.S. Agency for International Development through Family Health International have until now gone almost exclusively for prevention, even though the efficacy of these interventions among the poor is difficult to demonstrate.[22] The exception more recently has been to fund palliative care (sometimes under the euphemism "community-based care") or low-cost prevention of certain opportunistic infections.

By this point, readers may conclude that I am making an attack on prevention or public-health approaches to HIV. Not true. I am calling instead for a redoubling of our efforts to improve prevention, including vaccine development, and even more effective educational tools. Prevention, however, will be most effective as part of a comprehensive plan to meet widespread demands for treatment and health equity in general. And it is high time to admit the limitations of existing prevention strategies.

Prevention is cheap, compared to therapy of already infected people. But what is the cost of focusing *solely* on prevention, given our current limitations? First, we fail to represent the aspirations of those already infected or sick. They will number, soon enough, more than 100 million.[23] This large number represents parents, farmers, doctors, teachers, factory workers—the very fabric of a society as we know it. Second, let-

ting HIV disease run its course in high-burden countries will mean—
and has already meant—significant reductions in life expectancy, with
many drastic social consequences, even if new infections were to cease
immediately.[24] The number of AIDS orphans grows, with sober projections of 40 million orphans by 2010—on the continent of Africa alone.[25]
Many children left to fend for themselves will eventually turn to sex
work or crime, or perhaps become soldiers in some local conflicts. They
will almost certainly live out their lives in poverty. And if little is done,
they too are likely to die of AIDS, which is already killing ten times as
many Africans as war.[26] Third, other diseases will emerge. Throughout
sub-Saharan Africa and beyond, HIV is driving the frightening rise in
TB incidence. The wealthy country of South Africa shows rates of TB
two or three times higher than those registered in far poorer countries
in which HIV is not a ranking problem.[27]

Fourth, by focusing solely on prevention, we fail to engage fully the
medical and scientific community as partners in responding to this cat-
aclysmic epidemic. The medical and scientific community finds itself
unequipped to participate in the arena of primary and secondary prevention. By asking clinicians and bench scientists who wish to work in
or on behalf of poor countries to put all of their weight behind "information, education, and communication," we are undermining the
potential contribution of a highly skilled sector eager to help. This de-
prives us of sorely needed clinical and scientific abilities. Fifth, we fail
to recognize that existing AIDS-prevention strategies have their limitations. The most eloquent rebuke to optimism regarding their efficacy is
the rapidly rising HIV incidence in many nations. We are finally beginning to acknowledge this failure with honesty—fully twenty years into
the epidemic. Health education alone does not suffice. In some settings,
paradoxically, "the presence of health-education materials seemed to
lead to *lower* frequency of condom use."[28] Notes a recent, candid review: "Somewhat surprisingly, towards the end of the second decade of
the AIDS pandemic, we still have no good evidence that primary prevention works."[29]

Twenty years is a long time to wait for such candor. One of the reasons for this delay is that the social scientists who might have offered
critical assessments in a more timely fashion were too busy scrambling

for their piece of the pie, as is argued in the chapters of this book. We undermine faith in medicine and public health whenever we make unreasonable, excessive, or propagandistic claims. Arguing, for example, that "education is the only vaccine" is neither accurate nor wise: since we cannot show that cognitive interventions have been highly effective in preventing HIV infection among the poor—the global risk group—it is surely unwise to rely *exclusively* on such methods.

Having staked these claims, allow me to make several assertions that spring from the argument that we must move beyond weak prevention programs to develop a global HIV strategy that encompasses meaningful prevention efforts and treatment of those already afflicted. It should be obvious that each of these assertions also holds true for drug-resistant tuberculosis.

1. Treatment cannot be regarded as solely the province of wealthy countries.

There are many reasons for this, some of which will be examined below. But here I will underline the painful fact that, as AIDS deaths drop in North America and Europe (a welcome trend relating to increasingly effective therapies),[30] they continue to climb in Africa and in most other settings in the world. By the end of this decade, more than 95 percent of all AIDS deaths will occur in resource-poor settings.[31] Good but prohibitively expensive therapies can only heighten this trend of concentration unless global health equity becomes more than a slogan.

How are we to respond? One of the first things we should do is listen to those infected with HIV. They are forty million strong and growing, and they are not telling us to concentrate all of our AIDS activities on prevention. They are not reminding us that antiretroviral therapy is not cost-effective. They are not arguing that costly therapeutic interventions are not "sustainable" in poor settings, not "appropriate technology" for low-tech areas of the globe. Often enough, they are saying just the contrary, because the destitute sick remind us that sacrosanct market mechanisms will not serve the interests of global health equity.[32] Show us the data to support the assertion, widespread in international financial institutions, that the neoliberal economic policies now in favor will *ever* serve the interests of those living, already, with HIV. Show us the data to suggest that declining HIV incidence—and declining AIDS

deaths—in wealthy countries will not be followed by decreasing investment in the basic research necessary for new drug and vaccine development. No such data exist. If they did, new antituberculous agents, also
sorely needed, could not be termed "orphan drugs"[33]—a great irony,
since TB remains, along with AIDS, the leading infectious cause of
adult death in the world today.[34]

*2. Cost-effectiveness cannot become the sole gauge by which public-health inter-
ventions are judged.*

Market utilitarianism is a strange beast, since it seems to permit all
sorts of inefficiencies as long as they benefit the right people—namely,
the privileged. But if the goal is to heal or to ease the suffering of the
destitute sick, we are asked to jump through hoops to finance what was
once felt to be a public good. Show us the data to suggest that *any*
costly interventions serving the destitute sick will find favor in a world
in which corporate welfare goes unquestioned, but chiding rebukes follow the introduction of antiretroviral therapy to poor communities. But
again, examples from tuberculosis highlight the weaknesses of cost-
effectiveness argument in the arena of infectious disease: although rifampin causes orange tears, it is considered to be an integral part of
"cost-effective" treatment of tuberculosis in developing countries. A
couple of decades ago, however, an editorial in the *British Medical Journal* argued that the price of rifampin rendered its use "prohibitive in developing countries, certainly for routine treatment." [35] Confident claims
about what is cost-effective and what is not should be viewed with some
suspicion by those bent on providing quality care to the destitute sick.

3. AIDS research in developing countries must include a social-justice component.

It is clear that many in the community of researchers would just as soon
ignore poor people's bitter criticisms of our program priorities. But
what do we expect when we provide first-world diagnostics (viral-load
and genomic testing, which are used to contribute to data collection)
and third-world therapeutics (treatment of certain opportunistic infections or sexually transmitted diseases only, leaving HIV to progress un-
hindered) within the same research project? It sounds as if poor people
are excellent lab rats but unlikely patients. If the press for cheaper—or

even free—medications for HIV has had resonance, it's surely because something inside all of us recognizes the fundamental unfairness of this situation. Asking the destitute sick to wait for research to pay off is also unfair. The need for reciprocity is widely acknowledged in international public health, but it rings hollow to call people to participate in research for the greater good when the poor will rarely benefit from research outcomes.

Besides, people sick with AIDS need effective treatment now, and there are more and more of them. Which groups have led this charge? Not, alas, the international health experts and responsible officials, but rather the AIDS activists and the nongovernmental organizations.[36] The fundamentally remediative nature of their work is more appropriate to this problem because it addresses widespread demands for *social justice*. If we're embarrassed by this term, then perhaps we should invent another. But show us the data to justify an absence of social-justice initiatives in even the most basic research, a dimension that must be built into all human research that involves drawing blood—or sweat or tears—from the destitute sick.

4. We need more effective prevention strategies.

The countless Knowledge, Attitudes, and Practices surveys and AIDS educational interventions derived from them have not achieved their aim, and to say so is not to object to AIDS education. Not at all. Educating everyone, and especially the young, is our civic duty, part of being human. But show us the data to suggest that, in settings where *social conditions* determine risk for HIV infection, cognitive exercises can fundamentally alter risk. We know that risk of acquiring HIV does not depend on knowledge of how the virus is transmitted, but rather on the freedom to make decisions. Poverty is the great limiting factor of freedom. Indeed, gender inequality and poverty are far more important contributors to HIV risk than is ignorance of modes of transmission or "cultural beliefs" about HIV.[37] We can already show that many who acquire HIV infection do so *in spite of* knowing enough information to protect themselves, if indeed cognitive concerns were ever central to preventing HIV among the poor. Until we have effective, female-controlled prevention, whether a microbicide or another, and an effective vaccine, nothing we do should suggest that education can substitute for, or remove the necessity of, effective therapy for AIDS. These truths are just now beginning to be acknowledged, and they are late in coming.[38]

5. We can no longer accept whatever we are told about "limited resources."

We keep hearing that we live in "a time of limited resources." But how often do physicians, anthropologists, and other researchers, or public-health specialists challenge this slogan? The wealth of the world has not dried up; it has simply become unavailable to those who need it most. Show us the data to prove that there are fewer resources than in previous decades, when we did *not* have effective therapies for many diseases. The struggle for social and economic rights for the poor must become central to every aspect of AIDS research and treatment.

Our challenge, therefore, is not merely to draw attention to the widening outcome gap, but also to attack it, to dissect it, and to work with all our capacity to reduce this gap. One way to do this is to let it be known that the community of those concerned with preventing and treating HIV—and with making common cause with the sick—is not willing to stand by idly as wealth becomes ever more concentrated. Even a doctor without formal economic training soon starts to wonder if the neoliberal agenda of the international financial institutions might be driving up HIV risks even as these institutions slap the hands of those who dare to treat the destitute sick.[39]

Another challenge is to "harmonize" a global research and treatment ethic rather than to maintain the pretense that rich and poor live in two different worlds. There is no wall between the worlds, as any honest assessment of either microbial traffic or capital flows will show. Our imperative is to develop treatment components for all research or prevention programs that involve HIV testing. As Wood and colleagues note, even "limited use of antiretrovirals could have an immediate and substantial impact on South Africa's AIDS epidemic."[40]

To unite treatment and research in this way, we need drugs, diagnostics, and increased investment in health infrastructures. We need to forge novel alliances. We need to have easier access to drugs, especially those developed with public funds.[41]

Finally, we also need pilot projects to pioneer the use of antiretroviral therapy in settings with a heavy burden of HIV but without laboratories capable of performing CD4 counts or viral loads. We need to think ahead, to pioneer the use of new agents where they are needed most. On the basis of our experience of developing directly observed therapy for tuberculosis, we have developed such a program in one of the poorest parts of rural Haiti, the poorest country in the Western hemisphere. We are using three-drug regimens that are little more complicated than short-course chemotherapy for TB; other, simpler regimens will soon be available.[42] Our HIV Equity Initiative in rural Haiti has not replaced our prevention efforts. Rather, it has helped to revive them. At this juncture, facing catastrophe in Africa and beyond, we are asked to choose between treatment and prevention. But we cannot make this choice. We remain squarely behind efforts to prevent transmission— from vaccine trials to improved educational interventions—but believe that prevention and treatment are intimately linked. They belong together as planks of a single platform to halt AIDS.

So why is treatment *not* central to AIDS policy in resource-poor settings? Because we're told it's "not sustainable." Why? It costs too much. And why is that? To answer this question, we'd need to look at the manufacture and sale of pharmaceuticals—an industry that, as noted, has consistently had among the highest margins of profit.[43] "The pharmaceutical industry," observes Angell in a recent editorial, "is extraordinarily privileged. It benefits from publicly funded research, government-granted patents, and large tax breaks, and it reaps lavish profits. For these reasons, and because it makes products of vital importance to the public health, it should be accountable not only to its shareholders, but also to society at large."[44] A uniform ethic should become a condition for entry into any national and international marketplace, so that publicly funded research is not siphoned away for private gain or handicapped for the benefit of private-sector companies. A call for this uniform ethic has generated fear among pharmaceutical companies, leading some of them to avoid working with scientists who are funded by government agencies such as the National Institutes of Health.[45] These companies are aware that antiretrovirals manufactured without recourse to publicly funded research would be further sheltered from legislation attempting, however timidly, to make public research lead to public good.[46]

What, then, is not sustainable? It is not the cost of HIV treatment that is not sustainable; it's rather the opposition to treatment in high-burden areas that is not sustainable. It's not morally sustainable, it's not intellectually sustainable, it's not epidemiologically or socially sustainable.

If unequal standards are to be accepted as a fact of life, then why do I feel uncomfortable that, to do summer research projects in places like this one, medical students from Harvard, say, are now required to travel with doses of "triple therapy" on the off chance that they *might* be exposed to HIV? Why do I feel uncomfortable that researchers from the same institutions dismiss as "utopian" the possibility of treatment for locals who are *already sick*? How sustainable is that?

It's my hope that *Infections and Inequalities* might serve a pragmatic end by calling into question these and other logics that promise a future in which health equity will play a shrinking role. Only by struggling for higher standards for the destitute sick will we avoid another unappealing role—that of academic Cassandras who prophesy the coming plagues, but do little to avert them. Then will come the time for more universal tears, whether orange or clear, whether scant or copious. In the interim, shoring up double standards for the poor will be identified most closely with the shedding of crocodile tears.

Durban, South Africa
July 11, 2000

NOTES

1. Special thanks to Jen Singler, David Walton, Gilles Peress, Haun Saussy, and Joia Mukherjee for their contributions to this preface.

2. In an overview of anthrax public-health management, Inglesby and colleagues note that, although it is believed that "at least 17 nations have offensive biological weapons programs . . . it is uncertain how many are working with anthrax" (Inglesby, Henderson, Bartlett, et al. 1999, p. 1736). Furthermore, continues the overview, most experts agree that most groups lack the technology and funding necessary to "manufacture" anthrax. And yet officialdom seems to fan such fears: discussions of possible bioterrorist attacks include preparations for both civilian and military preparedness (Fidler 1999). The level of panic and lack of knowledge about the dangers posed by such attacks are both marked. For example, a hospital in Florida was closed recently while doctors examined several local airport baggage holders for possible anthrax exposure, suspected after the workers handled a box from Puerto Rico containing animal skins. Although none of the individuals showed signs of exposure, and an infectious-disease specialist noted that risk of exposure was extremely low, the hospital was effectively sealed off for several hours ("Anthrax Scare Shuts Hospital in Florida," *Boston Globe*, June 21, 2000, p. A13). The lead story in the "Health, Education & Science" section of *USA Today* announces that "new foam defeats biological weapons." "A government task force has unleashed its latest weapon in the fight against bioterrorism," a chemical foam that can "neutralize," among other substances, "anthrax, a pathogen widely recognized for its ease of production and mobility." Fortunately, the foam "will be available for about $10 per gallon as soon as commercial partners sign on" (*USA Today*, June 29, 2000, p. 9D).

3. During the 1999 surge in funding for antibioterrorism efforts, John Hopkins University opened a center devoted to the subject, infused with a $150 million "emergency" appropriation allocated from Congress. The center sponsored a packed conference on the subject, where researchers issued dire warnings and "reviewed frightening scenarios" of hypothetical bioterrorist attacks (Marshall 1999, p. 1234). For reviews of recent bioterrorism efforts and concerns, see Centers for Disease Control and Prevention 2000; Fidler 1999; Fox 1999; Kaufmann, Meltzer, and Schmid 1997; Leggiadro 2000.

4. Clinton 1999.

5. Cohen, Sidel, Gould 2000, p. 1211.

6. A Central Intelligence Agency report released earlier this year warned of the threat posed by infectious diseases and biological warfare to U.S. security and interests abroad (Central Intelligence Agency 2000), and in remarks before Congress, a leading National Intelligence Council official warned that infectious diseases such as tuberculosis, malaria, and pneumonia pose a threat to U.S. security and will continue in the coming decades to harm economic and social

development in those countries in which the United States has vested interests (Tang 2000). See Henry and Farmer 1999 for an exploration of emerging infectious diseases and "national security concerns." A more thorough exploration of the topic is found in our complete paper, which is posted at http://www.sidint.org/new/globalization/presentation.htm.

7.   Program in Infectious Disease and Social Change 1999; World Health Organization 2000a.

8.   Although today's short-memoried epidemiologists will not be quick to point out that we have no data suggesting that universal infection will ensue, they forget that people like the Joseph family—who were receiving what amounts to no effective therapy for their tuberculosis—are in effect transported back to the preantibiotic era. There one finds ample evidence of universal infection when a household contains an untreated, coughing tuberculosis patient. For example, when, in 1936 Long and Hetherington surveyed 530 Native Americans in southern Arizona, they found that, although only 20 percent of children under five were tuberculin-positive, by the time study participants reached adulthood, 100 percent had evidence of true infection. The authors also note that infection rates among Native Americans at boarding school were lower than those documented at day schools, which they argued again suggested the role of infection within households with high rates of active tuberculosis (Long and Hetherington 1936). Even in the postantibiotic era, failure to identify and remove an active tuberculosis case leads to new infections. One Canadian study carried out in the late 1960s found household infection rates ranging from 29 percent to 61 percent for those households with a smear-positive tuberculosis case (see commentary in Rouillon, Perdrizet, and Parrot 1976).

9.   I have discussed the use of substandard and frankly deleterious care among the destitute sick throughout this book, but it is discussed as a human-rights violation in Farmer 1999c. *Pathologies of Power: Structural Violence and the Assault on Human Rights*, is due from the University of California Press in 2001.

10.   García-García, Ponce-de-León, Jiménez-Corona, et al. 2000. Note that I believe this to be a very important paper. What I question is its relevance to modeling the future of epidemics of drug-resistant tuberculosis, which are seated not in rural regions, but rather in prisons, slums, and, ironically enough, health-care institutions.

11.   For a discussion of the problem of multidrug-resistant tuberculosis in prisons in the United States and Russia, see Farmer 1999; Coninx, Mathieu, Debacker, et al. 1999; Portaels, Rigouts, and Bastian 1999. The edited volume *Sentenced to Die? The Problem of TB in Prisons in East and Central Europe and Central Asia* (Stern 1999) also highlights the increasing spread of TB in prisons in the former Soviet Union, as do reviews in *The Global Impact of Drug-Resistant Tuberculosis* (Farmer, Kononets, Borisov, et al. 1999; Mitnick and Farmer 1999).

12.   Kimerling, Kluge, Vezhnina, et al. 1999; see also Farmer, 1999b.

13. Farmer and Kim 1998; Farmer, Furin, and Shin 2000; Farmer, Kim, Mitnick, et al. 1999; Farmer, Shin, Bayona, et al. 2000.

14. Iseman 1998; Farmer, Becerra, and Kim 1999.

15. An estimated 5.4 million people were infected with HIV during the course of 1999—4 million in sub-Saharan Africa, 800,000 in Southeast Asia, and 210,000 in Latin America and the Caribbean (Joint United Nations Programme on HIV/AIDS 2000). We have attempted to explore the dynamics of HIV's rapid concentration among the poor in Farmer, Walton, and Furin 2000.

16. Of the 18.8 million HIV/AIDS deaths registered globally from the beginning of the epidemic through the end of 1999, 14.8 million have been in sub-Saharan Africa (Joint United Nations Programme on HIV/AIDS 2000).

17. Any author's royalties for this volume will be contributed directly to Zanmi Lasante's HIV Equity Initiative.

18. Joint United Nations Programme on HIV/AIDS 2000.

19. The mechanisms of growing economic inequality, and its effect on the health of the world's poor, is explored in *Dying for Growth: Global Inequality and the Health of the Poor* (Kim, Millen, Irwin, and Gershman 2000).

20. Fauci 1999; Cohen and Fauci 1998. With the advent of more effective therapies, AIDS mortality has dropped precipitously since the late 1990s in industrialized nations such as the United States (See Centers for Disease Control and Prevention 1999).

21. Farmer and Walton 2000.

22. "AIDSCAP interventions were built on three strategies for reducing HIV transmission: communication to encourage people to avoid behaviors that put people at risk of infection, improving treatment and prevention of other sexually transmitted diseases (STDs), and increasing access to and correct use of condoms. These central technical strategies were supported by policy development, behavioral research, evaluation, gender initiatives and capacity building" (Family Health International 1997). There have been calls to expand the FHI portfolio to include treatment, and an "HIV care coordinator" was recently appointed (Eric von Praag, personal communication).

23. Do the math. As of the end of 1999, an estimated 34.3 million adults and children were infected with the HIV virus; 1999 alone saw 5.4 million infections, at a rate of 15,000 new infections per day (Joint United Nations Programme on HIV/AIDS 2000).

24. The latest projections are staggering: in Botswana, where an estimated 36 percent of adults is infected with HIV, impressive gains in life expectancy over the past forty years have been dramatically reversed in the past decade: life expectancy had plummeted to 47.4 years by 1997, a 14 percent drop compared to 1975 (United Nations Development Programme 1999). In countries with adult HIV prevalence rates of 15 percent and above, current projections suggest that more than one-third of boys now aged fifteen will die of AIDS; in even harder-

hit countries, such as those in southern Africa, this proportion may exceed two-thirds (Joint United Nations Programme on HIV/AIDS 2000). See also Boerma, Nunn, and Whitworth 1998; Stover and Way 1998.

25. International Federation of Red Cross and Red Crescent Societies 2000. Global estimates for the end of 1999 put the number of AIDS orphans since the beginning of the epidemic at 13.2 million, with over 90 percent of these children living in sub-Saharan Africa (see Joint United Nations Programme on HIV/AIDS 2000).

26. In 1998, 200,000 Africans died in war, while more than two million died of AIDS (Joint United Nations Programme on HIV/AIDS 2000).

27. Relatively prosperous South Africa has one of the highest rates of HIV infection in the world. In 1998, the TB case notification rate was 326 per 100,000 population (World Health Organization 2000a); true incidence is estimated at over 500 per 100,000 population (Weyer, Fourie, and Nardell 1999). In contrast, poorer Senegal, where 1.77 percent of the adult population is HIV-positive, had a TB case notification rate in 1998 of 94 per 100,000 population (Joint United Nations Programme on HIV/AIDS 2000; World Health Organization 2000b).

28. Egger, Pauw, Lopatatzidis, et al. 2000, p. 2103; emphasis added.

29. Mayaud, Hawkes, and Mabey 1998, p. S31.

30. Moore and Chaisson 1999; Palella, Delaney, Moorman, et al. 1998; Mocroft, Vella, Benfield, et al. 1998.

31. Joint United Nations Programme on HIV/AIDS 2000.

32. The market fails when it comes to research and development—in the case of tuberculosis, for example, the last novel treatment was developed more than thirty years ago (t'Hoen 2000). Over the past two decades (1975–1996), less than 1 percent of more than 1,200 new molecular entities sold worldwide were earmarked for tropical diseases (Trouiller and Olliaro, 1999)—this despite the fact that infectious diseases remain a major cause of mortality throughout the world: in 1998, infectious diseases accounted for 25 percent of deaths worldwide and 45 percent of deaths in low-income countries (World Health Organization 1999). One candid review of drug development notes that "few developments are need-driven"—the average cost of bringing a new drug to market is approximately $224 million, costs that pharmaceutical companies argue would not be recouped for diseases endemic in poor countries with few resources and no property rights laws to prohibit far cheaper generic products from entering the market (Trouiller and Olliaro 1999, p. 164).

33. An orphan drug is defined under the U.S. Orphan Drug Act (1983) as one that affects fewer than 200,000 individuals in the United States and would not recoup development costs for domestic sales (Anonymous 1995). For more information on the Orphan Drug Act, see Asbury 1992.

34. Dye, Scheele, Dolin, et al. 1999; World Health Organization, 2000b; Joint United Nations Programme on HIV/AIDS 2000.

35. Anonymous 1973.

36. Organizations such as Médecins Sans Frontières have been at the forefront of the movement to gain equal access to effective therapies for the poor (t'Hoen 2000). One MSF spokesman argued recently, "The global HIV/AIDS-crisis has provided us with a magnifying glass under which the inequity in access to treatment became painfully clear. . . . Medicines cannot be treated as mere commodities. Often access to medicines is a question of life and death. Yet in international trade they are regulated very much the same as any other consumer good" (t'Hoen 2000).

37. For a review of the data supporting this claim, see Farmer, Connors, and Simmons 1996, which reviews more than a thousand studies and papers relevant to both HIV transmission and disease progression among women.

38. "Failure to use STD and HIV incidence as the outcome measure constitutes a major weakness in the behavioural-intervention area. Another important weakness is our failure to evaluate basic social structural interventions. We cannot know the effectiveness of interventions that have not been addressed. There is overwhelming evidence that oppression contributes to STDs and many other maladies" (Aral and Peterman 1998, p. S35). In a randomized control trial of more than twelve thousand adults in Tanzania assessing the effect of treating STDs as a means of preventing HIV transmission, Gilson and colleagues found that treating STDs reduced transmission of HIV-1 by about 40 percent. They conclude, "From a societal standpoint, therefore, the cost of the intervention is likely to be substantially less than the cost of not intervening" (Gilson, Mkanje, Grosskurth, et al. 1997, p. 1808).

39. Lurie, Hintzen, and Lowe 1995.

40. Wood, Braitstein, Montaner, et al. 2000, p. 2095. One model of the effect of antiretroviral use on the AIDS epidemic in South Africa projected that the use of short course prophylaxis would reduce perinatal transmission by 40 percent, preventing 110,000 infant HIV infections by 2005—at a cost of less than 0.001 percent of the per-person health expenditure. In a more costly scenario, triple-combination treatment for merely 25 percent of the HIV-1 positive population would prevent both 430,000 incident AIDS cases and a 3.1-year decline in life expectancy (Wood, Braitstein, Montaner, et al. 2000).

41. For example, AZT and to a lesser extent 3TC have been developed with federal research dollars. See also comments in t'Hoen 2000.

42. Within months we will have a triple nucleoside RT inhibitor pill—AZT, 3TC and abacavir, the most potent NRTI. Such a fixed-dose combination would be easier to use and would preserve both protease inhibitors and nonnucleosides for cases of resistance. Using a nonnucleoside (e.g., nevirapine) in a three-drug regimen may be more risky than using a protease inhibitor because a single mutation confers resistance to the entire class of drugs as opposed to resistance to nucleoside analogs and protease inhibitors in which it takes multiple mutations to confer clinically meaningful resistance. (For more on readily-induced nevirapine resistance, see Becker-Pergola, Guay, Mmiro, et al. 2000.)

43. According to a report in *Fortune* magazine, in 1999 the pharmaceutical industry far exceeded all other U.S. industries in its profit margin, realizing on average an 18.6 percent return on revenues; second was commercial banking, at 15.8 percent, while other industries ranged from 0.5 percent to 12.1 percent ("How the Industries Stack Up," *Fortune*, April 17, 2000). Noting that the top ten drug companies have a 30 percent profit margin, Angell (2000, p. 1903) pointedly states, "An industry whose profits outstrip not only those of every other industry in the United States, but often its own research and development costs, simply cannot be considered very risky."

44. Angell 2000, p. 1904.

45. In a recent article in the *New York Times,* one drug-company spokesman underscored this point quite candidly: "The industry has never been philanthropic. It has always produced products with an aim to getting a return on investment" (McNeil 2000, p. 1). Some investigators charge that drug companies have stopped funding clinically important studies because of concerns that possible study results could reduce sales of the drug (Bodenheimer 2000).

46. The Bayh-Dole Act, for example.

REFERENCES

Angell, M.
    2000.   "The Pharmaceutical Industry: To Whom Is It Accountable?" *New England Journal of Medicine* 342 (25): 1902–4.
Anonymous.
    1995.   "Buying into the Orphan Drug Market." *Lancet* 346:917.
Anonymous.
    1973.   "Rifampicin or Ethambutol in the Routine Treatment of Tuberculosis." *British Medical Journal* 4 (892): 568.
Aral, S. O., and T. A. Peterman.
    1998.   "Do We Know the Effectiveness of Behavioral Interventions?" *Lancet* 351 (Suppl. 3): 33–36.
Asbury, C. H.
    1992.   "Evolution and Current Status of the Orphan Drug Act." *International Journal of Technology Assessment in Health Care* 8(4):573–582.
Becker-Pergola, G., L. Guay, F. Mmiro, et al.
    2000.   "Selection of the K103N Nevirapine Resistance Mutation in Ugandan Women Receiving NVP Prophylaxis to Prevent HIV-1 Vertical Transmission (HIVNET-006)." Abstract of the 7th Conference on Retroviruses and Opportunistic Infections, San Francisco, January 30–Feb 2.

Bodenheimer, T.
    2000.   "Uneasy Alliance: Clinical Investigators and the Pharmaceutical
           Industry." *New England Journal of Medicine* 342 (20): 1539–44.
Boerma, J. T., A. J. Nunn, and J. A. G. Whitworth.
    1998.   "Mortality Impact of the AIDS Epidemic: Evidence from Community
           Studies in Less Developed Countries." *AIDS* 12 (Suppl. 1): S3–S14.
Centers for Disease Control and Prevention.
    1999.   *HIV/AIDS Surveillance Report* 11 (2).
———.
    2000.   "Biological and Chemical Terrorism: Strategic Plan for Preparedness
           and Response. Recommendations of the CDC Strategic Planning
           Workgroup." *Morbidity and Mortality Weekly Report* 49 (No. RR-4):
           1–14.
Central Intelligence Agency.
    2000.   "The Global Infectious Disease Threat and Its Implications for the
           United States." NIE 99-17D, January. www.cia.gov/cia/publica-
           tions/nie/report/nie99-17d.html (accessed 26 July 2000).
Clinton, W. J.
    1999.   "Remarks by the President on Keeping America Secure for the 21st
           Century." National Academy of Sciences, 22 January. www.white-
           house.gov/WH/New/html/19990122-7214.html (accessed 26 July
           2000).
Cohen, H. W., V. W. Sidel, and R. M. Gould.
    2000.   "Prescriptions on Bioterrorism Have It Backwards. *British Medical
           Journal* 320:1211.
Cohen, O. J. and A. S. Fauci.
    1998.   "HIV/AIDS in 1998—Gaining the Upper Hand?" *JAMA* 280 (1):
           87–88.
Coninx, R., C. Mathieu, M. Debacker, et al.
    1999.   "First-line Tuberculosis Therapy and Drug-resistant *Mycobacterium
           tuberculosis* in Prisons." *Lancet* 353:969–73.
Dye C., S. Scheele, P. Dolin, et al.
    1999.   "Global Burden of Tuberculosis: Estimated Incidence, Prevalence,
           and Mortality by Country." *JAMA* 282 (7): 677–86.
Egger, M., J. Pauw, A. Lopatatzidis, et al.
    2000.   "Promotion of Condom Use in a High-risk Setting in Nicaragua:
           A Randomised Controlled Trial." *Lancet* 355:2101–5.
Family Health International.
    1997.   *Making Prevention Work: Global Lessons Learned from the AIDS Control
           and Prevention (AIDSCAP) Project 1991–1997.* Arlington, Va.: Family
           Health International and AIDSCAP.
Farmer, P. E.
    1999a.   "Cruel and Unusual: Drug Resistant Tuberculosis as Punishment."

In *Sentenced to Die? The Problem of TB in Prisons in East and Central Europe and Central Asia,* edited by V. Stern, pp. 70–88. London: International Centre for Prison Studies.

———.

1999b.   "Managerial Successes, Clinical Failures." *International Journal of Tuberculosis and Lung Disease* 3 (5): 365–7.

———.

1999c.   "Pathologies of Power: Rethinking Health and Human Rights." *American Journal of Public Health* 89 (10): 1486–96.

Farmer, P. E., M. C. Becerra, and J. Y. Kim.

1999.   "Conclusions and recommendations." In Program in Infectious Disease and Social Change, *The Global Impact of Drug-resistant Tuberculosis.* pp. 169–177. Boston, Mass.: Harvard Medical School and the Open Society Institute.

Farmer, P., M. Connors, and J. Simmons, eds.

1996.   *Women, Poverty, and AIDS: Sex, Drugs, and Structural Violence.* Monroe, Maine: Common Courage Press.

Farmer, P. E., J. J. Furin, and S. S. Shin.

2000.   "Managing Multidrug-resistant Tuberculosis." *Journal of Respiratory Diseases* 21 (1): 53–6.

Farmer, P. E., and J. Y. Kim.

1998.   "Community-based Approaches to the Control of Multidrug-resistant Tuberculosis: Introducing 'DOTS-plus.'" *British Medical Journal* 317 (7159): 671–4.

Farmer P. E., J. Y. Kim, C. Mitnick, and R. Timperi.

1999.   "Responding to Outbreaks of MDRTB: Introducing 'DOTS-Plus.'" In *Tuberculosis: A Comprehensive International Approach,* edited by L. B. Reichman and E. S. Hershfield, 2d ed., pp. 447–69. New York: Marcel Dekker.

Farmer, P. E., A. S. Kononets, S. E. Borisov, et al.

1999.   "Recrudescent Tuberculosis in the Russian Federation." In Program in Infectious Disease and Social Change, *The Global Impact of Drug-resistant Tuberculosis,* pp. 39–84. Boston, Mass.: Harvard Medical School and the Open Society Institute.

Farmer, P. E., S. S. Shin, J. Bayona, et al.

2000.   "Making DOTS-Plus work." In *Multidrug-resistant Tuberculosis,* edited by I. Bastian and F. Portaels, pp. 285–306. Dordrecht: Kluwer.

Farmer, P. E. and D. A. Walton.

2000.   "Condoms, Coups, and the Ideology of Prevention: Facing Failure in Rural Haiti." In *Catholic Ethicists on HIV/AIDS Prevention,* edited by J. F. Keenan, J. D. Fuller, L. S. Cahill, and K. Kelly, pp. 108–19. New York: Continuum.

Farmer P. E., D. A. Walton, and J. J. Furin.
    Forthcoming.   "The Changing Face of AIDS: Implications for Policy and
            Practice." In *The emergency of AIDS: the impact on immunology, micro-*
            biology, and public health, edited by K. Mayer and H. Pizer. Washing-
            ton, D.C.: American Public Health Association.
Fauci, A. S.
    1999.   "The AIDS Epidemic: Considerations for the 21st Century." *New*
            England Journal of Medicine 341 (14): 1046–50.
Fidler, D. P.
    1999.   "Facing the Global Challenges Posed by Biological Weapons."
            Microbes and Infection 1 (12): 1059–66.
Fox, J. L.
    1999.   "Adjusting FDA Policies to Address Bioterrorist Threat." *Nature*
            Biotechnology 17 (4): 323–4.
García-García, M. L., A. Ponce-de-León, M. E. Jiménez-Corona, et al.
    2000.   "Clinical Consequences and Transmissibility of Drug-resistant
            Tuberculosis in Southern Mexico." *Arch Intern Med* 160:630–36.
Gershman J., and A. Irwin.
    2000.   "Getting a Grip on the Global Economy." In *Dying for Growth: Global*
            Inequality and the Health of the Poor, edited by J. Y. Kim, J. V. Millen,
            A. Irwin, and J. Gershman, pp. 11–43. Monroe, Me.: Common
            Courage Press.
Gilson, L., R. Mkanje, H. Grosskurth, et al.
    1997.   Cost-effectiveness of Improved Treatment Services for Sexually
            Transmitted Diseases in Preventing HIV-1 Infection in Mwanza
            Region, Tanzania. *Lancet* 350:1805–9.
Henry C. and P. Farmer.
    1999.   "Risk Analysis: Infections and Inequalities in a Globalizing Era."
            Development 42 (4): 31–4.
Inglesby, T.V., D. A. Henderson, J. B. Bartlett, et al.
    1999.   "Anthrax as a Biological Weapon: Medical and Public Health
            Management." *JAMA* 281 (18): 1735–45.
International Federation of Red Cross and Red Crescent Societies.
    2000.   *World Disasters Report 2000.* Geneva: International Federation of
            Red Cross and Red Crescent Societies.
Iseman, M. D.
    1998.   "MDR-TB and the Developing World—a Problem No Longer to be
            Ignored: The WHO Announces 'DOTS Plus' Strategy." *International*
            Journal of Tuberculosis and Lung Disease 2 (11): 867.
Joint United Nations Programme on HIV/AIDS.
    2000.   *Report on the Global HIV/AIDS Epidemic, June 2000.* Geneva: Joint
            United Nations Programme on HIV/AIDS.

Kaufmann, A. F., M. I. Meltzer, and G. P. Schmid.
    1997.   "The Economic Impact of a Bioterrorist Attack: Are Prevention and
            Postattack Intervention Programs Justifiable?" *Emerging Infectious
            Diseases* 3 (2): 83–94.

Kim, J. Y., J. V. Millen, A. Irwin, and J. Gershman, eds. *Dying for Growth: Global
    Inequality and the Health of the Poor.* Monroe, Maine: Common
    Courage Press.

Kimerling M. E., H. Kluge, N. Vezhnina, et al.
    1999.   "Inadequacy of the Current WHO Re-treatment Regimen in
            a Central Siberian Prison: Treatment Failure and MDRTB."
            International Journal of Tuberculosis and Lung Disease 3 (5):
            451–453.

Leggiadro, R. J.
    2000.   "The Threat of Biological Terrorism: A Public Health and Infection
            Control Reality. *Infection Control and Hospital Epidemiology* 21 (1):
            53–56.

Long, E. R. and H. W. Hetherington.
    1936.   "A Tuberculosis Survey in the Papago Indian Area of Southern
            Arizona." *American Review of Tuberculosis* 33: 407–33.

Lurie P., P. Hintzen, and R. A. Lowe.
    1995.   "Socioeconomic Obstacles to HIV Prevention and Treatment in
            Developing Countries: The Roles of the International Monetary
            Fund and the World Bank." *AIDS* 9 (6): 539–46.

Marshall, E.
    1999.   "Bioterror Defense Initiative Injects Shot of Cash." *Science* 1999;
            283:1234–35.

Mayaud, P., S. Hawkes, and D. Mabey.
    1998.   "Advances in Control of Sexually Transmitted Diseases in Develop-
            ing Countries." *Lancet* 351 (Suppl. 3): S29–S32.

McNeil, D. G, Jr.
    2000.   "Drug Makers and the Third World: A Case Study in Neglect." *New
            York Times*, May 21.

Mitnick, C. D. and P. E. Farmer.
    1999.   "Promise and Peril: TB and MDR-TB in Azerbaijan." In Program
            in Infectious Disease and Social Change, *The Global Impact of Drug-
            resistant Tuberculosis,* pp. 85–106. Boston, Mass.: Harvard Medical
            School and the Open Society Institute.

Mocroft, A., S. Vella, T. L. Benfield, et al.
    1998.   "Changing Patterns of Mortality across Europe in Patients with
            Human Immunodeficiency Virus Infection." *Lancet* 352:1725–30.

Moore R. D. and R. E. Chaisson.
    1999.   "Natural History of HIV Infection in the Era of Combination Anti-
            retroviral Therapy." *AIDS* 13 (14): 1933–42.

Palella F. J., K. M. Delaney, A. C. Moorman, et al.
    1998.   "Declining Morbidity and Mortality among Patients with Advanced
             Human Immunodeficiency Virus Infection." *New England Journal of
             Medicine* 338:853–60.
Portaels F., L. Rigouts, and I. Bastian.
    1999.   Addressing Multidrug-resistant Tuberculosis in Penitentiary
             Hospitals and in the General Population of the Former Soviet
             Union." *International Journal of Tuberculosis and Lung Disease* 3 (7):
             582–8.
Program in Infectious Disease and Social Change.
    1999.   *The Global Impact of Drug-resistant Tuberculosis.* Boston, Mass.:
             Harvard Medical School and the Open Society Institute.
Rouillon, A., S. Perdrizet, and R. Parrot.
    1976.   "Transmission of Tubercle Bacilli: The Effects of Chemotherapy."
             Tubercle 57:275–299.
Stern, V. ed.
    1999.   *Sentenced to Die? The Problem of TB in Prisons in East and Central
             Europe and Central Asia.* London: International Centre for Prison
             Studies.
Stover, J. and P. Way.
    1998.   "Projecting the Impact of AIDS on Mortality." *AIDS* 12 (Suppl. 1):
             S29–39.
Tang, D.
    2000.   "Disease Called Threat to Security." *Washington Times,* June 30.
t'Hoen, E.
    2000.   Statement from Médecins Sans Frontières, Campaign for Access to
             Essential Medicines at the Health Issues Group DG Trade, Brussels,
             26 June.
Trouiller, P. and P. L. Olliaro.
    1999.   "Drug Development Output: What Proportion for Tropical Dis-
             eases?" *Lancet* 354 (9173): 164.
United Nations Development Programme.
    1999.   *Human Development Report 1999.* New York: Oxford University
             Press.
Weyer, K., P. B. Fourie, and E. A. Nardell.
    1999.   "A Noxious Synergy: Tuberculosis and HIV in South Africa." In
             Program in Infectious Disease and Social Change, *The Global Impact
             of Drug-resistant Tuberculosis,* pp. 127–148. Boston, Mass.: Harvard
             Medical School and the Open Society Institute.
Wood, E., P. Braitstein, J. S. G. Montaner, et al.
    2000.   "Extent to Which Low-level Use of Antiretroviral Therapy
             Could Curb the AIDS Epidemic in Sub-Saharan Africa." *Lancet*
             355:2095–99.

World Health Organization.
    1999.   *Removing Obstacles to Healthy Development.* Geneva: World Health Organization.

————.

    2000a.   *Anti-tuberculosis Drug Resistance in the World.* Report no. 2: *The WHO/IUATLD Global Project on Anti-Tuberculosis Drug Resistance Surveillance 2000.* Geneva: World Health Organization.

————.

    2000b.   *Global Tuberculosis Control: WHO Report 2000.* Geneva: World Health Organization.

Acknowledgments

The writing of any book incurs obligations to friends and colleagues. Because the essays presented in this book were written about the sick, however, my greatest debt is to patients and informants, two overlapping groups. Caring for persons with HIV disease and tuberculosis has been my greatest privilege; failing to avert unnecessary deaths, such as those of Annette Jean and others described in these pages, remains my greatest regret.

Most of my patients and informants live—or have died—in poverty. Perhaps as a point of order, I'd like to respond to the question, Who are "the poor"? The objectification of the poor is, of course, a risk run by anyone who employs some sort of class analysis, and I will be specific in these essays whenever possible. At the same time, I'm not skittish about using the term: striving to understand a commonality of constraint is hardly tantamount to denying the salience of personal experience. I've been impressed, in my work in Haiti and Peru, at how often people use the label "the poor" to describe themselves. These people do not share nationality or gender or language or culture; they share only their relative social positioning at the bottom of the ladder. And it is these people who have endured the sicknesses described in this book.

I would also like to acknowledge three sets of colleagues. My fellow clinicians at both the Clinique Bon Sauveur and the Brigham and Women's Hospital have not only shared responsibility for the care of these patients; they have also taught me a great deal about caring for the sick. I am especially grateful to Maxi Raymonville, Fernet Léandre, Jean Hughes Jérôme, Tony Francillon, Philomène Durosier, Johanna Daily, James Maguire, and Paul Sax, and also to Ed Nardell, Mike Iseman, Jennifer Furin, and Sonya Shin. It's difficult to convey to Marshall Wolf my gratitude for a decade of medical mentoring (and for being my doctor when my own foolishness and fondness for *ceviche* almost got me listed for a liver transplant), but I'll say it again: thank you.

For the skills necessary to understand why some people are sick and others are not, my greatest debt is to the Harvard Medical School's Department of Social Medicine, my intellectual roost since I was a first-year medical student. Arthur Kleinman combines analytic rigor and honesty even as he remains open to new approaches and new problematics; he's as inspirational a colleague as he was a teacher (and he was the best teacher I had). I'm grateful, too, to Ken Fox, Mary Jo Good, Byron Good, and Allan Brandt, who've been with me all along the way. For many years of good counsel, warm thanks to Dan Federman.

In previous publications, I've thanked the medical anthropologists who've been my teachers and colleagues; my debt to them remains enormous. But because this book is more an exercise in social medicine, I'd like to pay tribute to three physicians who've fought the good fight for decades: Leon Eisenberg, Howard Hiatt, and Julius Richmond. In a time in which many of the trends now registered are precisely those they have so valiantly resisted, I hope that each will take heart in knowing that many of us, inspired by their vision, are committed to continuing the fight for equity in health care. To Howard, I add special thanks for his hard work in advocating for our patients with drug-resistant tuberculosis.

Three community-based organizations—Partners in Health, Zanmi Lasante, and Socios en Salud—serve as the settings in which these patients' infections have been diagnosed and treated. Situated respectively in Cambridge, Massachusetts, in Haiti's Central Plateau, and in urban

Peru, these organizations (which I describe in greater detail in Chapter 1) are the tools with which we are able to intervene to prevent the embodiment of inequalities as pathologies or, failing that, to treat the pathologies. In this work, I'm most indebted to Tom White, Jim Yong Kim, and Ophelia Dahl, similarly obsessed with addressing the inequalities documented in this book. They are, most often, the other constituents of the "we" in these chapters. Colleagues and friends (happily, another overlapping group) in each of these organizations have made this work possible. Special and loving thanks are owed to Fritz and Yolande Lafontant and to Marie Flore Chipps. *Mesi anpil.* For coffee and encouragement and wise steering, I thank Jésula Pierre and Loune Viaud; for her ability to produce misplaced documents at midnight, I thank Anne Hyson. Special thanks to Jaime Bayona and the "TB team" in Peru, who have weathered the controversies born of our advocacy for those with tuberculosis, and to Jack Roussin, who paid the ultimate price for his own commitment to the poor.

Didi Bertrand deserves a thank-you paragraph all her own.

For help in preparing this volume, I am most indebted to Mercedes Becerra, Cassis Henry, and Aaron Shakow. Without their encouragement and assistance, I would not have undertaken the editing and updating necessary to make this collection as free of error and redundancy as possible. I thank, too, Jennifer Furin, Keith Joseph, David Walton, and Carole Mitnick, who read and commented on revisions of some of the chapters. For case studies from Bombay and Harlem, I'm indebted to Sarthak Das and Anitra Pivnick, respectively. Intellectual guidance was afforded by Carol and Noam Chomsky, Kwame MacKenzie, Vinh Kim Nguyen, Randall Packard, Lee Baker, and Bill Rodríguez; invaluable bibliographic assistance came from Virginia Farmer, Rebecca Wolfe, Mirjam van Ewyck, Paul Grifhorst, Annabelle McKnight, and Stephen Buttenweiser. For a wonderful place to live, I thank Kristine Forsgard and Stephen Mitchell. For stylistic revisions *and* illuminating discussions of social theory, I'd like to thank Catherine Bertrand Farmer.

I'm most grateful to the University of California Press, which afforded a physician-writer invaluable assistance in the persons of Mary Renaud, who edited every line of this book, and Mary Severance, who saw it through to completion. Stan Holwitz, also of the University of California Press, has been a friend since we first met, and I look forward to continued collaboration over the years. It was Stan who encouraged me to enlarge the scope of this book, to move from the specific case—AIDS and tuberculosis in Haiti—to some of the more general questions raised both by my work and by the emergence or reemergence of modern plagues. Further, it was Stan who encouraged me to incorporate some of the indignation that any physician feels when people die of readily treatable afflictions. What place, in scholarship, for passion? Is it truly "neutral" to remain dispassionate before unnecessary suffering? Or is such studied neutrality really a concession to the inevitability of inequalities of outcome?

One model of passionate engagement in the struggle to prevent unnecessary suffering died tragically as this book was going to press. Jonathan Mann was a staunch supporter of the organizations described in Chapter 1. We will miss him sorely.

Finally, I'm pleased to acknowledge a deep debt to Haun Saussy. For almost twenty years, we've been engaged in what might seem to be altogether unrelated endeavors. But Haun has taught me that being a critical reader of Chinese literature is not unrelated to being a critical reader of medical anthropology—or of any other discipline. This book is dedicated to Haun in celebration of a long and warm and instructive friendship.

Introduction

Medical statistics will be our standard of
measurement: we will weigh life for life and see
where the dead lie thicker, among the workers or
among the privileged.

RUDOLF VIRCHOW, 1848

WHAT KILLED ANNETTE JEAN?

Early on the morning of her death, Annette Jean was feeling well enough
to fetch a heavy bucket of water from a spring not far from her family's
hut. In the weeks prior to that day, she had been complaining of a "cold."
It was not serious, she thought, although night sweats and a loss of ap-
petite were beginning to trouble her. Annette's brothers later recalled that
she was cheerful, "normal," that morning. She made everyone coffee and
helped her mother load up the donkey for market. It was an overcast day
in October of 1994, and Haiti's rainy season was drawing to a close.

Shortly after Annette's brothers left for their garden, the young woman
abruptly began coughing up blood. A young cousin, watching from
across the yard, saw her throw off a bright red arc and then collapse on
the dirt floor of the tiny house. The child ran for Annette's three brothers,

1

who tried in vain to rouse her; the young woman could do no more than gurgle in response to their panicked cries. The brothers then hastily confected a stretcher from sheets and saplings. It would take them more than an hour, carrying their inert sister, to reach the nearest clinic, situated in the village of Do Kay far below their mountaintop garden.

Halfway there, it began to rain. The steep path became slippery, further impeding progress. Two-thirds of the way there, Annette coughed up clots of darker blood and then stopped gurgling. By the time they reached the clinic, it was raining heavily. The larger clots refused to melt, hardening on her soaked shirt, and Annette was motionless in a puddle of diluted blood. She was not yet twenty years old.

I was in the clinic on that rainy day, conversing with a patient near the building's main entrance when the Jean brothers and a fourth man passed into the clinic's courtyard with their terrible cargo. A single rivulet of blood was falling from somewhere under the stretcher onto the paved courtyard. They approached me wordlessly, and I, also silent, reached for the young woman's wrist. It was an easy, joyless diagnosis— death from massive hemoptysis due, almost certainly in a woman her age, to tuberculosis—and Annette was already cold. Her brothers, who had been numbed into silence by the hope that something might still be done, began wailing, each taking up in turn a shrill cry of grief as I pronounced her dead.

One of the women from Do Kay had been mopping the floor of the clinic, but she had stopped to stare. When the men began to weep, she lifted her apron to her eyes and turned away. She had never met Annette Jean or her brothers, but she had seen plenty of tuberculosis. Her own sister, the mother of five children, had died of the same disease in October of 1988. One of those children also died years later from complications of tuberculosis, but not before going stone deaf from one of the medications used to treat it.

I had seen a lot of tuberculosis, too, even though the little clinic in Do Kay was built to serve only a tiny region of the Central Plateau. In 1993 alone, we had diagnosed over four hundred cases of tuberculosis, more than were registered in the entire state of Massachusetts that same year. Diagnosing tuberculosis is something I expect to do on a daily basis. But I too was shaken by the blood, the rain, and by the brothers' sharp grief.

The story does not end with Annette's dramatic agony. Another sister, I learned, had also succumbed to tuberculosis. And a few months after Annette's death, one of her brothers, Marcelin, returned to the clinic with a case of shingles (herpes zoster). From our interview I soon learned that he—like Annette, the child of a peasant family—had been working as a servant in Port-au-Prince, Haiti's capital city. This employment history in a person with herpes zoster has come to suggest, for many of us, early HIV disease, a suspicion confirmed in Marcelin's case by a laboratory test. Although, unlike his sisters, Marcelin was fortunate enough to receive treatment for the active tuberculosis that he later developed, he has told his family that he will die.

I could tell that Annette's family did not—could not—comprehend why they should be so unfortunate. To lose two young, previously healthy members of a close-knit family seemed both insufferable and unfair; so did Marcelin's illness. But their incomprehension eventually gave way first to hypotheses and then to conclusions. They were the victims of sorcery, they surmised. Someone had it in for them, and that someone was likely to be another villager.

After a decade of medical practice in the same village, I was accustomed to ferreting out accusations of sorcery and had previously spent some years trying to make sense of them.[1] And that, paradoxically, is the primary function of such accusations: to make sense of suffering. The anthropologist within me is perfectly satisfied to analyze such explanations, but to a physician it is nothing less than punishing to see preventable or treatable pathologies chalked up to village-level squabbles.

The doctor in me insists that no one should die of tuberculosis today; it's completely curable. Yet it is, at the same time, the world's leading infectious cause of death among young adults. An estimated three million people are dying each year from tuberculosis.[2] This figure comes as a surprise to many, who read more frequently in their newspapers about Ebola or "flesh-eating bacteria" than about tuberculosis. Exacting its toll among the world's poor, tuberculosis has ceased to occasion much interest, either in scientific circles or in the popular press. Barry Bloom puts it even more strongly: tuberculosis, he writes, "has been virtually ignored for 20 years and more."[3]

Many are also surprised to learn that infectious diseases remain the world's single most common cause of death. In 1995, for example, a year in which an estimated 52 million people died worldwide, about 17.3 million of these deaths were due to bacterial, viral, or parasitic infections.[4] And although the majority of deaths occurred in the developing world, infectious diseases also remain a major killer of the U.S. poor. One study of New York City welfare recipients revealed staggeringly high rates of tuberculosis and AIDS: of 858 clients enrolled in 1984, 47 developed tuberculosis and 84 were diagnosed with AIDS. The study thus revealed tuberculosis and AIDS incidence rates well in excess of those found in many poor countries and seventy times higher than the U.S. national rate. In fact, simply being on welfare and having a history of drug or alcohol abuse were strongly associated with death: fully 183 clients—21.3 percent of the cohort—died within eight years. The mean age at death was less than fifty years.[5]

INFECTIONS AND INEQUALITIES

Amartya Sen has observed that the first question in any critical examination of equality is "equality of *what?*"[6] This book examines inequalities in the distribution and outcome of infectious diseases. It asks why people like Annette Jean and her siblings are likely to die of infections such as tuberculosis and AIDS and malaria, while others are spared this risk. It explores the creation and maintenance of such disparities, which are biological in their expression but are largely socially determined. This book also explores social responses to infectious diseases, responses ranging from quarantine to accusations of sorcery.

This exploration leads me to examine various, often discrepant explanations for these disparities of risk and outcome, including those proffered by officialdom and by academics. I argue that scholars often weaken their contributions to an understanding of infectious diseases by making "immodest claims of causality" regarding the distribution and course of these disorders. These claims are immodest because they are wrong or misleading. They are immodest because they distract attention from the modest interventions that could treat and, often enough, cure people like Annette Jean. And they are immodest because they distract attention from the preventable social disorder that exacerbates biological disorders.

Using data from Haiti, the United States, Peru, and elsewhere, this volume calls into question many such claims. *Infections and Inequalities* is intended as a corrective and a complement to the growing literature on "emerging infectious diseases." Although many who study the dynamics of infectious disease will concede that, in some sense, disease emergence is a socially produced phenomenon, few have examined the contribution of specific social inequalities. Yet such inequalities have powerfully sculpted not only the distribution of infectious diseases but also the course of health outcomes among the afflicted.

Strikingly patterned outbreaks of HIV, tuberculosis, and even Ebola—and the social responses to these outbreaks—all suggest that models of disease emergence need to be dynamic, systemic, and critical. They need to be critical of facile claims of causality, particularly those that scant the pathogenic roles of social inequalities. Critical perspectives on emerging infections must ask how large-scale social forces come to have their effects on unequally positioned individuals in increasingly interconnected populations; a critical epistemology needs to ask what features of disease emergence are obscured by dominant analytic frameworks. Such models must strive to incorporate change and complexity and must be global in scope, yet alive to local variation.

This critique leads inevitably to questions about my own disciplinary perspectives. Although this book is the work of a full-time clinician who is also an anthropologist, these essays are neither clinical nor ethnographic. They are instead lodged between medicine and anthropology, drawing freely on both disciplines and on several others, including the sociology of knowledge. This willed "interdisciplinarity" is not meant to free the author from the responsibilities of discipline. Rather, it is clear to me that the disparities of risk and outcome described here are embedded in complex *biosocial* realities. To understand these realities, nothing less than a biosocial analysis will do—an analysis that draws freely on clinical medicine and on social theory, linking molecular epidemiology to history, ethnography, and political economy. Of course, such a synthesis is easy to demand but harder to produce; Fineberg and Wilson have termed it the "Holy Grail" of epidemiology.[7]

Finally, this book is lodged as a protest. The inequalities of outcome I describe are, by and large, biological reflections of social fault lines.

Annette Jean's death could and should have been averted; effective interventions might have ranged from the clinical to the political. To conclude otherwise is to engage, wittingly or unwittingly, in delusion or obfuscation.

VISUAL-FIELD DEFECTS
IN ANTHROPOLOGY AND MEDICINE

In reexamining anthropology and medicine from the vantage point of Haiti, there often seems to be no shortage of delusion and obfuscation. At the very least, a good deal of selective blindness exists. The exact nature of the visual-field defect seems to depend on what sort of anthropologist or physician one is. The histories of both anthropology and medicine show these disciplines to be notable for their lack of attention, respectively, to oppression (and, perhaps, to human suffering in general) and to the sicknesses of the poor.[8]

Take anthropology, for starters. Not too long ago, in her study of hunger in Brazil, Scheper-Hughes wrote that "everyday violence, political and domestic horror, and madness . . . are strong words and themes for an anthropologist."[9] Why is this so, if anthropologists work in the same regions from which television exports its images of famine and strife? The killing fields described by journalists were the training fields for generations of anthropologists. What exactly *were* we talking about when we were not talking about "everyday violence, political and domestic horror, and madness"? We were talking a lot about "culture," and part of the problem lies in the ways this term was used. "The idea of culture," explained one authority approvingly in a 1975 book on the subject, "places the researcher in a position of equality with his subjects: each 'belongs to a culture.'"[10]

The tragedy, of course, is that this equality, however comforting to the anthropologist, is entirely illusory. Anthropologist and informant are not separate and equal; both are caught up in a global web of unequal relations. But such illusions reveal an important means by which key misreadings are sustained. A blindness to inequality and structural violence, often the local manifestation of transnational (or at least extraregional) forces, has long marred anthropology.

In a much-quoted essay, "Missing the Revolution," Orin Starn examines the ethnographies coming from highland Peru on the eve of the country's guerrilla war. Working in the very same villages that would later
prove sympathetic to the Shining Path (Sendero Luminoso), how was it
that anthropologists failed to see what was happening? Following Said,
Starn writes of an "Andeanism" that appreciatively stressed the highland
peasants' continuity with Incan ancestors. Concerned with ecology and
ritual, with depicting remoteness rather than discerning links, a generation of anthropologists seemed to have missed the revolution:

> Ethnographers usually did little more than mention the terrible infant
> mortality, minuscule incomes, low life expectancy, inadequate diets, and
> abysmal health care that remained so routine. To be sure, peasant life
> was full of joys, expertise, and pleasures. But the figures that led other
> observers to label Ayacucho a region of "Fourth World" poverty would
> come as a surprise to someone who knew the area only through the
> ethnography of Isbell, Skar, or Zuidema. They gave us detailed pictures
> of ceremonial exchanges, Saint's Day rituals, weddings, baptisms, and
> work parties. Another kind of scene, just as common in the Andes, al-
> most never appeared: a girl with an abscess and no doctor, the woman
> bleeding to death in childbirth, a couple in their dark adobe house cry-
> ing over an infant's sudden death.[11]

A more systemic view of highland Peru, and its many economic and
administrative links to Lima and beyond, might have corrected this
myopia. But, as Starn points out, "this economic nexus was one that most
anthropologists—largely depending on the categories of 'culture' and
'community'—were unprepared to explore."[12]

A decade earlier, many of the classic ethnographies of anthropology—
including those by Evans-Pritchard, Malinowski, and Lévi-Strauss—
were critiqued as similarly shortsighted. But more recent studies have
also shown a disturbing tendency to offer misreadings of oppression and
suffering. Common indeed are the ethnographies in which poverty and
inequality, the end result of a long process of impoverishment, are reduced to a form of cultural difference. We were sent to the field to look
for different cultures. We saw oppression; it looked, well, *different* from
our comfortable lives in the university; and so we called it "culture." We
came, we saw, we misdiagnosed.

These omissions were the result, it's been argued, of theoretical fashions, of the ways in which anthropology "makes its object," and of the ways in which ethnography was written.[13] Most now agree that the omissions were also the result, in part, of anthropologists' relations with colonial or neocolonial power. On the level of the individual researcher, however, the visual-field defects of anthropology are rarely a question of motives but rather, as Asad suggests, a question of our "mode of perceiving and objectifying alien societies."[14] Three decades ago, today's truisms triggered acrimonious debate within anthropology. But debates that focused on the image of the anthropologist as the willing stooge of power often failed to address the more subtle effects of hegemony. This book suggests that the myths and mystifications surrounding these issues often serve powerful interests, in spite of the best intentions of researchers.

The extent to which these critiques of anthropology are still valid is a matter of some debate. Perhaps Marcus and Fischer were correct when, more than a decade ago, they argued that "our consciousness has become more global and historical: to invoke another culture is to locate it in a time and space contemporaneous with our own, and thus to see it as a part of our world, rather than a mirror or alternative to ourselves, arising from a totally alien origin."[15] Perhaps scores of students are this minute studying, say, the plight of women like Annette Jean. Perhaps several Fulbrights have been awarded to study the effects of recent political and economic policies on health outcomes among the poor of Latin America and Africa. But I don't think we're battering down wide-open doors here, if working in Haiti and dealing with AIDS and tuberculosis are at all instructive.

In my first years of reading anthropology, I certainly "missed the revolution." But what better remedial training than that to be found in Haiti? Although I went there in the spring of 1983 with a host of pre-fab research questions, each tightly linked to a sanctioned desire to "contribute to theory," I gradually developed a quite different set of questions, the ones addressed in this book. And in the course of a decade of research, reading, and writing, much of it in collaboration with very ecumenical colleagues, I came to discern disturbing patterns in much social-science writing on AIDS and tuberculosis.[16] For example, when we were face to face with sexual practices or AIDS outcomes that were manifestly linked to poverty and inequality, we wrote instead about the exotic reflections of cultural difference. Animal sacrifice, zoophilia, ritualized homosexuality, scarification, and ritual beliefs all figure prominently in the early anthropology of AIDS. The only problem was that none of this had any demonstrable relevance to HIV transmission or AIDS outcomes, and claims to the contrary were eventually revealed to be mistaken—not, however, before a certain amount of damage was done, as several of the chapters that follow suggest.

This conflation of structural violence and cultural difference has marred much commentary on AIDS, especially when that commentary focuses on the chief victims of the disease: the poor. A related trend is the exaggeration of the agency of those most likely to become infected. Often such exaggeration is tantamount to blaming the victim.[17] Explorations of AIDS have involved intense scrutiny of local factors and local actors, including the natives' conceptions and stated motives. But is it possible to explain the distribution of HIV by discussing only attitude or cognition? After more than fifteen years in Haiti, I would not hazard to comment on the psychological makeup specific to Haitians with AIDS, and I suspect that quests for psychological "predispositions" are fundamentally misguided. On the makeup of Haiti's changing social conditions and their relation to AIDS, however, much can be said. On the nature of inequality and on the structure of poverty—increasingly a global process—much can be said. On the mechanisms by which these forces come to alter sexuality and sexual practices, much can be said. On Haitians' lack of access to both AIDS prevention and treatment, again, much *must* be said. It is thus unfortunate that these topics have been neglected in the social science and clinical literature on AIDS.

What about medicine's blind spots? If the anthropologist working in Haiti is faced with a host of theoretical and methodological dilemmas, it would seem, at first blush, that the physician's task would be somewhat easier. To a certain extent, it is. There is, first, the wonderful simplicity of the patient-healer dyad. The doctor's allegiance, goes the saw, is always to his or her patient. There is thus little need for angst over social theory: this allegiance holds whether that patient is an elderly, overweight U.S. businessman with coronary artery disease or a thin, coughing Haitian woman, still in her twenties and dying of tuberculosis and malnutrition.[18] Having had the privilege of caring for both of these patients, I can say only that a warm and caring rapport is possible, indeed necessary, in both cases. Furthermore, the warmth of clinical exchanges—the vitality of practice—can serve as a powerful corrective to the "experience-distant" models of economics, political science, and sociology.

That said, it is important to add, though perhaps not to one's patients, that North American men with coronary artery disease are apt to live much longer than Haitian women with tuberculosis. North American men with coronary artery disease are apt to live longer than Haitian women, period. And the former, even those who are uninsured, clearly have much greater access to top-quality care than do the latter: indeed, it may be true that few Haitian peasants have received state-of-the-art care for pulmonary tuberculosis or any other serious illness—ever.[19]

A warm patient-doctor relationship is surely indispensable to quality care. So too is a familiarity with the biomedical literature. The vast, if still largely potential, power of modern medicine stems in great measure from its focus on the biological sciences. No one who has access to the vast array of drugs and diagnostic tools of a modern hospital could fail to appreciate the century's remarkable return on investments in bench science. No one who confidently prescribes a new medication could fail to appreciate the double-blinded controlled trial. But the narrow or uncritical use of these tools is one reason for physicians' blindness to the large-scale forces that generate sickness. Such pathogenic forces were once the focus of social medicine, as the work of Rudolf Virchow and others can remind us:

> Virchow understood, as we his successors have not, that medicine, if it is to improve the health of the public, must attend at one and the same time to its biologic *and* to its social underpinnings. It is paradoxic that, at the very moment when the scientific progress of medicine has reached unprecedented heights, our neglect of the social roots Virchow so clearly identified cripples our effectiveness.[20]

Physicians again need to think hard about poverty and inequality, which influence *any* population's morbidity and mortality patterns and determine, especially in a fee-for-service system, who will have access to care. In short, all of the forces that bring a patient to a doctor (or keep a patient from a doctor), all of the processes leading to sickness and then to diagnosis and treatment, are related to a series of large-scale social factors. The diagnostic dilemma, in thinking about the health of populations, is not so very different from that faced by the anthropologist.

So how might humane and compassionate physicians work such perspectives into their practice? Many of the finest clinicians I know have neither the time nor the inclination to consider such large-scale questions. Obligated to keep up with the explosion of medical knowledge and increased administrative demands, they are (or feel) consumed by the task at hand—to see a patient through an acute illness or to diminish the suffering of the chronically ill. Their patients might prefer such an approach, I suspect, to the one advanced in this book; no one who is ill wants the doctor visibly distracted by the problems of others.

In a utopia, perhaps this would be enough. Others would make sure that everyone had access to high-quality medical services. Someone else would enforce standards of care and monitor the forces that generate sickness in a society. Others would make sure that medical care, broadly conceived, was designed to promote the full development of each member of society.

Alas, we live in a society that encompasses both Haiti and the United States. It is a society that includes both Harlem and the Lower East Side of Manhattan, Paris and Kinshasa, London and Bombay. Further, we live in a society that is poorly defined by national boundaries. Nowhere is this clearer than in the case of HIV, as I've tried to show in previous work:

> The ties that bind Haiti to urban North America have a historical basis, and they continue to change. These connections are economic and affective; they are political and personal. One reason this study of AIDS in rural Haiti returns again and again to urban Haiti and the United States is that the boundaries separating them are, at best, blurred. The AIDS pandemic is a striking reminder that even a village as "remote" as Do Kay is linked to a network that includes Port-au-Prince and Brooklyn, voodoo and chemotherapy, divination and serology, poverty and plenty. Indeed, the sexual transmission of HIV is as eloquent a testimony as any to the salience—and complicated intimacy—of these links.[21]

Such arguments are not inappropriate to the analysis of other diseases, including tuberculosis. Is it mere polemic to argue that in terms of social causation the coronary artery disease of millions of overfed northerners is linked to the tuberculosis of malnourished Haitian women?

Our society ensures that large numbers of people, in the United States and out of it, will be simultaneously put at risk for disease and denied access to care. In fact, the spectacular successes of biomedicine have in many instances further entrenched medical inequalities. This necessarily happens whenever new and effective therapies—from antituberculous drugs to protease inhibitors—are not made readily available to those in need. Perhaps it was in anticipation of late-twentieth-century technology that Virchow argued that physicians must be the "natural attorneys of the poor."

In any setting where medical injustice is a given, it is incumbent upon physicians and other healers to respond to the troubling questions posed by the destitute sick. These issues cannot be left to the leaders of the insurance and pharmaceutical industries, whose bottom line is not relief of suffering. Until doctors ask other types of questions—Who becomes sick and why? Who becomes a patient? Who has access to adequate services? How might inequalities of risk and outcome be addressed?—they will remain at least as blind as the anthropologists who "missed the revolution."

ON CLAIMS OF CAUSALITY

Responses to these questions demand much more than careful phenomenology, a cornerstone of both good ethnography and clinical medicine. Studies compiled from the twelfth century onward show that the poor, quite simply, are sicker than the nonpoor and that this is true in both rich and poor countries.[22] In a 1969 volume of papers addressing the issues of poverty and health, we read: "Clearly the poverty population is considerably less healthy than the rest of the population of [the United States]. It still experiences substantially higher rates of overall mortality (all ages and by age, and especially from the communicable diseases), infant mortality, and severe illness."[23] A more recent review argues that studies continue to point to the same conclusion:

> One of the most striking features of the relationship between [socioeconomic status] and health is its pervasiveness and persistence over

time. This relationship is found in virtually every measure of health status: age-adjusted mortality for all causes of death as well as specific causes, the severity of acute disease and the incidence of severe infectious conditions, the prevalence and severity of nearly every chronic disease, and measures of disability and restricted activity.[24]

But how, precisely, are these inequalities of outcome explained? Also writing of the U.S. poor, Ryan puts it trenchantly: "The facts are plain: their health is bad. The cause is plain: health costs money, and they don't have money."[25] In the years since Ryan made this claim, we have learned that the relationship between poverty and health is more complicated.[26] But the complexities are often found in the diverse ways in which the health of the disenfranchised may be made to suffer. That is, poverty and other social inequalities come to alter disease distribution and sickness trajectories through innumerable and complicated mechanisms.

Take tuberculosis, with its persistence in poor countries and its resurgence among the poor of many industrialized nations. We cannot understand its markedly patterned occurrence—in the United States, for example, afflicting those in homeless shelters and in prison—without understanding how social forces, ranging from political violence to racism, come to be embodied as individual pathology.

Initially, poverty and racism increase the likelihood that one will become infected by *Mycobacterium tuberculosis*. The mechanisms by which this occurs include the prevalence of the disease among the poor and the fact that the poor are more likely to live together, often in the cramped, airless quarters that once characterized the "lung blocks" of industrializing cities and now describe the urban ghettoes in which tuberculosis is endemic. Various institutions designed to serve or contain the poor have in many instances been the settings for amplified outbreaks of tuberculosis. Nardell and Brickner argue, for example, that homeless shelters have become the lung blocks of the late twentieth century.[27] Poverty and racism surely increase the likelihood that one will end up in a shelter, just as these forces arrange the chances that one will wake up in a crack house or a prison.

Once infected, the poor are more likely to progress to active disease. Again, the mechanisms are myriad. Cell-mediated immunity, which keeps tuberculosis quiescent in most persons, may be compromised by malnutrition, HIV infection (or other concurrent disease), or addiction to drugs or alcohol. Addiction, in turn, is usually not comprehensible without an understanding of subjugation and racism, at least not if historical and population-based studies are to be believed. Even reinfection with *M. tuberculosis* might play a role in ensuring that tuberculosis infection will progress to disease; the risk of reinfection is strongly influenced by the social factors just described.

These same factors determine outcomes among those with active tuberculosis disease. Poverty and racism increase the likelihood of dire outcomes among the sick by restricting access to effective therapy or rendering it less effective if patients are malnourished or addicted. Poverty clearly decreases the ability of patients to "comply" with demanding, lengthy regimens. Indeed, the advent of truly effective therapies only brings into starker relief the centrality of social inequalities, when unequal access to these therapies heightens the inequalities of infection and reactivation already described.

Thus do *fundamentally social forces and processes come to be embodied as biological events*. Throughout this book, I will make similar arguments in considering HIV and other infectious pathogens.

While underlining the essentially social nature of unequal health outcomes, I also want to avoid what might be termed the "Luddite trap." Addressing the social roots of disease is sometimes held to be incompatible with advocating the delivery of high-quality, high-tech care—an opinion often voiced by critics of private-sector medicine. But the facts are otherwise, as Paul Wise observes in a subtle discussion of racial disparities in infant mortality: "Too often, those who elevate the role of social determinants indict clinical technologies as failed strategies. But devaluing clinical intervention diverts attention from the essential goal that it be provided equitably to all those in need. Belittling the role of clinical care tends to unburden policy of the requirement to provide equitable access to such care."[28]

Nothing is wrong with high-tech medicine, except that there isn't enough of it to go around. It is, in fact, concentrated in precisely those areas where it will have the most limited effects. We need more and better clinical services for those marginalized by poverty and by discrimination. Annette Jean would no doubt be alive today had she been diagnosed and treated in a timely fashion. Combination antiretroviral therapy would—and, I hope, will—no doubt prolong her brother's life. The poor need access to the best clinical interventions available, and we are living in a time when double standards of care must be questioned. Indeed, this is one of the messages to be distilled from the voices cited in this book.

Another message is that, with effective clinical interventions, we can often hope to efface the embodied manifestations of social inequalities. This has certainly been the goal of many health care providers working in settings of great privation.[29] We can show that tuberculosis outcomes can be as good among the rural Haitian poor as they are anywhere else.[30] Others working in U.S. inner cities have shown that inequalities of survival among those living with HIV can also be erased if high-quality AIDS care is afforded to all, regardless of ability to pay.[31]

Nevertheless, we must remember that effacing the inequality of outcomes is not the same as eliminating the underlying forces of inequality itself. And studying inequality is perhaps even further removed from this goal. But a desire for equality, whether avowed or hidden, often underpins such studies, as Sen points out: "When we assess inequalities across the world in being able to avoid preventable morbidity, or escapable hunger, or premature mortality, we are not merely examining differences in well-being, but also in the basic freedoms that we value and cherish."[32]

In a very real way, inequality itself constitutes our modern plague. The burdens of inequality are primarily borne by the poor and marginalized, for not everyone can claim victimhood, despite the self-serving identity politics and "soft relativism" of our times. But it is worth noting that even wealthy societies riven by great inequalities are bereft of social cohesion. This lack of cohesion is tightly linked to increased rates of morbidity and mortality: "It is now clear," writes Wilkinson in an important study of inequality in industrial societies, "that the scale of income differences in a society is one of the most powerful determinants of health standards in different countries, and that it influences health through its impact on social cohesion."[33]

In the United States, where this correlation is pronounced, one notes with alarm the widening income gap between worker and management: at this writing, the average CEO of a major company makes more than two hundred times what the average factory worker earns.

This disparity, five times greater than it was thirty years ago, is growing. "You can almost hear the proletariat sharpening the guillotine," warned *Newsweek* in an article on the subject; but in truth there seems to be a monopoly of violence from above, not below.[34]

    .   .   .   .   .

This book consists of ten chapters. The first, written at the behest of an anonymous reviewer who commented on an earlier incarnation of the book, offers an overview of my own engagement in efforts to remediate inequalities of access to potentially life-saving interventions. It is the story of an expanding group of people—some of them chroniclers of the modern plagues, others absorbed in combating them—for whom pragmatic engagement in the clinic and the field lends to life a vitality all too uncommon in the modern university.

Chapter 2, which is necessarily less personal, takes a closer look at the concept of "emerging infectious diseases" and in so doing elaborates the analytic framework used in the rest of the book. The general argument it presents is that social inequalities often determine both the distribution of modern plagues and clinical outcomes among the afflicted. Thus does inequality itself become a pathogenic force. Like the introduction, these two chapters are critical of rigidly disciplinary approaches to complex biosocial phenomena such as epidemic disease. And, like the rest of this volume, these chapters draw unabashedly on methodologies ranging from ethnography to molecular epidemiology.

Subsequent chapters seek to apply this framework to specific diseases—primarily AIDS and tuberculosis—and specific settings. But the perspective here is neither epidemiologic nor sociologic; rather, it is my hope that a deep concern with individual experience suffuses every page. All of the chapters tell the stories of people afflicted by these plagues.[35]

In examining these deadly epidemics, the chapters move from a broad sociology-of-knowledge approach to an in-depth look at the dynamics of infectious disease and, finally, to pragmatic interventions designed to improve outcomes. An "ethnographic interlude" links the chapters on AIDS and tuberculosis, underscoring the perils of relying overmuch on a single discipline.

   Chapter 10, the book's conclusion, is as much a warning as a plea. The further entrenchment of social inequality has dire implications in a time of rapid advancement in science and technology. If I am correct, the plagues of our times require as "co-factors" such inequalities—that is, steep grades of inequality fuel the persistence or emergence of epidemic disease. Greater access to effective medical services is but a necessary first step in stanching these epidemics.

1 The Vitality of Practice

ON PERSONAL TRAJECTORIES

One learns, I would hope, to discover what is

right, what needs to be righted—through work,

through action.

DANIEL BERRIGAN, 1971

As I prepared this book, an anonymous reviewer of an early draft suggested that, since the book reflects a personal journey, it should make explicit the itinerary taken. The idea of a confessional cast to a book about the plagues of the poor made me shudder, at least initially. But it is nonetheless true that my experiences in Peru and, especially, in Haiti have shaped my interpretations every bit as much as has training in anthropology and medicine.

Curiously, perhaps, I knew early—at twenty years of age, before I went to Haiti—that I wanted to be a physician-anthropologist. But my experience in central Haiti helped me decide what kind of medicine to practice. In my first year there, I witnessed preventable deaths from malaria, tuberculosis, and postpartum infections. That was enough to make me decide to specialize in infectious disease. Haiti also strengthened my interest in social theory, particularly in the relationship between structural constraints and personal agency. How do life conditions restrict any individual's capacity to make choices? The constraint part of the formula was critical, for poverty was the central fact of life for the Haitians with whom I lived and worked. It seemed at times as if their every move was trammeled by the hard surfaces of economic want. "Life for the Haitian peasant of today," observed anthropologist Jean Weise over twenty-five years ago, "is abject misery and a rank familiarity with death."[1]

Accordingly, lack of access to effective biomedical services was the most salient feature of the Haitian health system. The country had only one medical school, and its graduates usually sought to remain in Port-au-Prince after graduation—or, better yet, to leave Haiti altogether. In the decade following the ascent of Dr. François Duvalier to power, for example, 264 physicians graduated from the state medical school, and all but 3 left the country.[2] In the eighties, Haiti's nationwide physician-to-population ratio was 18 physicians per 100,000 inhabitants, compared to 250 physicians per 100,000 in the United States—and 364 per 100,000 in neighboring Cuba.[3] This figure varied substantially between the country's four administrative districts. The Haitians whose stories are presented in this book live in the Région Transversale, which is by far the most underserved region, with about 5 physicians per 100,000 inhabitants.[4] That made me, from the time I was a medical student, something of a novelty in rural Haiti.

By the spring of 1984, a year after my arrival, I'd cast my lot with a group of landless peasants who were working with a dynamic Haitian priest. He knew nothing about health care, he told me. Since I was going to be a doctor—he never evinced much interest in my anthropology studies—it would be my job to oversee health-related projects. So get cracking, he said; find the necessary resources. Wouldn't it be better, I objected, to conduct a preliminary "needs assessment" of the region, one that would ask those living in the communities to be served what they'd like to see come from our efforts? "Fine," replied the priest. "Do as you wish. But they're just going to tell you they want a hospital."

He was right. Although they also mentioned schools and water and land, most people surveyed said that a hospital was what the region needed. (Notably, we never heard requests for research.) Although we knew better than to wait to hear demands for, say, vaccinations against tetanus and measles, we decided to act as if we meant it when we insisted that their opinions mattered to us. At the same time that we sought to establish preventive services, we built a clinic.

Founded in 1985, the Clinique Bon Sauveur has since served the rural poor of Haiti's Central Plateau. My experiences there further shaped my medical interests. Within a year of opening the clinic, we saw our first case of AIDS, in a young man who presented with disseminated tuberculosis. His drama became mine too, since no one knew, really, what was going on, and I, a physician-in-training, was often the most "medical" person around. Manno became a central figure in my dissertation and the book it engendered—and forced me to come to terms with the nature of my own involvement in the lives of my "informants." My priority, I knew, was not analytic; it was pragmatic.

From the early eighties, I commuted between Haiti, with its dearth of medical services, and Harvard, where there were innumerable doctors and veritable thickets of hospitals. The experience has been jarring, certainly, but also illuminating. Haiti became a sort of interpretive grid for what I was hearing in medical school. First, I paid special attention to information that would be useful there—and soon became aware of a striking lack of interest in tuberculosis and parasitology on the part of U.S. academic medicine.[5] Second, my experience in Haiti made me skeptical of certain claims of causality. I found precious little discussion of how poverty affects disease distribution and outcome and virtually no mention of the pathogenicity of social inequality. Even in social medicine classes, which did discuss social forces, much of the debate did not ring true for me.

The people I'd been working with in Haiti, hungry and sick, were completely absent from consideration and so, of course, was their plight. For example, we heard and read of enormous resources poured into "technological fixes," such as neonatal intensive care units, that yielded, in the view of some, few discernible results. Critics of the status quo, including many public health activists, seemed content to call for less funding for these fixes and more for the interventions of their choice (which were usually "low-tech" and grounded in preventive medicine).

I knew that Harvard Medical School was merely a brief airplane ride away from a setting in which markedly unheroic interventions would indeed have been lifesaving. But didn't the dilemmas of the Haitian sick call for a full range of high-tech *and* low-tech interventions? Why, I wondered anxiously, was it so manifestly impolitic, in Harvard's rarefied circles, to press for the former as well as the latter? Certainly the people of central Haiti were not specifically requesting low-tech solutions for their grave medical problems. When asked what *they* wanted, they had replied unhesitatingly, "A hospital." Not a clinic, a health post, or a dispensary. Not vaccines or prenatal care. They wanted a hospital.

Although experiences in Haiti made me a fairly discerning consumer of the literature on medical futility, it slowly became clear that I'd been taken in by some of the pieties of development work. Talk of "appropriate technology" and "sustainability" had sounded good to me, at least initially. The problem was that these sounded silly, even sinister, to the landless peasants with whom I worked and to many of their staunchest advocates. Early in my stay in Do Kay, during a year of transformative experiences, I ran head-on into the fundamental disjuncture between "expert views" on these matters (as promulgated, for example, in scholarly journals and in schools of public health) and the views of those whose commitment was to more radical changes in the circumstances endured by the poor.

Take an exchange between myself and the aforementioned Haitian priest, who had for decades devoted himself to improving the lot of the rural poor. It was late 1984, and I had returned to the Central Plateau after months away in medical school. The priest was anxious to show me the new latrines they'd built in the village. The latrines were made of cement; they were solid and square and tin-roofed, and they looked faintly incongruous next to the thatched and lopsided shacks in which so many of the villagers lived.

Unwisely, I asked whether the latrines were really "appropriate technology" for such a poor village. The priest was furious. "Do you know what 'appropriate technology' means?" he finally answered. "It means good things for rich people and shit for the poor." He wheeled away, fuming, and refused to speak to me for a couple of days.

With the help of my (sometimes stern) Haitian hosts, I've since come to believe that the hypocrisies of development are not only morally flimsy but in fact analytically shallow.[6] Many of the positions advanced in the development field are underpinned by a zero-sum approach: only exceedingly limited funds are available for "sustainable" projects, goes this logic, and so those who work for the poor must choose between, say, high-tech interventions and preventive services. Such Luddite critiques of technological advancement treat poor villages like Do Kay as if they were cut off from the rest of the world.[7]

I knew, however, that we were living not in two different worlds but in the same world. This was brought home repeatedly on an experiential level by the brevity of my trip back to Miami. More to the point, it was brought home on an analytic level by actually taking the trouble to study the historical record. The truth was that Do Kay was a squatter settlement of self-described "water refugees." Their misery had begun, they said, when a U.S.-financed hydroelectric dam, itself the centerpiece of a "development project," flooded the valley where they had farmed for years. The project had been signed into existence in Washington, D.C.[8]

To better understand the Harvard-Haiti axis, I turned to anthropology. Although my mentors were mostly engaged, at the time, in symbolic anthropology, they encouraged me to read widely. I found what's known as "world-systems theory" to be exceedingly helpful as I attempted to simultaneously complete medical school and a doctorate in anthropology. Perhaps less a theory than a call for analytic rigor, the world-systems approach was a challenge to ferret out connections.[9] Reading the works of Immanuel Wallerstein, Sidney Mintz, and Eric Wolf was invigorating as I explored the historical links between Haiti and the United States. In addition, studying these connections and their construction over time wasn't a bad way to learn to think about a new epidemic caused by an intracellular organism.[10] Other illnesses then said to be "emerging" or "reemerging" were clearly caught up in these same transnational systems. Laurie Garrett, whose excellent book *The Coming Plague* contains an ominous forecast, puts it this way:

> Rapid globalization of human niches requires that human beings everywhere on the planet go beyond viewing their neighborhoods, provinces, countries, or hemispheres as the sum total of their personal ecospheres. Microbes, and their vectors, recognize none of the artificial boundaries erected by human beings. Theirs is the world of natural limitations: temperature, pH, ultraviolet light, the presence of vulnerable hosts, and mobile vectors.[11]

AIDS, I learned through research, brought connections, not discontinuities, into relief. In the midst of this quest for connections, I was becoming disenchanted with a certain type of disconnected anthropology.[12] This brand of inquiry had as its goal the search for "thick" local meaning unhinged from history and political economy. In rural Haiti, nothing much seemed unhinged from history and political economy; the connections, historically deep and geographically broad, came into view with minimal effort.

If my experience there estranged me from static cultural analyses, AIDS drove a final nail in the coffin. When Nancy Scheper-Hughes wrote about "the mountain of uninspiring social science literature on AIDS, a morass of repetitive, pious liturgies about stigma, blaming, and difference," I knew just what she meant.[13] During the years of my training, anthropology joined the other social sciences in carving out "turf" in the study of AIDS, and there followed a spate of disconnected studies of "cultural" phenomena related, in one way or another, to AIDS. Very often, these phenomena were much more tightly linked to poverty and inequality than to the specific culture in question—a classic example of the conflation of structural violence and cultural difference.

What claims did this mountain of literature make? What functions did it subserve? For what audiences was it written and disseminated? What canonical concerns framed this inquiry so that certain "cultural" exotica would be sharply in focus while other considerations—poverty and inequality and the feckless, sometimes deadly policies of the powerful— rarely appeared in the frame of analysis? Work on AIDS and tuberculosis posed such questions forcefully and often.

I soon learned that scholars trained in different disciplines could examine the very same topic (the spread of HIV, say, or the reason why millions die of a disease as treatable as tuberculosis) and come up with altogether incompatible conclusions. What's more, these scholars could advance such completely discrepant assessments with great confidence. These "immodest claims of causality" became one of my central interests, even though such inquiry was generally viewed as more appropriate to the sociology of knowledge than to either anthropology or medicine. To explore these causal claims, one needed to regard as cultural artifacts not only the popular press but also the scholarly journals. My doctoral dissertation, subsequently published as *AIDS and Accusation* (1992), claimed to be an interpretive ethnography accountable to history and political economy and informed by a critical epidemiology.[14] I also tried to tackle many of the sociology-of-knowledge questions that had arisen as the scientific and medical communities scrambled to make sense of AIDS.

Immodest claims of causality, the hypocrisies of development, crazy theories about the origins of AIDS, and other ideologies posing as analysis—all were run through the interpretive grid that grew out of these travels along the Harvard-Haiti axis. But what sounds like some great intellectual adventure was in fact often painful. A mountain of doctoral dissertations would not, I suspected, allay the awful suffering I'd witnessed in Haiti. And things were going from bad to worse. Medical services for the people I'd come to care about were simply not "cost-effective" in the increasingly dominant framework of neoliberalism; nor were their proposed projects, however modest, sustainable according to the criteria imposed by the development set that at times seemed to be running Haiti.

And yet health care for the poor struck me, early on, as the noblest goal a physician could have. The unarguable immediacy of their needs, and the vitality of practice of those seeking to meet them, was sufficient rejoinder to both the uninspiring social science and the ultimately punitive policies favored by the burgeoning development bureaucracies.

Where was I going to work, if I found existing institutions, or at least their confidently advanced ideas, so distasteful? By the time I'd started asking these questions, I'd struck up with Jim Yong Kim. We shared more or less the same academic background and the same concerns. What were we to make of our "ridiculously lavish educations," we who had received so much?[15]

Staying put in Boston was not an option, not after all we'd seen. World-systems theory, perhaps, helped us to see people like ourselves, with one foot in Harvard and another in Haiti, as possible conduits for resources. These conduits would have valves that could lead resources to flow against the current, back to the poor communities we had studied. This was a moral commitment, certainly, but careful analysis seemed to lead to the same conclusions. Understanding AIDS called for a systemic approach, so why shouldn't responses to such diseases be transnational and, given the transnational nature of HIV's spread, make a claim on a commensurate share of the world's wealth? Business was conducted globally; so was U.S. foreign policy—often with disastrous results, if outcomes among the poor are deemed in any way important to an assessment of such policies. Why not medicine?

Jim Kim and I, working largely with friends from outside the academy, felt sure that our own quest for the vitality of practice needed to be transnational, rooted in social justice (we followed liberation theology in making a "preferential option for the poor"), and informed by what we'd learned at Harvard and in Haiti. We proceeded in precisely this manner, even though we never assumed, initially, that our projects would matter much to the academic community that had nourished us so unstintingly. We were wrong on that score.

PRAGMATIC SOLIDARITY IN HAITI

To do this work—which we termed, rather grandly, "pragmatic solidarity"—we first established two organizations: Zanmi Lasante, a community-based organization in Haiti led by the priest and his coworkers; and Partners in Health, a Massachusetts-based, nongovernmental organization with a mission to remediate inequalities of access to health care. In the intervening decade, we've been able to provide services to hundreds of thousands of people, almost all of them living in poverty.[16]

Although I initially worked as a community health worker and something akin to a fundraiser, in recent years most of my time has been consumed in direct clinical care. The HIV and tuberculosis clinic in Do Kay eventually grew to see up to 20 percent of all ambulatory patients (some thirty thousand a year) who arrive at the Clinique Bon Sauveur. This combined HIV and tuberculosis unit is simply called "the TB clinic," in part because AIDS is more stigmatized than tuberculosis but also because most of our patients with HIV disease fall ill with TB. Since roughly a third of the world's population carries quiescent tuberculosis infection, tuberculosis is probably the world's most common AIDS-associated opportunistic infection.[17] It's certainly the most important opportunistic infection in Haitians with HIV infection, a finding noted as early as 1983.[18]

On a busy day, the Clinique Bon Sauveur receives 250 patients, which can mean 40 or 50 patients in the TB clinic. They are seen by myself or a generalist, a licensed practical nurse, and a placid young man with a grade-school education whose job it is to greet and weigh the patients and to collect their chest films. (His name, fittingly, is Seraphim.) The patients come early in the morning and spend most of the day waiting, since turnaround on chest films or labs is slow.

In rural Haiti, the clinic is hot and stuffy and overcrowded, often rendered even noisier by the nearby dentist's drill. An average day in the clinic is in some ways similar to a day in the clinic of a Boston teaching hospital: the day is split between highs and lows. The highs usually involve sick patients' prompt response to therapies. Failure to respond to therapies accounts for many of the lows, but these are just as frequently the result of a lack of something: a medicine, a diagnostic test, a bit of already published information, or cash for families who need food and housing more than they need medicines. Moving along the Harvard-Haiti axis keeps nerve endings raw, since I know, as my Haitian co-workers often do not, just what—or, often as not, just how little—we are missing to clinch a diagnosis or to ensure a good outcome. This regret is heightened by the fact that I spend four months a year at the Brigham and Women's Hospital in Massachusetts, where the latest treatments are readily available, even for patients without insurance.

Sometimes we're able to provide state-of-the-art care at the Clinique Bon Sauveur, if by accident and epidemiologic happenstance. Take the case of Marie, a twenty-eight-year-old mother of four. She was diagnosed with HIV disease in January 1996, when she presented with herpes zoster. She'd had, she said, no fever, chills, or cough. A chest radiograph at that time was remarkable only for changes consistent with quiescent tuberculosis infection. Laboratory studies revealed mild anemia but a normal white blood cell count. Marie was placed on isoniazid prophylaxis—since the prevention of "reactivation tuberculosis" is one of the best services we can provide our patients—and an iron supplement and was asked to return in one month with her partner and their children. Instead, she returned two weeks later after a witnessed seizure. When I saw her, she was still groggy but clearly had weakness in her left hand and arm. A lumbar puncture was more or less normal, as were other screening lab studies. Her chest film was unchanged.

We felt sure that Marie had a mass lesion in her brain, and the most common mass lesions in the brains of our patients with early HIV disease are tuberculomas. But we had no way to prove it; Haiti's only CT scan, in far-off Port-au-Prince, had long been out of commission, and Haiti's neurosurgeons were practicing in Canada or the United States. Marie was placed on seizure medications and that day began treatment for tuberculosis of the brain. We reasoned that she had early HIV infection: zoster is often the harbinger of HIV disease in Haiti. Even without a CD4 count, we felt that toxoplasmosis, cryptococcosis, and lymphoma—the usual culprits, in the United States—were less likely than a tuberculoma.

Marie responded clinically: her neurological defect resolved, and her seizures did not recur. After nine months of therapy, both her antituberculous medications and her seizure medications were stopped. She remains asymptomatic to this day.

Such stories abound. But as I reflect on the past several years, it's easy to discern both successes and failures in our clinical work in Haiti. Under the former rubric we can include early detection and aggressive therapy for tuberculosis among the HIV-infected; the use of AZT during pregnancy to prevent vertical transmission of HIV (from mother to baby); improved services for sexually transmitted diseases; and screening for cervical cancer. We've also improved our laboratory capacity, standardized certain treatment algorithms, and trained physicians and nurses from throughout Haiti's Central Plateau. We've conducted research that we hope may influence how the medical community comes to understand the complex interplay between gender inequality, poverty, and the distribution of HIV. We've countered incorrect stereotypes about Haitians and incorporated these insights into a broad array of prevention materials. Finally, and most important, we've eased the pain of tuberculosis and HIV disease exacerbated by poverty.

But we've also been plagued by the problems specific to settings such as ours—an impoverished rural backwater in an impoverished country. The Clinique Bon Sauveur has experienced rapid turnover of medical staff, which inevitably results in gaps in continuity of care. We have patients who for lack of access to other facilities (as well as lack of roads and vehicles) walk for days to seek care in our clinic and, once seen, never return for follow-up visits. We also experience what we term *ruptures de stock*—an interrupted supply of key drugs—which can have implications in terms of drug resistance. It's demoralizing for the staff, to say nothing of the patients.

Because poverty is the central fact of life for the people of Haiti, so too is it the central fact of our lives as their physicians and their advocates. If I've learned anything during the AIDS years, it's that, no matter who you are or what you earn, it's always difficult to live with HIV. But living with both HIV disease and poverty is brutally painful. This insight triggers angst. We're plagued by a nagging sense of failure as we attempt to raise the funds necessary to pay community health workers and lab technicians what they deserve—and doctors what they demand. We can't help wanting better drugs and better laboratory facilities. And, yes, we need indices of viral load, and we need protease inhibitors and other highly active antiretroviral therapy. At the AIDS conference held in Vancouver, many from the Third World saw the meeting motto—"One World, One Hope"—as disingenuous because what was missing were serious efforts to alleviate the crushing inequalities that make HIV infection a very different experience depending on where you have the misfortune to contract it.

Often enough, though, this angst fades away in the course of a busy day at the clinic. Often enough, one is satisfied with small victories: a patient whose painful oral candidiasis "miraculously disappears" with a few antifungal troches; another who is relieved of chronic diarrhea when the etiology is revealed by stool studies; yet another whose shortness of breath, due to miliary tuberculosis, is relieved by adding steroids to a standard antituberculous regimen.

And, occasionally, small victories are reclassified by patients as *gwo mirak*—big miracles. In these instances, the gratitude of a patient is more reward than one could ever deserve. This came to mind recently, when the mother of an eighteen-month-old baby broke into tears of relief when I announced that, two years after a difficult course of AZT during her pregnancy, her baby had now proven seronegative. "Thanks be to God," said the mother, who before her pregnancy had barely survived miliary tuberculosis, "for another *gwo mirak*."

None of this medical service, miraculous or otherwise, would have been possible without the organizations we founded to keep our solidarity pragmatic.[19] A substantial network of friends came to constitute Partners in Health, and we set off to address inequalities of access and outcome. At times this meant setting off to places such as Haiti or Chiapas; at other times, to places such as Roxbury, a part of inner-city Boston. I lived in Roxbury during my medical school years, and I knew it to be an attractive enough neighborhood. But other indices revealed it to be a nexus of the petty drug trade, an area afflicted by high rates of unemployment, by racism, and by excess morbidity and mortality.[20] At one point, frustrated residents had announced their intention to rebaptize the borough as "Mandela" and secede from the city of Boston. This did not come to pass, but it was through our Roxbury connections that we came to have a keener understanding of how relative poverty (relative since, after all, the malnutrition of rural Haiti is not the same as, say, the addiction or violence seen in Roxbury) comes to have its pathogenic effects.

It was also through Roxbury connections that we became involved in Peru. One of our number, after seventeen years of work in Roxbury, left for Lima, Peru. Our friend went to Carabayllo, a rapidly growing slum on the northernmost reaches of the sprawling capital city. In the setting of growing political violence, and with diminishing harvests and economic dislocations in the world markets, millions of rural Peruvians had "invaded" Lima.[21] Carabayllo, and indeed the entire northern reach of the metropolis, was one part of the city most affected by these *invasiones*, as they are termed locally. Looking around the dusty, desert slum, it was impossible not to think of the relative beauty of the places the migrants had left behind. It was also possible, however, to see some of Carabayllo's attractions: one merely had to look up at the electric pylons or to talk to the squatters. They would be quick to tell you that they'd come for better schools and medical care, for water and electricity, and to be out of the way of the violent conflict between the Sendero Luminoso guerrillas and the Peruvian army. In the confused swirl of these trends, old social typologies were breaking down, as Orin Starn has noted:

> The distance between thatch-roofed adobe Andean peasant dwellings and city shacks of tin, cardboard, and straw mats was not that between

"indigenous" Andean society and "Western" modernity. Rather it was the space between different points on a single circuit that was integrated by family ties, village loyalties, and constant circulation of goods, ideas, and people. Indian, cholo, and mestizo were not discrete categories, but partly overlapping positions on a continuum.[22]

During our co-worker's first years in Peru, Partners in Health became involved in a number of small projects, founding in the process a third sister organization, Socios en Salud. One of these projects was the construction of a community pharmacy—a *botiquín*—that would make medications available to the destitute sick. Shortly after the building was completed, it was destroyed by a bomb. Sendero, everyone said, and the motive was held to be the usual: if we were reformers, patching up the wounds of the poor, we were, in Sendero's eyes, palliatives, delaying the necessary radical transformation of Peruvian society. A couple of years earlier, a Sendero communiqué had ordered nongovernmental organizations out of Peru because "you give crumbs to the people to entertain them and fail to realize that the correct path is that of the people's war."[23]

It seems cheap to say that we appreciated neither the logic nor the methods of our detractors. Cheap because it's been said so many times, by anthropologists as well as by the pillars of the Peruvian state. Sendero's analysis, though riddled with inconsistency and undermined by arbitrary violence, was less easy to dismiss. We *were* patching up wounds. Such interventions would not, it's true, alter the overall trends registered in the slums of Lima, settlements growing at a rapid rate.

With a certain degree of angst, we continued our modest attempts (including rebuilding the *botiquín*) and planned to keep our projects small. But in the spring of 1994, our co-worker became ill. He began to cough, to experience diarrhea and night sweats. As he continued to lose weight, we asked him to come home. He did return to Boston, where, right off the plane, he was diagnosed with disseminated tuberculosis. In keeping with standard practice, he was placed on empiric therapy with four drugs. These drugs are the most powerful antituberculous agents available, and they are usually rapidly effective. But our friend worsened on this regimen. Less than a month after his return, he died without knowing what was, in fact, killing him: his strain of tuberculosis was resistant to all four of the drugs. He had what's usually called "MDRTB"—multidrug-resistant tuberculosis.

In the course of treating cases of MDRTB in Haiti, I'd read a good deal of the clinical and epidemiologic literature on this very modern phenomenon. After all, organisms become resistant to drugs only after selective pressures created by us humans, the manufacturers and prescribers of the drugs. I'd learned that drug resistance must be diagnosed quickly and that treatment regimens must be based on the results of drug-susceptibility testing—that is, they must consist of drugs with a demonstrated ability to kill the particular strain infecting the patient. These regimens need to include multiple drugs and to last far longer than the empiric regimens that contain the more powerful, "first-line" drugs. This means, of course, that treating MDRTB is more expensive than treating susceptible disease. But treatment is the only way to prevent ongoing transmission, which can occur whenever a patient with pulmonary MDRTB coughs viable organisms into the air. Some believe that a person with active pulmonary tuberculosis infects, on average, between ten and twenty persons per year.[24] Thus the cornerstones of managing MDRTB are rapid identification of active cases through an aggressive search and the prompt initiation of individualized therapy.

At Partners in Health, we were faced with more than our own grief. What were our obligations, knowing as we did that our friend had died of MDRTB acquired in a Peruvian slum? Had he died while working in Roxbury, the public health department would have initiated an aggressive quest for contacts and cases. But the state of Massachusetts was in no way prepared to embark on a transnational effort to trace contacts, and it was even less likely that any U.S. agency would be prepared to treat any active cases revealed through such an effort.

For years, from Haiti and in the context of the AIDS pandemic, we'd been arguing for a systemic and critical look at the transnational nature of epidemics. We'd been arguing, too, for the remediation of inequalities of access, calling for the sort of pragmatic solidarity that the Haitian poor had demanded. Wasn't our friend's death a sort of test case for both our analysis and our convictions? Wasn't it a sign?

After a good deal of soul-searching, we went to Lima in an effort to identify and treat active cases of MDRTB. Working with Socios en Salud, we first contacted the local public health authorities, who sharply reminded us that Peru had a model tuberculosis program, as anyone who worked in the field should know. The World Health Organization (WHO) and the Pan American Health Association had declared as much, and so Peru needed no help in dealing with its tuberculosis problem. In other words, we were sent packing.

In the crowded barrio shantytowns of Carabayllo, a very different response awaited us. In every clinic we visited, nurses and technicians told us about patients who had failed to respond to directly observed therapy with first-line drugs. Many had died before suspected resistance could be confirmed, said the providers, but other patients had laboratory-confirmed MDRTB. How were individuals in this latter group responding to therapy, we asked? Most were not on therapy at all, came the response, or they were slated to receive "isoniazid for life." Since these patients were all resistant to isoniazid, we knew we were in for trouble if our goal was to identify and treat patients with MDRTB. And in the context of Peruvian officialdom's rapt embrace of "free market principles," support for public health programs had ebbed.

Where would small organizations like Partners in Health and Socios en Salud find the resources and backing to tackle a problem as weighty as MDRTB? Because we knew that the World Health Organization had in recent years become the world leader in effective management of tuberculosis, we contacted the WHO. We also knew that the WHO and other international health organizations were using the specter of "an untreatable form of tuberculosis"—termed "Ebola with wings" by the popular press—in an overt effort to frighten donor nations into funding tuberculosis control.[25] In addition, after careful study of deadly outbreaks of MDRTB in U.S. hospitals and jails, the U.S. Centers for Disease Control and Prevention (CDC) had concluded that only aggressive contact tracing and prompt initiation of therapy would interrupt transmission of resistant strains.[26] Since a third of U.S. tuberculosis patients are foreign-born, we thought we'd get a sympathetic hearing from the CDC.[27]

When we contacted these organizations, however, we quickly learned that the Peruvian position had in fact come from them: it was not "cost-effective" to treat MDRTB in developing countries, went the argument. The number of resistant cases in Peru was too small to warrant individualized treatment regimens, said the experts; all energies must be directed to treating the far larger number of drug-susceptible cases.

Wait a minute, we objected; what's the threshold for a public health emergency? We quickly documented a hundred cases of pulmonary MDRTB in the northern reaches of Lima alone and collected reports of hundreds more elsewhere in the city.[28] Because none of these people were receiving appropriate therapy, all were to be considered infectious. Didn't their presence in the midst of a city of six million constitute a public health emergency?

The "constant circulation of goods, ideas, and people" mentioned by Starn referred to intranational linkages, but we had also documented transnational cases—that is, cases of MDRTB contracted in Peru but diagnosed elsewhere. Our friend's case was one example, but a more spectacular one was offered by a woman from the Carabayllo region who fell ill with MDRTB while working as a maid in wealthy Westchester County, New York. Little could be done for those exposed to such highly resistant strains: there was no agreed-upon course of action for this woman's asymptomatic contacts, since the standard preventive approach—prophylaxis with isoniazid—was useless in these cases.[29]

Unable to find partners in this endeavor, we sought to treat these patients ourselves. Initially, our efforts were blocked, and we stood by as people, including those you will encounter in Chapters 7 and 9, died. Eventually, pressure from the afflicted communities led to an agreement with the local public health authorities, and our treatment effort began in earnest. Not surprisingly, MDRTB proved no more "untreatable" in urban Peru than in New York. In fact, our results seemed to be significantly better than those obtained in some of the early efforts documented in Denver and New York.[30]

The entire quarrel—whose myths and mystifications are examined in Chapters 7, 8, and 9—afforded rich material for an anthropologist. But what really struck me was, again, the pathogenic role of inequality. The contribution of inequality to the genesis of resistance was certainly clear. The steep grades of social inequality in Lima meant that the second-line antituberculous drugs necessary to treat MDRTB were available on the market but that the people most at risk for MDRTB were unable to purchase these drugs in a reliable manner. And surely differential valuation of human life underpinned the public health community's ready acquiescence to cost-effectiveness models that made MDRTB a treatable disease in some communities and "untreatable" in others. Where were the Virchows of modern public health? Where were the "natural attorneys of the poor"?

The cost-effectiveness models used to argue against treatment for MDRTB in Peru were also based on faulty analysis. Analyses confined within the framework of the nation-state ignore both transnational microbial traffic and the movement of massive amounts of capital in and out of Peru—amounts that dwarfed what would have been needed to treat every case of active disease in the country. But woe to those who had the cheek to observe that the fact that close to 20 percent of all Peru's governmental outlays were going to finance its external debt might be related to a lack of funding for public health.[31]

Once again, we discern the pernicious effects of the two-worlds myth. Although they might be regarded by U.S. free marketeers, for instance, as potential consumers or laborers, poor Peruvians are deemed "untreatable" when ill with a disease that calls for aggressive therapy in New York City. Recent debates about the ethics of international medical research are highly specific reflections of the same general problem. In September 1997, two physicians, Peter Lurie and Sidney Wolfe, argued that U.S.-financed research projects in Africa and Asia were unethical if, in exploring mother-to-infant transmission of HIV, they compared the efficacy of AZT to a placebo. Because previous research had already answered the question, they pointed out, such an investigation would not have been approved by ethics review boards in U.S. universities and hospitals. Marcia Angell, the editor of the *New England Journal of Medicine*, went a step further, arguing that "the justifications [for a placebo group] are reminiscent of those for the Tuskegee study: Women in the Third World would not receive antiretroviral treatment anyway, so the investigators are simply observing what would happen to the subjects' infants if there were no study."[32]

Lurie and Wolfe touched off a furor by observing, as had millions of apparently inaudible poor people, that such trials were unethical. But one implication of the debate went largely unremarked, in part because most medical ethicists—entranced by the quandary ethics of the individual—

had little interest in questions of poverty, inequality, and access to care.[33] The human-rights community also had little to add, since social and economic rights had not been central to its agenda. Yet what is missing from the debate is acknowledgment that the growing inequalities of the global era—the context, after all, of research conducted in a poor country but sponsored by a rich one—constitute, in and of themselves, a sort of "global Tuskegee experiment," to quote Jim Yong Kim. After all, we have the treatments for the afflictions of the poor, and yet for most we do nothing, leaving a vast "control group" of unfortunates to exhibit the natural history of untreated disease.

A conflation of structural violence and cultural difference inhabits the reasoning of this debate over medical ethics.[34] Take, for example, an article published on the op-ed page of the *New York Times*. Responding with some heat to Angell's criticisms—they described comparisons to Tuskegee as "inflammatory and wrong"—the writers explained that cultural differences were at the heart of the problem. This *New York Times* piece ran under the title "A Cultural Divide on AIDS Research," with the divide in question being between "American values" and "African realities." Who would fail to conclude that these were two different worlds? Although the authors of the piece may not have chosen the title affixed to it, they closed by arguing that "Americans should not impose their standards of care on developing countries. Local health experts, bioethicists and affected groups are best qualified to judge the risks and benefits of any medical research."[35]

Impose their standards of care. The irony will not be lost on those whose experiences are described in this book. Americans may impose—through the World Bank or the International Monetary Fund, say, or through foreign policy writ large—social and economic policies that drive up inequalities, leaving the destitute sick out of the frame of analysis. But heaven forfend that we should require that the Third World poor be subject to "culturally inappropriate" medical standards.

The AIDS research debates rankle because, deep down, many know that such obscenely disparate standards of care must be addressed. Equality of access to the fruits of science is the only acceptable goal. The poor, as we've learned—in Haiti and Peru and Roxbury—demand it. As a teacher, I've also learned that medical students become frustrated when confronted by the enormity of the problems before us. It's hard not to give up. And yet solutions are within our grasp if we have sufficient vision and will to demand something better for the poor, wherever they live. In constructing an alternative vision, we will all be acting unreasonably— that is, without the certainty of success. "Nonetheless," notes Wallerstein, "we are condemned to act." He continues: "Therefore, we must first be clear about what is deficient in our modern world-system, about what it is that has made so large a percentage of the world's population angry, or at least ambivalent as to its social merits. It seems quite clear to me that the major complaint has been the great inequalities of the system, which means the absence of democracy."[36]

2 Rethinking "Emerging Infectious Diseases"

However secure and well-regulated

civilized life may become, bacteria,

Protozoa, viruses, infected fleas, lice,

ticks, mosquitoes, and bedbugs will

always lurk in the shadows ready to

pounce when neglect, poverty,

famine, or war lets down the

defenses. And even in normal times

they prey on the weak, the very

young and the very old, living along

with us, in mysterious obscurity

waiting their opportunities.

HANS ZINSSER, 1934

The microbe is nothing; the terrain,

everything.

LOUIS PASTEUR, 1822–1895

AIDS. Ebola. Flesh-eating bacteria. With newspaper and television reports rife with references to mysterious and lethal outbreaks caused by new (or newly virulent) pathogens, perhaps it's safe to conclude that we're living in a time of unprecedented popular interest in infectious diseases. Yet medical historians might be quick to discern, in this most recent wave of hysteria and genuine interest, but a small peak in that jagged line charting the course of popular concern with epidemic disease.

That's not to say that there's nothing new under the sun. This most recent surge of interest comes at a time when novel technologies can reveal a level of detail—about both pathogens and hosts—unimagined by our recent forebears. And this past decade has surely been one of the most eventful in the long history of the study of infectious diseases. There are multiple indices of these events, and also of the rate at which our knowledge base has grown. We have only to follow, for example, the sheer number of relevant publications to perceive the explosive growth in this knowledge base. We have developed new methods of monitoring antimicrobial resistance patterns. And we have new ways to promote the rapid sharing of information (and also, unfortunately, speculation and misinformation) through means such as the Internet that barely existed even ten years ago.

Then there are the microbes themselves. One of the most significant events of the past ten or fifteen years, and perhaps the most remarked upon, is the explosion of "emerging infectious diseases." Some of these disorders—such as AIDS and Brazilian purpuric fever—can be regarded as genuinely new. Others were clinically identified some time ago but have newly identified etiologic agents or have again burst onto the scene in dramatic fashion. For example, the syndromes caused by Hantaan viruses have been known in Asia for centuries, but they now seem to be spreading beyond that continent as a result of ecological and economic transformations that increase contact between humans and rodents. The phenomenology of neuroborreliosis had been tackled long before the monikers "Lyme disease" and *Borrelia burgdorferi* were coined, and before suburban reforestation and golf courses complicated the equation by creating an environment agreeable to both ticks and affluent humans. Hemorrhagic fevers, including Ebola, were described long ago, and their etiologic agents were in many cases identified in previous decades. Still other diseases grouped under the "emerging" rubric are ancient and well-known foes that have somehow changed, either in pathogenicity or distribution. Multidrug-resistant tuberculosis and invasive or necrotizing Group A streptococcal infection—the "flesh-eating bacteria" of the popular press—are cases in point.

Popularizing the concept of "emerging infectious diseases" has helped to marshal a sense of urgency, notoriously difficult to arouse in large bureaucracies. Funds have been channeled, conferences convened, articles written, and a dedicated journal founded. The research and action programs elaborated in response to the perceived emergence of new infections have, by and large, been sound.

But the concept also carries complex symbolic burdens—as do some of the diseases most commonly associated with it. Such burdens have certainly complicated and, in some instances, hampered the laying down of new knowledge. If certain populations have long been afflicted by these disorders, why are the diseases considered "new" or "emerging"? Is it simply because they have come to affect more visible—read, more "valuable"—persons? This would seem to be an obvious question from the perspective of the Haitian or African poor.

In the emerging literature on emerging infectious diseases, some questions are posed while others are not. A subtle and flexible understanding of emerging infections would be grounded in critical and reflexive study of how our knowledge develops. Units of analysis and key terms would be scrutinized and regularly redefined. These processes would include regular rethinking not only of methodologies and study design but also of the validity of causal inference, and they would allow reflection on the limits of human knowledge.

The study of such processes, loosely known as epistemology, often happens in retrospect. To their credit, however, many of the chief contributors to the growing literature on emerging infectious diseases, accustomed to debate about microbial nomenclature, have shown exceptional self-awareness in examining the epistemologic issues surrounding their work. Many are also thoroughly familiar with the multifactorial nature of disease emergence. In a 1995 review, one of the prime movers in the field (a virologist) noted that the emergence of a newly recognized or novel disease is rarely a purely virological event without identifiable causative co-factors: "Responsible factors include ecological changes, such as those due to agricultural or economic development or to anomalies in the climate; human demographic changes and behavior; travel and commerce; technology and industry; microbial adaptation and change; and breakdown of public health measures."[1] Similarly, the Institute of

Medicine's influential report on emerging infections does not even categorize microbial threats by type of agent, but rather according to major factors held to be related to their emergence: "human demographics and behavior; technology and industry; economic development and land use; international travel and commerce; microbial adaptation and change; and breakdown of public health measures."[2]

Many students of emerging infectious diseases thus distinguish between a host of phenomena directly related to human actions—ranging from improved laboratory techniques and scientific discovery to economic development, global warming, and failures of public health—and another set of phenomena, much less common and deriving more directly from changes in the microbes themselves. Even in cases of microbial mutations, however, we often find signs that human actions have played a large role in enhancing pathogenicity or increasing resistance to antimicrobial agents. In one long list of emerging viral infections, for example, only the emergence of Rift Valley fever is attributed to a possible change in virulence or pathogenicity; and this cause is enumerated after other, social factors for which better evidence exists.[3]

No need, then, to launch a campaign calling for a heightened awareness of the sociogenesis, or "anthropogenesis," of disease emergence. Ironically, perhaps, some of the bench scientists involved in the field are both more likely to refer to a broad range of social factors and less likely to make immodest claims of causality about any one of them than are behavioral scientists who study infectious diseases.

Yet a *critical* epistemology of emerging infectious diseases is still in the early stages of development. A key task of this endeavor is to take our existing conceptual frameworks and ask, What is obscured in this way of conceptualizing disease? What is brought into relief?

For example, a first step in understanding the epistemologic dimension of disease emergence involves, as Eckardt argues, developing "a certain sensitivity to the terms we are used to."[4] When we think of "tropical diseases," for instance, malaria comes quickly to mind. But not too long ago, malaria was a significant problem far from the tropics. Although there is imperfect overlap between malaria as currently defined and the malaria of the mid-nineteenth century, some medical historians agree with contemporary assessments that this illness "was the most important disease in the United States at that time."[5] In the Ohio River Valley, according to Daniel Drake's 1850 study, thousands died in seasonal epidemics.[6] A million-odd soldiers were afflicted with malaria during the U.S. Civil War.[7] During the second decade of the twentieth century, when the population of twelve southern states was about twenty-five million, the region saw an estimated one million cases of malaria per year. Malaria's decline in this country was "due only in small part to measures aimed directly against it, but more to agricultural development and to other factors some of which are still not clear."[8]

One responsible factor that is clear enough, if little discussed in the literature, is the reduction of poverty, including the development of improved housing, land drainage, mosquito repellents, nets, and electric fans—all of which have been (and remain) beyond the reach of those most at risk for malaria.[9] In fact, many "tropical" diseases predominantly afflict the poor; the groups at risk for these diseases are often bounded more by socioeconomic status than by latitude. In Haiti, for example, my patients with malaria are almost exclusively those living in poverty. None have electricity; none take prophylaxis; many have lost kin to malaria. This aspect of disease emergence is thus obscured by an uncritical use of the term "tropical medicine," which implies a geographic rather than a social topography.[10]

Any modern practitioner dealing with infectious disease knows this well, even if he or she sits in a travel clinic in New England. Those who come in for malaria prophylaxis and to ask about appropriate vaccinations are students, professionals, and tourists. When practitioners are called into the emergency room for an imported case of malaria, however, we usually see a very different patient shuddering on a damp gurney. In Boston, at least, the patient with malaria is likely to have been born in an endemic region—Haiti, say, or West Africa—and to be working as a laborer in the U.S. service economy. And that patient is also likely to tell us the diagnosis, for it will not be the first time that he or she has had malaria.

Similarly, the concept of "health transitions" is influential in what some have termed "the new public health" and also among sectors of the international financial institutions that so often control development efforts.[11] The "health transitions" model suggests that nation-states, as they develop, go through predictable epidemiologic transformations. Death due to infectious causes is gradually supplanted by death due to malignancies and complications of coronary artery disease; the latter deaths occur at a more advanced age, reflecting progress. Although it describes broad patterns now apparent throughout the world, the concept of national health transitions also masks other realities, including morbidity and mortality differentials *within* nationalities, which show that health conditions are often more tightly linked to local inequalities than to nationality.

For example, much was made of the fact that noncommunicable pathologies such as coronary artery disease and malignancies caused the majority of all world deaths in 1990. A very different picture emerges, however, when we compare causes of death among the wealthiest fifth of the world's population to the afflictions that kill the poorest fifth: although only 8 percent of deaths among the world's wealthiest were caused by infections or by maternal and perinatal mortality, fully 56 percent of all deaths among the poorest were caused by these pathologies, with infectious diseases at the head of the list.[12] How do the variables of class and race fit into such paradigms? In Harlem, where age-specific mortality in several groups is higher than that in Bangladesh, leading causes of death are infectious diseases and violence.[13]

The units of analysis are similarly up for grabs. When Surgeon General David Satcher, writing of emerging infectious diseases, reminds us that "the health of the individual is best ensured by maintaining or improving the health of the entire community,"[14] we should applaud his clear-sightedness. But we should also go on to ask, What constitutes "the entire community"? In a few instances—the 1994 outbreak of cryptosporidiosis in Milwaukee, say—the answer might be part of a city.[15] In other instances, "community" may mean a village or a group of passengers on an airplane. But the most common unit of analysis referred to in public health, the nation-state, is not all that meaningful to organisms such as dengue virus, *Vibrio cholera* O139, HIV, penicillinase-producing *Neisseria gonorrhoeae*, multidrug-resistant tuberculosis, and hepatitis B virus. Such organisms often proudly disregard political boundaries, even though a certain degree of "turbulence" in their dynamics may be introduced at national borders. The dynamics of disease emergence are not captured in nation-by-nation analyses any more than the diseases are contained by national boundaries, which are themselves emerging entities. (Most of the world's nations are, after all, twentieth-century creations, which might also give pause to those buying into the two-worlds myth.)

The limitations of these three important ways of viewing the health of populations—the concepts of tropical medicine, health transitions, and national health profiles—demonstrate that models and even assumptions about infectious diseases need to be *dynamic, systemic,* and *critical.* That is, models with explanatory power must be able to track rapidly changing clinical, even molecular, phenomena and link them to the large-scale (often transnational) social forces that shape the contours of disease emergence. I refer here to questions less on the order of how pig-duck agriculture might be related to the antigenic shifts central to influenza pandemics and more on the order of the following: Are World Bank policies related to the spread of HIV, as some have recently claimed?[16] What is the connection between international shipping practices and the spread of cholera from Asia to South America and elsewhere in this hemisphere?[17] How is genocide in Rwanda related to cholera in Zaïre?[18]

The study of anything said to be "emerging" tends to be *dynamic.* But the very notion of emergence in heterogeneous populations poses analytic questions that are rarely tackled, even in modern epidemiology, which, as McMichael argues, "assigns a primary importance to studying interindividual variations in risk. By concentrating on these specific and presumed free-range individual behaviors, we thereby pay less attention to the underlying social-historical influences on behavioral choices, patterns, and population health."[19]

Systemic analyses of disease emergence are not hemmed in by political or administrative borders. New tools based on DNA analysis allow us to rethink comfortable conclusions regarding treatment for some but not for others. The notorious "W strain" of MDRTB, for example, spread quickly through New York City but then moved on to Atlanta, Miami, and Denver.[20] New data suggests that the W strain's family tree has roots in Asia and Russia.[21] If these are transnational pandemics, spread through sharing air, then surely responses must be transnational—although, thus far, such responses have been hobbled by short-sighted parochialism. Genetic subtyping of HIV leads to the same conclusions.

A *critical* (and self-critical) approach would ask how existing frameworks might limit our ability to discern trends that are related to the emergence of diseases. Not all social-production-of-disease theories are equally alive to the significance of how relative social and economic positioning—inequality—affects the risk of infection. For example, neither poverty nor inequality appears as a "cause of emergence" in the self-described "catalog" of emerging infections compiled by the Institute of Medicine.

Further, a critical approach would push the limits of existing academic politesse in order to ask more difficult and rarely raised questions, questions that still need to be answered if we are to better understand disease emergence. Examples might include issues such as these: By what mechanisms have international changes in agriculture shaped recent outbreaks of Argentine and Bolivian hemorrhagic fever, and how do these mechanisms derive from international trade agreements such as GATT and NAFTA? How might institutional racism be related to both urban crime and the epidemics of multidrug-resistant tuberculosis registered in New York prisons? Does privatization of health services buttress social inequalities, increasing risk for certain infections—and poor outcomes—among the poor of sub-Saharan Africa and Latin America? How do the colonial histories of Belgium and Germany, and the neocolonial histories of France and the United States, tie in to genocide in Rwanda—which was itself related to an epidemic of cholera? We can productively pose similar questions about many of the diseases now held to be emerging, as a few examples will suggest.

EMERGING HOW AND TO WHAT EXTENT?
THE CASE OF EBOLA

Hemorrhagic fevers have been known in Africa since well before the continent was dubbed "the White man's grave" (an expression that, when used to refer to a region with such high rates of premature death, speaks volumes about the differential valuation of human lives). Ebola itself was isolated more than two decades ago.[22] Its appearance in human hosts has at times been insidious but more often takes the form of explosive eruptions.

In accounting for recent outbreaks, it is unnecessary to postulate a change in filovirus virulence through mutation. For filoviruses, the Institute of Medicine catalog lists a single "factor facilitating emergence": "virus-infected monkeys shipped from developing countries via air."[23] Other factors can be easily identified, however. As with many infectious diseases, the distribution of Ebola outbreaks is tied to regional trade networks and other evolving social systems. And, as with most infectious diseases, Ebola explosions afflict—researchers aside—certain groups (people living in poverty, health care workers who serve the poor) while largely sparing others in close physical proximity.

Take, for example, the 1976 emergence of Ebola in the Sudan. This epidemic was anything but random, for it was amplified by substandard medical practices in a mission hospital. Richard Preston recounts the story in his best-seller *The Hot Zone:* "It hit the hospital like a bomb. It savaged patients and snaked like chain lightning out from the hospital through patients' families. Apparently the medical staff had been giving patients injections with dirty needles."[24] Two months later, the better-known and more virulent outbreak in the region drained by Zaïre's Ebola River gave the disease its name and its fame.

The story was almost identical in both instances. The nuns who ran the Yambuku Mission Hospital started their busy day, notes Preston in his dramatic account of the Sudanese outbreak, by laying out five hypodermic syringes. These were used on the hundreds of patients who each day sought care there. "The nuns and staff occasionally rinsed the needles in a pan of warm water after an injection, to get the blood off the needle, but more often they proceeded from shot to shot without rinsing the needle."

> The virus erupted simultaneously in fifty-five villages surrounding the hospital. First it killed people who had received injections, and then it moved through families, killing family members, particularly women, who in Africa prepare the dead for burial. It swept through the Yambuku Hospital's nursing staff, killing most of the nurses, and then it hit the Belgian nuns.[25]

The 1976 Zaïre outbreak afflicted 318 persons. Although much speculation about respiratory spread arose at the time, it has not been conclusively demonstrated as a cause of human cases. Most expert observers felt that the cases could be traced to failure to follow contact precautions as well as improper sterilization of syringes and other paraphernalia—measures that, once taken, terminated the outbreak.[26]

It would be a grave error, however, to conclude that poor nursing practices were central to Ebola's emergence. Such simplifications desocialize our understanding by masking the contributions of social inequalities to the shape of these epidemics. On closer scrutiny, such an "explanation" suggests that Ebola does not emerge randomly: in Mobutu's Zaïre, one's likelihood of coming into contact with, say, unsterile syringes was inversely proportional to one's social status there. Local elites and sectors of the expatriate community with access to high-quality biomedical services (namely, the European and American communities and not the Rwandan refugees) were quite unlikely to contract such a disease.

The changes involved in the disease's *visibility* are equally embedded in social context. The "emergence" of Ebola has also been partly a question of our consciousness. Modern communications, including print and broadcast media, have been crucial in the casting of Ebola—a minor player, statistically speaking, in Zaïre's long list of fatal infections—as an emerging infectious disease.[27] Through CNN and other television networks, names such as "Kikwit" became, however briefly, household words in parts of Europe and North America. Journalists and novelists wrote best-selling books about small but horrific plagues, which in turn became profitable cinema. Thus, symbolically if not epidemiologically, Ebola spread like wildfire—as a danger potentially without limit. It emerged.

EMERGING FROM WHERE?
THE CASE OF TUBERCULOSIS

Tuberculosis is considered another emerging disease, although in this case, "emerging" is synonymous with "reemerging." Some attribute its recrudescence to the advent of HIV—the Institute of Medicine's catalog lists "an increase in immunosuppressed populations" as the sole named factor facilitating the resurgence of tuberculosis[28]—and to the development of drug resistance. In a book subtitled *How the Battle Against Tuber-*

culosis Was Won—and Lost, Ryan states that "throughout the developed world, with the successful application of triple therapy and the enthusiastic promotion of prevention, the death rate from tuberculosis came tumbling down."[29] A more recent piece in the *Washington Post* observes that "the invention of antibiotics quickly tamed the epidemic and most Americans put it out of mind."[30]

But can these claims of causality be taken seriously on the merits of the evidence? To be sure, the discovery of effective antituberculous therapies has saved hundreds of thousands afflicted with the disease, primarily in developed countries. But deaths from tuberculosis—once the leading cause of mortality among young adults in Europe and North America—were already declining there well before the 1943 discovery of streptomycin. In the rest of the world, and in small pockets of the United States and Europe, tuberculosis remains undaunted by ostensibly effective drugs, which are used too late, inappropriately, or not at all. From our clinic in central Haiti, it is impossible not to regard the notion of "tuberculosis resurgence" as something of a cruel joke—or yet another reminder of the invisibility of the poor.

Not all U.S. specialists are deaf to the persistent hack of patients far away. "It is sufficiently shameful," writes Michael Iseman, "that 30 years after recognition of the capacity of triple-therapy . . . to elicit 95%+ cure rates, tuberculosis prevalence rates for *many* nations remain unchanged."[31] Some estimate that over 1.7 billion persons are currently infected with quiescent but viable *Mycobacterium tuberculosis*, and, failing dramatic shifts in local epidemiology, a global analysis does not project major decreases in the importance of tuberculosis as a cause of death. Tuberculosis has retreated in certain populations, maintained a steady state in others, and surged forth in still others, remaining, at this writing, the world's leading infectious cause of preventable deaths.[32]

At mid-century, tuberculosis was still acknowledged as the great white plague. What explains this killer's invisibility by the 1970s and 1980s? Again, one must look to the study of disease *awareness*—that is, of consciousness and publicity—and its relation to power and wealth. "The neglect of tuberculosis as a major public health priority over the past two decades is simply extraordinary," wrote Murray in 1991. "Perhaps the most important contributor to this state of ignorance was the greatly reduced clinical and epidemiological importance of tuberculosis in the wealthy nations."[33]

Perhaps more telling was the lack of official concern evinced over persistently high, then rising, rates of tuberculosis among U.S. citizens living in poverty. TB's resurgence in the United States has occasioned more commentary than trends elsewhere, and it merits special scrutiny. The resurgence was initially signaled by an alteration in the trend of steady decline. Beginning in 1985, national data revealed a slowing of this trend: the decline was only 0.2 percent in 1985, while 1986 saw a 2.6 percent increase in reported cases. In 1987, the decline was 1.1 percent. This failure to improve was described by the term "excess cases," but the true dimensions of the problem, concealed in national statistics, are revealed by breaking down the "excess cases" according to other variables.

For the CDC, the salient variables are race, age, and geography. Basing an analysis on these variables reveals a much more disturbing pattern. During the years 1985–87, we find no mere "failure to decline," but rather a sharp increase in tuberculosis case rates among certain people in certain places. For example, nationwide the case rate increased 6.8 percent among blacks and 12.7 percent among Hispanics, although it *decreased* 4.8 percent among non-Hispanic whites. The increases were largest among young adults of color. Among blacks and Hispanics in the age group 25–44, increases in tuberculosis were reported at 17 and 27 percent, respectively.[34]

It is thus clear that some groups—ethnic minorities—account for the majority of excess cases in the United States. Snider, Salinas, and Kelly estimate that 85 percent of cases among minorities can be defined as "excess," and in 1987 the absolute number of cases among blacks exceeded that among non-Hispanic whites for the first time. But we find striking geographic focus as well. Two-thirds of tuberculosis cases among blacks were reported from nine states. Between 1980 and 1987, New York City experienced a 45 percent increase in the number of persons with tuberculosis, with the burden again borne by people of color: "Increases have been most pronounced in blacks (79 percent) and in Hispanics (115 percent), especially in the 25- to 44-year age group where increases of 152 percent in blacks and 216 percent in Hispanics have been observed."[35]

In a sense, then, this "race-and-space" approach yields great insights. What at first appeared to be relatively insignificant changes in national data—a decline in the decline, as it were—were in fact significant focal outbreaks of a transmissible disease. But since race and place are largely proxies for poverty, a variable not recorded in national data on tuberculosis, there is still more to the story. As described in the Introduction, one study of welfare recipients in New York City found rates of tuberculosis that were seventy times the national average.[36] Clearly, the "resurgence" of tuberculosis has been felt largely by those who were already living with elevated tuberculosis risks. "Tuberculosis is not 'resurgent,'" writes Katherine Ott, "to those who have been contending with and marginalized by it all their lives."[37] In the communities most affected by tuberculosis, the disease in fact had never disappeared. Ott continues: "The story ends up as 'Tuberculosis is Back' rather than, more appropriately, 'Tuberculosis is Back in the News.' It is not its return that is extraordinary, but that its decline was to a great extent an artifact of socially constructed definitions."[38]

When complex push-pull forces move more poor people into the United States, or reduce the standard of living of many people in the country, an increase in U.S. tuberculosis incidence is likely. A 1995 study of tuberculosis among foreign-born persons in the United States essentially credits immigration with the increased incidence of tuberculosis morbidity in this country. The authors observe that in some of the immigrants' countries of origin the annual rate of infection is up to two hundred times that registered in the United States; they further observe that those sampled included many living in homeless shelters, prisons, and camps for migrant workers. But the study contains no discussion of poverty or inequality, even though these are, along with war and political disruption, leading reasons for both high rates of tuberculosis *and* for immigration to the United States. "The major determinants of risk in the foreign-born population," conclude the authors, "were the region of the world from which the person emigrated and the number of years in the United States."[39]

Mycobacteria do not respect national boundaries. The fact that endemic areas are the settings from which will come many future North American tuberculosis cases argues for a more systemic approach to treatment and prevention as well as to our understanding of TB's reemergence. For this reason, at the very least, cooperation between industrialized nations and poor communities hard-hit by tuberculosis should be a new priority in tuberculosis-control efforts in North America.

GOING WHERE? THE CASE OF HIV

To grasp the complexity of the issues—medical, social, and communicational—that surround the emergence of a disease into public view, consider AIDS. In the early 1980s, health officials informed the public that AIDS had probably emerged from Haiti. As Chapter 4 describes, this speculation proved incorrect, but not before doing significant damage to Haiti's tourist industry and economy. The result: more desperate poverty, and a yet steeper slope of inequality and vulnerability to disease, including AIDS. The label "AIDS vector" was also a heavy burden for the million or so Haitians living elsewhere in the Americas and certainly hampered public health efforts among them.[40]

HIV disease has since become the most spectacularly studied infection in human history. But some questions have been much better studied than others, and among those too well studied are a number of utter dead ends. Nonetheless, error is worth studying, too. Careful investigation of the mechanisms used to propagate immodest claims is an important part of a critical epistemology of emerging infectious diseases. As regards Haiti and AIDS, these mechanisms included the "exoticization" of Haiti, the existence of influential folk models about Haitians and Africans, and the conflation of poverty and cultural difference. Critical epidemiologic studies might well reveal such folk models and half-baked cultural generalizations as unfortunate co-factors in the disease's spread.

HIV may not have come *from* Haiti, but it certainly went *to* Haiti. A critical reexamination of the Caribbean AIDS pandemic reveals that the distribution of HIV disease does not follow the outlines of nation-states but rather matches the contours of a transnational socioeconomic order. As Chapter 4 shows, much of the spread of HIV in the 1970s and 1980s moved along international "fault lines," tracking along steep gradients of inequality, which are also the paths of labor migration and sexual commerce.[41]

Also lacking, then, are considerations of the multiple dynamics of AIDS. In an important overview of the pandemic's first decade, Mann, Tarantola, and Netter observe that its course "within and through global society is not being affected—in any serious manner—by the actions taken at the national or international level."[42] HIV has emerged, but where is it going? Why, how, and how fast? The Institute of Medicine catalog lists several factors facilitating the emergence of HIV: "urbanization; changes in lifestyles/mores; increased intravenous drug abuse; international travel; medical technology."[43] Much more could be said. HIV has spread across the globe, often wildly but never randomly. Like tuberculosis, HIV is entrenching itself in the ranks of the poor and marginalized.

Take, as an example, the rapid increase in AIDS incidence among women. In a 1992 report, the United Nations observed that "for most women, the major risk factor for HIV infection is being married."[44] It is not marriage per se, however, that places young women at risk. Throughout the world, most women with HIV infection, married or not, are living in poverty. The means by which confluent social forces—here, gender inequality and poverty—come to be embodied as risk for infection with this emerging pathogen have been neglected in the biomedical, epidemiologic, and even social science literature on AIDS. As recently as October 1994—fifteen years into an ever-emerging pandemic—editorialists writing in Lancet could comment concerning a new study: "We are not aware of other investigators who have considered the influence of socioeconomic status on mortality in HIV-infected individuals."[45] Thus AIDS follows the general rule that the effects of certain types of social forces on health outcomes are less likely to be studied.

Yet AIDS has always been a strikingly patterned pandemic. Despite the message of public health slogans—"AIDS Is for Everyone"—some groups are at high risk of HIV infection, whereas others clearly are shielded from risk. Furthermore, although the terminal events have been grimly similar across the board, the course of HIV disease has been highly variable. These disparities have sparked the search for hundreds of cofactors, from Mycoplasma and ulcerating genital lesions to voodoo rites and psychological predispositions. To date, not a single one of these associations has been convincingly shown to explain disparities in distribution or outcome of HIV disease. The most well-demonstrated co-factors

are *social inequalities*, which structure not only the contours of the AIDS
pandemic but also the nature of outcomes once an individual is sick with
complications of HIV infection.[46] And a "cure," though eminently desir-
able, will not change the prognosis for the vast majority of AIDS sufferers. The advent of more effective antiviral agents promises to heighten
those disparities even further: a three-drug regimen including a protease
inhibitor costs $12,000 to $16,000 a year.[47] The formulators of health policy have already declared antiviral therapy to be "cost-ineffective" in the
very regions in which HIV is most endemic.

TAKING A SECOND LOOK
AT EMERGING INFECTIOUS DISEASES

Writing of the emerging infectious diseases of the century, Zinsser observed in 1934 that "the appraisal of the appearance of a so-called 'new'
disease is fraught with many pitfalls."[48] Even a cursory reading of the
emerging literature on emerging diseases makes it clear that the examples cited here—Ebola, tuberculosis, HIV—are in no way unique in demanding contextualization through approaches offered by the social sciences. Ethnographic work is often a powerful corrective for tendencies to
generate flimsy hypotheses and to rely on outmoded or inappropriate
categories.[49] For example, an anthropologist working in Haiti in the early
1980s would have quickly questioned the hypothesis that voodoo was
somehow related to the occurrence of the new disease known as AIDS.
The "risk groups" identified by slipshod epidemiologic research would
have been called into question by an intimate acquaintance with the
emerging epidemic in Haiti—an epidemic that was, in fact, transnational
in nature and tightly linked not to voodoo but to high grades of inequality between Haiti and the nearby United States.

Such approaches also include the grounding of case histories and local epidemics in the larger biosocial systems in which they take shape—
which calls, most of the time, for the exploration of social inequalities.
Why, for example, were there ten thousand cases of diphtheria in Russia
from 1990 to 1993? It is easy enough to answer, as did the CDC, that the
excess cases were due to a failure to vaccinate.[50] But only if we link this
distal (and, in sum, technical) cause to the much more complex socioeco-

nomic transformations altering the region's morbidity and mortality patterns will we discover compelling explanations.[51]

An epidemiology that is narrowly focused on individual risk and short on critical contextualization will not reveal these deep transformations, nor will it connect them to disease emergence. "Modern epidemiology," observes one of its leading contributors, is "oriented to explaining and quantifying the bobbing of corks on the surface waters, while largely disregarding the stronger undercurrents that determine where, on average, the cluster of corks ends up along the shoreline of risk."[52] Nor will standard journalism add much: "Amidst a flood of information," complains one of the chief chroniclers of disease emergence, "analysis and context are evaporating. . . . Outbreaks of flesh-eating bacteria may command headlines, but local failures to fully vaccinate preschool children garner little attention unless there is an epidemic."[53]

For understanding and eventually controlling emerging infectious diseases, the research questions identified by various blue-ribbon panels are uncontestably important; they are, no doubt, the primary issues raised by the epidemics in question.[54] Yet there exists a series of corollary questions posed both by the diseases and by popular and scientific commentary about them. These questions pose, in turn, a series of research questions that are the exclusive province neither of social scientists nor of bench scientists, neither clinicians nor epidemiologists. Indeed, we will need genuinely transdisciplinary collaboration to tackle the problems posed by emerging infectious diseases. As prolegomenon, four areas of corollary research, outlined in the following sections, are easily identified. In each is heard the recurrent leitmotiv of inequality.

1. Emerging Infectious Diseases and Social Inequalities

Study of the reticulated links between social inequalities and emerging disease would not construe the poor simply as "sentinel chickens" or mineshaft canaries. Instead it would ask, What are the precise mechanisms by which these diseases come to afflict some bodies but not others? What propagative effects might inequality per se contribute?[55] Similar queries were once major research questions for epidemiology and social medicine, but they have fallen out of favor, leaving a vacuum in which scholars and officials can easily stake immodest claims of causality.

Studies that examine the conjoint influence of social inequalities are virtually nonexistent; Krieger, Rowley, Herman, Avery, and Phillips, in a magisterial review, conclude that "the minimal research that simultaneously studies the health effects of racism, sexism, and social class ultimately stands as a sharp indictment of the narrow vision limiting much of the epidemiological research conducted within the United States."[56] And yet social inequalities shape not only the distribution of emerging diseases but also the health outcomes of those afflicted—a fact that is often downplayed: "Although there are many similarities between our vulnerability to infectious diseases and that of our ancestors, there is one distinct difference: we have the benefit of extensive scientific knowledge," wrote David Satcher in 1995.[57] True enough, if one is willing to gloss over the all-important question of who "we" are. The persons most at risk for emerging infectious diseases generally do not, in fact, have much of the benefit of scientific knowledge. We live in a world where infections pass easily across borders—social and geographic—while resources, including cumulative scientific knowledge, are blocked at customs.

2. Emerging Infectious Diseases in Transnational Perspective

"Travel is a potent force in disease emergence and spread," as Wilson reminds us, and the "current volume, speed, and reach of travel are unprecedented."[58] Although the smallpox and measles epidemics accompanying the European colonization of the Americas were early and deadly reminders of the need for systemic understandings of microbial traffic, recent decades have seen a certain reification of the notion of the "catchment area." A useful means of delimiting a sphere of action—a district, a county, a country—has been erroneously elevated to the status of explanatory principle whenever the geographic unit of analysis is other than that defined by the disease itself.

Almost all diseases held to be emerging—from increasing drug resistance to the great pandemics of HIV and cholera—stand as modern rebukes to the parochialism of this and other public health constructs, as those who study such diseases are well aware.[59] Nevertheless, a critical sociology of liminality—of both the advancing, transnational edges of pandemics and the impress of human-made administrative and political boundaries on disease emergence—has yet to be attempted. But this sort of pragmatic solidarity, even if born of self-interest, seems unlikely to occur without new and aggressive advocacy. "Unless there is a clear and substantial immediate local need," notes a recent *Lancet* editorial, the "long-term implications of transnational disease spread are rarely addressed."[60]

The study of borders qua borders means, increasingly, the study of social inequalities. Many political borders serve as semipermeable membranes, often quite open to diseases and yet closed to the free movement of cures. Thus inequalities of access can be created or buttressed at borders, even when pathogens cannot be so contained. Research questions might include, for example, the following: How does the interface between two very different types of health care systems affect the rate of advance of an emerging disease? What turbulence is introduced when the border in question lies between rich and poor nations? Writing of health issues at the U.S.-Mexican border, for example, Warner notes: "It is unlikely that any other binational border has such variety in health status, entitlements, and utilization."[61] Among the infectious diseases registered at this border are multidrug-resistant tuberculosis, rabies, dengue, and sexually transmitted diseases including HIV (said to be due, in part, to "cross-border use of red-light districts"). As Russia's epidemic of multidrug-resistant tuberculosis continues to grow, wealthy Scandinavia—and eventually other parts of Europe—will be hard-pressed to argue that the treatment of the disease is not "cost-effective" in Russia.

As increased air and sea travel change our notion of shared borders, steep grades of transnational inequality become more significant. Methodologies and theories relevant to the study of borders and emerging infections can come from disciplines ranging from the social sciences to molecular biology; mapping the emergence of diseases is now more feasible with the use of DNA fingerprinting and other new technologies.[62] Again, such investigations will pose difficult questions in a world where plasmids move freely but compassion is often grounded.

3. Emerging Infectious Diseases and the Dynamics of Change

As we elaborate lists of the factors that influence the careers of infectious diseases, we need conceptual tools that will perforce be historically deep, geographically broad, and at the same time *processual*, incorporating concepts of change. Above all, these tools must allow us to incorporate complexity rather than merely dissect or dismiss it. As Levins argues, "effective analysis of emerging diseases must recognize the study of complexity as perhaps the central general scientific problem of our time."[63]

But the complexity of operators is convincing only when the variables on which it operates are well chosen. Can integrated mathematical modeling be linked to new ways of configuring systems, avoiding outmoded units of analyses such as the nation-state in favor of the more fluid biosocial networks through which most pathogens clearly move? Can our embrace of complexity also encompass social complexities, including the unequal positioning of groups within larger populations? Such perspectives could be directed toward mapping the progress of diseases ranging from cholera to AIDS and would be suited to analysis of more unorthodox research subjects—for example, the effects of World Bank projects and policies on diseases ranging from onchocerciasis to plague.

4. Emerging Infectious Diseases and Critical Epistemology

I have argued that when we ask, "What qualifies as an emerging infectious disease?" we should understand that we are also asking, "What is meant by 'emerging'?" This is no trivial shift of topic. It leads to other questions: Why do some persons constitute "risk groups," while others are "individuals at risk"? Why are some approaches and subjects considered appropriate for publication in influential journals, while others are dismissed out of hand? A critical nosology would explore the boundaries of polite and impolite discussion in science, interrogating the ways in which *perceptions* of a disease might contribute to its career. A trove of complex, affect-laden issues—the attribution of blame to perceived vectors of infection, the identification of scapegoats and victims, the role of stigma—though rarely discussed in academic medicine, are manifestly part and parcel of many of the epidemics in question.

Finally, why are some epidemics visible to those who fund research and services, while others are invisible? As we will see in examining multidrug-resistant tuberculosis, the degree to which this disease is seen as a threat varies with the degree to which the powerful—or, at least, the nonpoor—are deemed to be "at risk." In its recent statements on tuberculosis and emerging infections, the World Health Organization manifestly attempts to use fear of contagion to goad wealthy nations into investing in disease surveillance and control out of self-interest—an age-old public health ploy acknowledged as such in the Institute of Medicine report on emerging infections: "Diseases that appear not to threaten the United States directly rarely elicit the political support necessary to maintain control efforts."[64]

The rhetoric of immediacy has been central to professional commentary on emerging infectious diseases, a strategy that is not without risk for those who have been silently suffering with these diseases, often for generations. In fact, differential valuation of human life runs throughout this commentary and throughout much of the policy designed to address epidemic disease. Critical reexamination of the impact of such differential valuation and its effect on the allocation of resources must figure in discussion of emerging infections. That it does not is a marker more of analytic failures than of editorial standards.

.   .   .   .   .

More than ten years ago, the sociologist of science Bruno Latour reviewed hundreds of articles appearing in several Pasteur-era French scientific reviews in order to constitute what he called an "anthropology of the sciences" (he objected to the term "epistemology"). Latour cast his net widely. "There is no essential difference between the human and social sciences and the exact or natural sciences," he wrote, "because there is no more science than there is society. I have spoken of the Pasteurians as they spoke of their microbes."[65] Here, perhaps, is a reason to engage in a proactive effort to explore themes usually relegated to the margins of scientific inquiry: those of us who describe the comings and goings of microbes— feints, parries, emergences, retreats—may one day be subjected to the scrutiny of future students of the subject.

But there are more compelling reasons to seek a sounder analytic grasp of disease emergence. The Pasteurians' microbes remain the world's leading cause of death.[66] In an essay entitled "The Conquest of Infectious Diseases: Who Are We Kidding?" two researchers from the CDC argue that "clinicians, microbiologists, and public health professionals must work together to prevent infectious diseases and to detect emerging diseases quickly."[67] Clearly such transdisciplinary work is necessary if we aspire to a sound analytic purchase on disease emergence—a prerequisite of effective control measures.

My intention is ecumenical and complementary. A critical framework would not aspire to supplant the methodologies of the many disciplines, from virology to molecular epidemiology, that now concern themselves with emerging diseases. "The key task for medicine," argued the pioneers Eisenberg and Kleinman almost two decades ago, "is not to diminish the role of the biomedical sciences in the theory and practice of medicine but to supplement them with an equal application of the social sciences in order to provide both a more comprehensive understanding of disease and better care of the patient. The problem is not 'too much science,' but too narrow a view of the sciences relevant to medicine."[68]

The rest of this book brings this biosocial framework to bear on the diseases that have wreaked such havoc on the lives of my patients. The focus is thus on the two diseases—tuberculosis and AIDS—that have caused the greatest number of deaths. Along the way, it becomes clear that malaria, typhoid, and the other plagues of the poor must be subjected to similar scrutiny. But the goal of this rethinking is never merely to come up with a better model. The goal, all along, has been to allay the unnecessary suffering caused by inequality and its embodied forms.

3 Invisible Women

CLASS, GENDER, AND HIV

These days, whenever someone says

the word "women" to me, my mind

goes blank. What "women"? What is

this "women" thing you're talking

about? Does that mean me? Does

that mean my mother, my

roommates, the white woman next

door, the checkout clerk at the

supermarket, my aunts in Korea,

half the world's population?

JEEYEUN LEE, 1995A

The close of the 1980s found me sitting in a new clinic in a small village in Haiti's Central Plateau. What awaited us outside in the noisy courtyard was not entirely what we'd expected. Certainly we should have anticipated the crowd, since ours was the first facility in the region to declare a special interest in the destitute sick. And we should have expected that many would be gravely ill by the time they reached our doorstep. Granted, we did expect patients with tuberculosis. But we were nevertheless surprised by just how many rural families were affected by a disease popularly associated with overcrowded cities. We also knew, sitting in the clinic, that people with AIDS would come to us; we knew that many of them would be returning from Port-au-Prince. But why, we wondered, were so many of these patients young women?

On a trip back to the United States, I turned to the massive and expanding literature on AIDS. A search of a computerized AIDS database revealed that more than one hundred thousand references were instantaneously available. But when I restricted the search by adding the term "women" to "AIDS," I found only two thousand references. Seeking to further restrict my search by adding the word "poverty" as a third qualifier, I was informed that there were "no references meeting these specifications."

This knowledge gap was the impetus for a collective effort to review the scholarly literature, such as it was, on women and AIDS.[1] But it was the "invisible" suffering of the young women in the clinic courtyard that fueled both our reanalysis and a series of programs designed to remediate—or at least to ease—this suffering.

.   .   .   .   .

AIDS was first recognized as a distinct clinical syndrome in the summer of 1981, when physicians in California and New York noted clusterings of unusual infections and cancers in their patients, almost all of whom were young, gay men. The story has been, by now, told often. Less well known is the chronicle of the disease among women. In August, a mere two months after the first cases were reported in men, doctors identified the same syndrome in a woman.[2] Within a year, AIDS cases were also being registered among men and women who injected drugs, among hemophiliacs and some of their sexual partners, and among women and men from poor countries, including Haiti, who seemed to share few of the "risk factors" identified in the other patients.

Since that time, both AIDS and commentary about it have swept the globe. Never before has a single sickness been the subject of such intense and sustained scrutiny. Given the intensity of public awareness and fear of AIDS, it is not surprising that so many myths and misunderstandings about the disease have thrived and even proliferated and that fantasies and junk science have often dominated public discussions of AIDS.

The initial misunderstanding—that AIDS was a disease of men—can perhaps be attributed to historical accident: the new disease was first characterized in the technologically advanced United States, where it did, initially at least, primarily afflict men.[3] But from the outset of the world pandemic, it was apparent that women were also vulnerable to

AIDS; and, within in a year or two, data suggested that women were at least as likely to become infected as men.

Evidently, however, AIDS cases involving women did not count for much. In 1985, a cover story in *Discover*, a popular science magazine, dismissed the idea of a major epidemic among women. The story claimed that because the "rugged vagina," unlike the "vulnerable anus," was designed for the wear and tear of intercourse and birthing, it was unlikely that large numbers of women would ever be infected through heterosexual intercourse. AIDS, we were informed, "is now—and is likely to remain—largely the fatal price one can pay for anal intercourse."[4]

Such mistaken verdicts were slowly called into question. By late 1986, it was becoming clear that AIDS incidence was declining among gay men even as it was climbing among those classed as the "heterosexual exposure group."[5] "Suddenly," proclaimed the cover of *U.S. News and World Report* in January 1987, "the disease of *them* is the disease of *us*." The accompanying illustration depicted the "us" in question (accurately enough, as far as the journalistic stance went) as a white, yuppie couple.[6]

In her study of the gradual evolution of AIDS discourse in the United States, Paula Treichler discerns a "diversification" of commentary about women and AIDS in the spring of 1987.[7] Nonetheless, one still heard voices maintaining that women would never constitute a significant proportion of AIDS victims. *The Myth of Heterosexual AIDS*, first released in 1990, typifies that sort of thinking: "Among the great wide percentage of the nation the media calls 'the general population,' that section the media and the public health authorities has [*sic*] tried desperately to terrify, there is no epidemic. AIDS will pick off a person here and there in this group, but the original infected partner will be one of the two groups in which the disease is epidemic. Most heterosexuals will continue to have more to fear from bathtub drowning than from AIDS."[8]

If there is irony here, it is not the easy irony of false predictions. Even as such projections were being written, millions of women—whose partners were neither bisexual men nor intravenous drug users—had *already* been "picked off" by HIV. Even in the United States, where the epidemic among women had initially been closely linked to injection (intravenous) drug use, the proportion of women who were reported to have been exposed by a partner whose risk was not specified—in other words, not an injecting drug user and not bisexual or gay—quintupled from 1983–84 to 1989–90. In the five years preceding the publication of *The Myth of Heterosexual AIDS*, the percentage increase in annual AIDS incidence was greater among the "heterosexually acquired" exposure group than in any other.[9] By 1991, AIDS was the leading killer of young women in most large U.S. cities.[10] Rates of bathtub drowning remained low.

The mismatch between reality and representation led Paula Treichler to pose the following question in 1988: "Given the intense concern with the human body that any conceptualization of AIDS entails, how can we account for the striking silence, until very recently, on the topic of women in AIDS discourse (including biomedical journals, mainstream news publications, public health literature, women's magazines, and the gay and feminist press)?"[11] In other words, why did many continue to think of AIDS as a men's disease? More poignantly, perhaps, why were the voices of women with AIDS absent from scientific and popular commentary a full decade into the pandemic?[12]

One explanation is that the majority of women with AIDS had been robbed of their voices long before HIV appeared to further complicate their lives. In settings of entrenched elitism, they have been poor. In settings of entrenched racism, they have been women of color. In settings of entrenched sexism, they have been, of course, women.

If it is finally recognized that AIDS poses enormous threats to poor women, this wisdom comes too late. Throughout the world, millions of women are already sick with complications of HIV infection. In the United States and in Latin America, the epidemics among women are increasing at a rate much higher than that registered among other groups: AIDS is already the leading cause of death among young African American women living in the United States.[13] In Mexico, the male:female ratio of HIV infection went from 25:1 in 1984 to 4:1 in 1990. In São Paulo, Brazil, positive HIV tests (seroprevalence) among pregnant women increased sixfold in the three years from 1987 to 1990.[14]

Similarly disturbing trends are registered elsewhere in the world, particularly in developing countries, where 90 percent of all adults and 98 percent of all children infected with HIV live.[15] Many sub-Saharan African nations already report more new infections among women than among men. In 1992, the United Nations Development Program estimated that "each day a further three thousand women become infected, and five hundred infected women die. Most are between 15 and 35 years old."[16] The World Health Organization has predicted that, during the course of the 365 days of the year 2000, between six and eight million women will become infected with HIV.[17]

Once we begin to see the extent of the problem, further questions emerge. By what mechanisms do most seropositive women come to be infected with HIV? If not all women are at high risk, which groups of women are most likely to be exposed to the virus? How are women's risks similar—and different—in vastly different settings? Has scholarly research—whether clinical investigation, epidemiology, or social science—kept pace with the advancing AIDS pandemic? Finally, what effects have persistent misunderstandings about women and AIDS had on the allocation of resources for prevention, detection, or treatment of HIV infection?

Throughout this book, I will return to these questions. But let us begin by examining the experience of three women living with HIV. These women are from very different backgrounds: "Darlene" is an African American woman from Harlem; "Guylène" is the daughter of poor peasants from rural Haiti; "Lata" was living in a rural Indian village when, at the age of fifteen, she was sold into prostitution in Bombay. Their stories, similar in some ways and different in others, speak to many of the questions raised here.

DARLENE

Darlene Johnson was born in Central Harlem in 1955, one of three children born to a mother who was chronically homeless, leaving her husband and children for long periods of time.[18] Darlene remembered her parents having terrible fights in which her father hit her mother and her mother "cried for days." When Darlene was five, her mother sent her to Alabama to live with her maternal grandmother.

Darlene was shuttled back to New York City when she was eleven and was left to the care of her brother, who was ten years older. Darlene's brother, angry that this new burden narrowed his own life chances, beat her frequently. With no other means of support, Darlene lived with her abusive brother until after eleventh grade, when she married a "hardworking man." The couple soon had two children. "No welfare," she said later. "We never did it, not even when things were hard."

Things were often hard. The couple had many problems. Chief among them was their mutual passion, not for each other but for heroin. "I didn't love him," she recalled. "He beat me, sometimes in front of the kids. It was drugs." After six years of abuse, Darlene found a way to leave. She and her children went to live with her estranged father.

A short while after moving in with her father, Darlene met her second husband. This marriage was for love. Her husband, also a heroin user, worked. They had two sons. Her two older children also loved this man, and things were looking up. Although she used heroin, Darlene insisted that it didn't interfere with taking care of her children. "It just made things smooth," she claimed.

In 1987, her stepbrother, also a heroin user, was diagnosed with AIDS. "He just died," said Darlene; no mess, no fuss. Everyone in the family was stunned. Shortly thereafter, Darlene's stepfather, whom she saw fairly frequently, had a fatal heart attack. An autopsy found that he too had been HIV-infected.

Darlene grieved, but she was determined to keep her family together. Then her husband began to have high fevers and night sweats. He refused to go to the doctor, but Darlene knew it must be AIDS. She was tortured by the memory of all the times that she, her husband, and her stepbrother had shared needles. Darlene was tested and learned that she was indeed HIV-positive.

Her husband died two months later. Alone with four children, Darlene was heartbroken; she had lost her husband, her stepbrother, and her stepfather in a single year. Two women who were her baby's godparents and who had also shared needles had become ill, and they too had died.

Darlene was not only heartbroken. She was also broke, forced to add the constant struggle to make ends meet to the struggle to overcome her grief. Her children, she recalled, kept her going. She suspected that her youngest son, sick from birth with one thing or another, was also infected. His first serious bout with pneumonia made everything clear: "I didn't know he had it till they took my baby to the hospital." Darlene was, by her own account, in a state of shock. "Too many close people" had died.

ἐne decided to set up her home to care for her son. She didn't want

don him in the hospital, and so she learned to do everything she could for him. When her older children began to misbehave, cutting school and hanging out in the streets, Darlene tried to get help, to no avail. There was nothing for them. The counselors in their schools couldn't be trusted not to divulge information about her illness.

Soon the children were completely out of hand. By this time, the baby had begun to stare at Darlene as if he didn't know who she was. Crack, she explained, came to be the only way she could find to ease her pain. But, as always, there was a price to pay. She began to lose patience with her children. She yelled often; she didn't cook regular meals for them. She was relieved when they were away. No formal supports were available for her. Darlene had nothing but pain:

> This social worker was telling everybody I had the virus. . . . The police came looking for me when my little son ran away, he ran away with my big son; my big son brought him home. When I came downstairs, the cops jumped all the way down the stairs. "Oh, you supposed to be in the hospital cause you got AIDS." Everybody on the street was looking at me. . . . [The social worker] told my kids' friends, their parents. A little boy was up in the fire escape, he said, "Oh, look—there's David's mother; she got AIDS."

Darlene concluded that her children were suffering and neglected. She felt they had no family; everyone had died. So she turned to the Department of Social Services and asked that her three oldest children be placed in foster care while she tried to care for the youngest, now dying of AIDS. "I just didn't want to live any more and I didn't want the kids to be running in the street, to be hungry."

The department placed the three children in separate homes. The oldest was sent to a home in the Bronx, but he ran away to live with a friend of Darlene's who wanted him and who was willing to support him. Darlene also wanted the child to be with her friend, but she knew that city authorities would never grant custody to this woman, so she said nothing. Darlene's daughter was placed with a woman whom Darlene knew to be a drug user: "They put my daughter in a house where they sell drugs, crack. My daughter watches this lady's kids." Darlene had no power to change the placement.

Her third child was placed in New Jersey with a family that Darlene likes. He is well cared for, and she expects the family to adopt him when she dies. She is grateful for them and wants the adoption to happen. She attends family therapy sessions with this family. This son, she feels, will be all right.

Having given her children to foster care, and left alone with her youngest, Darlene found it painful to care for him. The little boy suffered terribly. His stomach became more and more distended, and he stopped responding to her. Finally one night, as he lay in bed with her, he stopped breathing. This death "took me out completely," Darlene recalled. "He was three years old. It took him six months to die." Six of the main people in her life had died in a single year.

Darlene gave in to crack completely and hit rock bottom. She lived on the streets for three months, but she was desperate "not to die that way." The children counted on seeing her. She went into the hospital to detoxify from crack and enrolled in a methadone program. Once in the program, she saw a doctor. All during the year of deaths, she had never gone to a doctor for herself. She thinks she must have been very depressed.

Darlene, too, has been diagnosed with AIDS, but mostly she worries about her two oldest children. She could have used some help with them when all the deaths began. Darlene sees the two children who live near her every day. She visits the son who lives in New Jersey every week. She says she'll see them this way until she dies. She only hopes she doesn't linger.

GUYLÈNE

Guylène Adrien was born in Savanette, a dusty village in the middle of Haiti's infertile Central Plateau. Like other families in the region, the Adriens fed their children by working a small plot of land and selling produce in regional markets. Like other families, the Adriens were poor; but Guylène recalled that, when she was small, they "had enough to get by." Times would get harder, however, as the eighties brought resurgent political unrest and a death in the family.

Guylène was the third of four children, a small family by Haitian standards. It was to become smaller still: Guylène's younger sister died in adolescence of cerebral malaria. Guylène's oldest sister is said to be somewhere in the Dominican Republic, where she has been living, if she is living, for over a dozen years. Guylène's other surviving sister lives with her mother and two children, working the family plot of land for ever-diminishing returns.

Guylène recounts her own conjugal history in the sad voice reserved for retrospection. When she was a teenager—"perhaps fourteen or fifteen"—a family acquaintance, Occident Dorzin, took to dropping by for visits. A fairly successful peasant farmer, Dorzin had two or three small plots of land in the area. In the course of these visits, he made it clear to Guylène that he was attracted to her. "But he was already married, and I was a child. When he placed his hand on my arm, I slapped him and swore at him and hid in the garden."

Dorzin was not so easily dissuaded, however, and eventually approached Guylène's father to ask for her hand—not in marriage, but in *plasaj,* a potentially stable form of union widespread in rural Haiti.[19] Before she was sixteen, Guylène moved with Dorzin, a man twenty years her senior, to a village about an hour away from her parents. She was soon pregnant. Occident's wife, who was significantly older than Guylène, was not at all pleased. Friction between the two women eventually led to dissolution of the newer union. In the interim, however, Guylène gave birth to two children, a girl and then a boy.

After the break with Dorzin, Guylène and her nursing son returned to her father's house. She remained in Savanette for five months, passing through the village of Do Kay on her way to the market in Domond or to visit her daughter, who remained in Occident's care. It was during these travels that she met a young man named Osner, who worked intermittently in Port-au-Prince as a laborer or a mechanic. One day he simply struck up a conversation with Guylène as she visited a friend in Do Kay. "Less than a month later," she recalled, "Osner sent his father to speak to my father. My father agreed." Leaving her toddler son in her parents' household, Guylène set off to try conjugal life a second time, this time in Do Kay.

The subsequent months were difficult. Guylène's father died later that year, and her son, cared for largely by her sister, was often ill. Guylène was already pregnant with her third child, and she and Osner lacked almost everything that might have made their new life together easier.

Osner did not have steady work in Port-au-Prince, although he occasionally found part-time jobs as a mechanic. After the baby was born in 1985, they decided to move to the city; Osner would find work in a garage, and Guylène would become involved in the marketplace. Failing that, she could always work as a maid. In the interim, Osner's mother would care for the baby, as Do Kay was safer than Port-au-Prince for an infant.

Osner and Guylène spent almost three years in the city. These were hard times. Port-au-Prince was wracked by political violence, especially in their neighborhood of Cité Soleil, a vast and notorious slum on the northern fringes of the city. The couple was often short of work: he worked only irregularly as a mechanic; she split her time between jobs as a maid and selling fried food on the wharf in Cité Soleil. Guylène much preferred the latter:

> Whenever I had a little money, I worked for myself selling, trying to make the money last as long as I could. When we were broke, I worked in ladies' houses. . . . If the work is good, and they pay you well, or the person is not too bad, treats you well, you might stay there as long as six or seven months. But if the person treats you poorly, you won't even stay a month. Perhaps you only go for a single day and then you quit. . . . Rich women often hate poor women, so I always had trouble working for them.

When asked what she meant by decent pay, Guylène stated that the equivalent of $20 a month was passable as long as you were able to eat something at work.

In 1987 (Darlene Johnson's year of losses), three "unhappy occurrences" came to pass in quick succession. A neighbor was shot and killed during one of the military's regular nighttime incursions into the slum; bullets pierced the thin walls of Guylène and Osner's house. A few weeks later, Guylène received word that her son had died abruptly. The cause of death was never clear. And, finally, Osner became gravely ill. It started, Guylène remembered, with weight loss and a persistent cough.

Osner returned to the clinic in Do Kay a number of times in the course of his illness, which began with pulmonary tuberculosis, a disease that we saw frequently at the clinic we'd recently founded there. In the case of a young man returning from Port-au-Prince with tuberculosis, it was routine practice to consider HIV infection in the differential diagnosis, and we suggested it as a possibility at that time. In the clinic, Osner reported a lifetime total of seven sexual partners, including Guylène. With one exception, each of these unions had been monogamous, if short-lived.

When Osner did not respond, except transiently, to biomedical interventions, many in the village began to raise the possibility of AIDS. At his death in September 1988, it was widely believed that he had died from the new disease. As his doctors, we concurred.

Guylène subsequently returned to Savanette, to a cousin's house. She tried selling produce in local markets, but she could not support even herself, much less the child she had left in the care of Osner's mother. She was humiliated, she says, by having to ask her mother-in-law for financial assistance, even though she informed the older woman that she was pregnant with Osner's child. Finally, a full year after Osner's death, the fetus "frozen in her womb" (as she put it) began to develop. It was, she insisted, Osner's baby. (Others identified a man from her hometown of Savanette as the child's father.) She had the baby, a girl, in November of 1989. Osner's mother always referred to the child as her granddaughter.

A month after her confinement, Guylène returned to Savanette with the baby. She was unemployed; her mother and sister were barely making ends meet. Guylène and others in the household often went hungry. Believing herself to be a burden, Guylène finally went to the coastal town of Saint-Marc, where she had cousins. She worked as a servant in their house until the baby became ill; Guylène, too, felt exhausted. Since free medical care was readily available only in Do Kay, she returned again to the home of Osner's mother. Guylène and Osner's first child had already started school there, and Osner's mother allowed that she could always find food for two more.

By early June 1992, Guylène was ill: she had lost weight, and her periods had ceased. Later that month, I listened to her story with some alarm. Yes, Guylène replied, she had heard of AIDS; some even said that Osner had died from it, but she knew that was not true. After reviewing Osner's chart, I suggested that she be tested for HIV. She was leaving for Port-au-Prince, Guylène informed me, but would return for the results. The child's physical exam was unremarkable except for pallor and a slightly enlarged liver. The baby was treated, empirically, for worms and also for anemia and then sent home.

The next day, Guylène returned to Port-au-Prince. She worked a few days as a maid but found the conditions intolerable. She tried selling cigarettes and candy but remained hungry and fatigued. The city was in the throes of its worst economic depression in recent decades. "I was ready to try anything," she later noted.

Although it seemed as if things couldn't get any worse, they soon did. In the early afternoon of a sweltering summer day, Osner's mother came running to us in a panic: the baby couldn't breathe, she reported, and she was in the clinic with one of the health workers. Another doctor and I ran just as quickly back to the clinic, where we found the baby struggling for every breath. Her lips went blue as we were obtaining an X-ray. With two stethoscopes applied to her chest, we both heard her heart go still. There was nothing we could do.

The chest film gave us a clue about what had happened—it revealed that the baby's heart had been twice the expected size—but it was Guylène's laboratory results that made everything clear. Because the mother was infected with HIV, it was very likely that the baby daughter had died of HIV cardiomyopathy.

Guylène was informed of her positive serology on the day following her return. She listened impassively as I went through the likely significance of the test and made plans to repeat it. Careful physical examination and history suggested that Guylène had not yet had a serious opportunistic infection. Her chief manifestations of HIV infection at that time were severe anemia, amenorrhea, weight loss, occasional fevers, and some swelling of her lymph nodes.

Guylène began visiting the clinic regularly after the confirmation of her positive HIV serology. We spoke with her regularly—"too often," she once remarked—about HIV infection and its implications. She was placed on prophylactic isoniazid, an iron supplement and multivitamins, and also a protein supplement. Instead of returning to Port-au-Prince, Guylène rented a house with the financial aid she received through an AIDS treatment program based in the clinic.

Although Guylène experienced significant improvement in less than a month, she remained depressed and withdrawn. A young man named René had been visiting her, but Guylène discouraged him, and he disappeared—"he went to Santo Domingo, I think, because I never heard from him again." In mid-November, however, Guylène responded to the advances of a soldier stationed in the town of Péligre. A native of a large town near the Dominican border, with a wife and two children there, the soldier had been in the region only about a month. Although residents of Péligre said that he had a regular partner there as well, Guylène insisted that she was his only partner in the region:

> He saw me here, at home. He saw me only a couple of times, spoke to me only a couple of times, before announcing that he cared for me. After that, he came to visit me often. I didn't think much of it until he started staying over. I got pregnant at about the time they announced that he was being transferred back to [his home town]. He said he'd be back, but I never saw or heard from him again.

As Guylène's physicians, we had gone to some trouble to discourage unprotected sexual intercourse. We were therefore anxious to know how conversations about this subject might have figured in her decision to conceive another child, if indeed the pregnancy was the result of a decision. That Guylène understood what it meant to be an asymptomatic carrier of HIV seemed clear from a metaphor she used to describe herself: "You can be walking around big and pretty, and you've got a problem inside. When you see a house that's well built, inside it's still got ugly rocks, mud, sand—all the ugly, hidden things. What's nice on the outside might not be nice on the inside."

Guylène understood, too, that her child might well be infected with HIV, and she opted to take AZT during the latter part of her pregnancy. She understood the rationale for such a measure and even recommended it to another woman. But she was impatient with questions, tired of talking about sadness and death. "Will the baby be sick?" she remarked during a prenatal visit. "Sure, he could be sick. People are never *not* sick. I'm sick . . . he might be sick too. It's in God's hands."

Now, two years after the birth of a son, Guylène says she is pleased that he has recently been declared free of HIV. In truth, however, she sees her life as ruined. Two of her children are dead; two others have long looked to a father or grandmother for most of their parenting. Guylène's own sisters are dead, missing, or beaten into submission by the hardness of Haiti. Few of her nephews and nieces have survived into adulthood.

Guylène assures her physicians that she is without symptoms, but she seems inhabited by a persistent lassitude.

LATA

When Lata first entered the world somewhere in rural Maharastra, in a small thatched hut lit only by lanterns, her mother began weeping—tears not of joy but of shame that she had brought yet another daughter into the world.[20] "God must not have been very happy with me that day," she said. Lata does not know what month she was born into her untouchable *Harijan* family of two sisters and three brothers, but the year was 1967. Her father farmed a very small plot in Solapur, a small agricultural village. As Lata remembers it, her mother did nearly all of the remaining work:

> So much of my childhood is a blur to me. I remember when my father would return home he would beat my mother for her cooking or because one of us was crying. And if he had drunk too much he would beat my sister and me, the whole time my mother running around to prepare better food or make us quiet so father could eat. It seems every day passed like this, the only difference being that father got meaner as he grew older.

Never permitted to attend school, Lata was tilling and weeding with her father by the age of six. "Years passed like this," she remarked, examining her hands as if for traces of blisters. Her two elder sisters were married at the ages of fifteen and sixteen, respectively, and both weddings came at a heavy price to Lata's family. One sister's dowry totaled 10,000 rupees, almost twice her father's earnings for that year. Predictably, both marriages forced the family to turn to the local moneylender, a man who maintained interest rates as high as 25 percent—compounded quarterly. Lata's father, already faced with selling off more of his tiny plot in order to service his debt, lived in fear of another wedding.

Lack of rainfall during the 1982 monsoon season brought a poor harvest, leaving the family in the worst financial state it had ever experienced. "My father was drinking more every day," recounted Lata. "Sometimes I recall him not even going out to the fields, yet forcing us to go, and

beating us more than he ever had. I know he was worried about my getting married, and when he was drunk he would curse my mother, blaming her for bringing him yet another daughter."

In this context, the arrival of a man who would take Lata from the de-
spair of her village life was regarded as a godsend. Like so many other
dalals ("middlemen," many of whom are women) who come from Bombay, Prasant had for some years been making a "decent" living in the
flesh trade. As he worked a route from the villages of southern Maharastra to the bordellos of Bombay, his scheme was identical in almost every
settlement. Upon arriving in a village, Prasant would seek out a local
moneylender and, often with the help of a small bribe, extract information about area families who had young daughters and heavy debt. Prasant, like other *dalals,* then approached the male heads of families, claiming to have work for their daughters as servants or seamstresses in
Bombay. In Lata's case, Prasant told her father that she would be given
work as a dishwasher:

> After [Prasant] arrived, my father took my mother aside and told her
> that jobs were available in Bombay, and this man would give him 11,000
> rupees as a payment for me washing dishes and housecleaning. He said
> I would be able to mail money home every month and allowed to visit
> Solapur after six months of work. Not for one moment did anyone sus-
> pect or question what he told us.

Desperate, hungry, facing the most acute poverty his family had ever
experienced, Lata's father saw opportunity and relief in his daughter's
departure. A few hours after he and Prasant had spoken, Lata was told to
pack her two cotton saris, her bangles, and sandals. She would leave for
Bombay in the morning.

A frail and frightened fifteen-year-old, Lata had difficulty holding
back tears as she waved goodbye. Her father's gaze was stoic, while tears
streamed down her mother's face. It was the last time she would ever see
her parents.

She remembered nothing of her trip to Bombay, although it was her
first train ride. Her inability to recollect, she later suspected, was the result of a drug she had been given. The next memory she had was of a taxi
in Bombay. Lata was entering the city's red-light district. Barely awake,

she was brought to Number 27 Falkland Road, where Prasant sold her to a pimp for 15,000 rupees (about $500). His tidy profit of 4,000 rupees was more than enough to carry him through the month.

Lata had arrived in the Kamathipura district of Bombay, and she was about to become one of its thirty thousand sex workers. Lata recalled that she came to complete consciousness in a "cage"—a cramped room full of girls putting on makeup, oiling their hair, and tightening their petticoats and blouses. Lata had no comprehension of where she was:

> I saw all of these girls wearing nothing but colored blouses, makeup, and skirts, and asked the madam, "What is this?" She told me it was a place for working girls. I still didn't understand, frightened by the very clothes these women wore. . . . Sapna, the madam, told me I would be staying with her and ordered me to put on clothes that lay on the floor for me and then stand outside. I began crying and told her I couldn't stay. She slapped me hard, and I remember I couldn't stop crying. I told her to let me go, and she looked me straight in the eye and said, "You want to leave, fine. Give me 15,000 rupees and you're free. Until then, get dressed and start paying back your *kurja*."

Lata's *kurja* was her debt, the mechanism by which she was indeed trapped as if in a cage. She did not join the other girls on the street that day, nor the day after. She slept and lay in the corner of the room, pretending to be ill, eating the food she was given, and listening to the other girls call out to customers on Falkland Road. She watched the parade of men and girls in and out of the adjacent room, furnished only with a bed. On Lata's third day in Bombay, Sapna's patience had been exhausted: she ordered one of her managers to "break Lata in."

No matter how many years pass, Lata still has trouble recounting this part of her story. Arun, a manager whose main responsibility was to bring in new customers, also had the duty of making sure the girls were bringing in enough money and "working" hard. As one madam put it, "There are times when they won't listen to us, so the managers and pimps keep the girls in line." Lata recalled:

> I had been sitting in the same corner for days, pretending I was not feeling well, frightened, and wishing Sapna would let me go. Finally Arun came to me and pulled me by my ear, telling me to put on the clothes and stand outside. I was a fifteen-year-old village girl and didn't even know what sex was, let alone prostitution. How could I understand

what was going on? He took me to the room with the bed and closed the door and forced me to have sex with him. Afterwards, he said, "Now do you understand?" and laughed and told me to get to work. I remember being silent while the other girls stared at me when I came out. I'm sure they knew what he did. And for the first time I began to accept that there was no way out—I was here to stay.

That day Lata, clad in a purple blouse and pink petticoat, nervously joined the thousands of prostitutes of Bombay's red-light districts. It was her first night on the streets and the beginning of a long and painful career.

Unlike most other girls, who stand in front of the cages beckoning to passing men, Lata stood quietly, receiving no business during her first three days out. The days were long: bathing at around 10 in the morning, out on Falkland Road by 11, lunch at 4 P.M., and back on the street until 2 or 3 A.M., with dinner if she was lucky. On an average day, a Bombay prostitute may see four to five customers a day. Times may vary, but generally late evening is when they are busiest. Early in the afternoon of her fourth day, Lata was finally approached:

An Arab man came and after seeing me spoke with the madam for some time and wanted to take me to the Taj Hotel for three days. I saw him give her many hundred rupee notes, and then he took me into his taxi and to the hotel. I was terrified of being alone with him; you have to remember that he was my first customer and I had no idea what to do. The first night we slept in separate beds, and the next day he took me to sari and jewelry shops, buying me clothes and gold. When he would go out in the day, he would lock me in the room. But the more he bought, the more scared I became of what he would expect. On the second night, he told me to dress in all of the clothes he bought for me. Frightened as I was, I knew that I had no choice. At that moment, I remember saying to myself, "This is now my life," truly accepting it for the first time. . . . No longer willing to fight him or my own self, I had sex with him.

Upon her return to Falkland Road, Lata settled into the routine of a Bombay prostitute. Slowly she came to know the stories of the girls in her brothel and others nearby. Although they hailed from many villages and even from Nepal, most had similar experiences. Like the others, she gave half of her daily earnings to the madam as repayment for her *kurja*. Yet Lata knew that she, and all girls sold into prostitution, had little hope of ever buying their freedom; her initial debt of 15,000 rupees was accruing interest at a rate of 20 to 25 percent a month. If a pimp brought a customer to her, she owed him 25 percent. And in most areas, police regularly extorted money from sex workers with the threat of jail. With an average of four or five customers per day, each paying about 20 to 30 rupees, she could be left with as little as 20 rupees to cover food, clothing, and other basic needs.

At this writing, Lata has been in Bombay for many years. She is a well-known figure at Number 27 Falkland Road, a small brothel sandwiched between a tea stall and a large pink building brimming with Nepali girls. Proudly wearing her gold bangles, her hair always neatly oiled and braided, Lata is now a respected veteran of the red-light community. At twenty-eight years of age, she continues to see an average of four or five customers a day.

Rumors of AIDS did not reach the red-light district of Bombay until 1989 or so—surely well after the virus itself had arrived. "Back then I and other people on Falkland Road started to know about AIDS, but we did not take it seriously. Then the Indian Health Organization people came and gave us free condoms."

In 1991, Lata became one of the first sex workers to volunteer as an AIDS peer educator, and she pushes her fellow prostitutes to demand that their clients use condoms: "I tell the girls, it's your life. If he refuses to wear one, send him away. And even if he offers you one million for sex without a condom, you don't do it. But I know this is hard. There are too many hungry girls. Too many scared girls. And the madams are always watching, putting on pressure."

Preventive messages came too late for Lata, who now knows that she is infected with HIV. She continues to work as both an AIDS outreach worker and a prostitute.

SEX, DRUGS, AND STRUCTURAL VIOLENCE

The stories of Darlene, Guylène, and Lata—recounted in detail in order to shed light on the forces that have constrained their options—reveal both differences and commonalities. But how locally representative is each of these histories?

Darlene Johnson's experiences are all too commonplace among African American women living in poverty. As a heroin user, a habit clearly tied to a poverty structured by racism, her chances of avoiding HIV were slim, even if she had wanted to quit the drug before her diagnosis. In 1987, the year that Darlene's world was burst asunder by AIDS, only 338,365 treatment slots were available to the nation's estimated four million addicts, and most of these programs predominantly served men. As a pregnant woman, Darlene would have found it next to impossible to find treatment for her addiction.[21] Writing about women of color who are also addicted and living in poverty, Janet Mitchell and her co-workers point out that "access to care and services has traditionally been *marginal* for women with any one of these three criteria. Any two of these . . . essentially put women in the *extremely limited* access category. Women with all three of these characteristics fall into the *no access* category."[22]

In the United States, HIV has moved almost unimpeded through poor communities of color. By 1991, African Americans, who constitute approximately 12 percent of the U.S. population, accounted for 30 percent of all reported AIDS cases. During the 1980s, the cumulative incidence of AIDS was more than eleven times higher for black women than for white women. Although many early cases occurred among those who injected drugs, the epidemic is fast expanding among women with no such history. As noted earlier, AIDS is the leading cause of death among African American women of ages 25 to 44; for Latinas in this age group, it is now the third leading cause of death.[23] When the first multicenter study of AIDS among U.S. women was funded, almost 78 percent of the more than 1300 patients recruited were women of color.[24]

Understanding the contours of the U.S. epidemic is less a matter of knowing one's geography and more a matter of understanding a limited number of events and processes that range from unemployment to the destruction of housing by fires—the "synergism of plagues" discussed by Rodrick Wallace.[25] "Urban poverty in the United States has created the perfect machinery for the continued propagation of HIV," Robert Fullilove argues. "Inner-city poor neighborhoods often shelter a vigorous drug trade, numerous opportunities for strangers to engage in drug-mediated, unprotected sex, and numerous locations where these and other risk behaviors go virtually unchallenged."[26]

In Haiti, similarly, little about Guylène's story is unique. We hear a deadly monotony in the stories told by rural Haitian women with AIDS. In a study we conducted at the Clinique Bon Sauveur, where Guylène receives her care, the majority of new AIDS diagnoses are registered among women, most of them with a trajectory similar to Guylène's. As young women—or teenage girls—they had been driven to Port-au-Prince by the lure of an escape from the harshest poverty. Once in the city, each worked as a domestic, but none managed to find the financial security so elusive in the countryside. The women we interviewed were straightforward about the nonvoluntary aspect of their sexual activity: in their opinions, they had been driven into unfavorable unions by poverty.[27] Indeed, such testimony calls into question facile notions of "consensual sex."

Lata's painful experience also exemplifies that of hundreds of thousands of poor girls in India, Nepal, and elsewhere. It has been estimated that up to 50 percent of Bombay's prostitutes were recruited through trickery or abduction.[28] Although few population-based surveys have yet been conducted, it is quite likely that most of India's prostitutes have high rates of HIV infection. In the late 1980s, some seven hundred sex workers were arrested and forcibly taken to the city of Madras; 70 percent of these women were found to have antibodies to HIV. Many of them were jailed or subjected to other forms of harassment, including having their names publicly listed.[29]

In short, the experiences of Darlene, Guylène, and Lata are all too typical. One clear lesson we can draw from their stories is that both immediate and systemic causes of increased risk need to be elucidated. For example, heroin use and needle sharing put Darlene at increased risk of HIV infection. Sex work—or, rather, unprotected sex work—put Lata at risk. But in both Harlem and Bombay, it seems fair to assert that the decisions these women made were linked to their impoverishment and to their subordinate status as women. Furthermore, it is important to remember that Darlene and Guylène and Lata were *born* into poverty. Their attempts to escape poverty were long bets that failed—and AIDS was the ultimate form their failure took.

The stories recounted here force a difficult question: how many girls are, from birth, at inordinate risk of AIDS or some other terrible destiny? "For some women," explains the founder of an AIDS support group for women, "HIV is the first major disaster in their lives. For many more, AIDS is just one more problem on top of many others."[30] In fact, attentiveness to the life stories of most women with AIDS usually reveals that it is the latest in a string of tragedies. "For poor women," as anthropologist Martha Ward describes, "AIDS is just another problem they are blamed for and have to take responsibility for. They ask, 'How am I going to take care of my family?' 'I have to put food on the table now.' 'You think AIDS is a problem! Let me tell you—I got real problems.'"[31]

Millions of women living in similar circumstances—but with very different psychological profiles and cultural backgrounds—can expect to meet similar fates. Their sickness is a result of structural violence: neither culture nor pure individual will is at fault; rather, historically given (and often economically driven) processes and forces conspire to constrain individual agency. Structural violence is visited upon all those whose social status denies them access to the fruits of scientific and social progress.

If we are to present meaningful responses to AIDS, we must examine the differential political economy of risk. Structural violence means that some women are, from the outset, at high risk of HIV infection, while other women are shielded from risk. Adopting this point of view—that we can describe a political economy of risk and that this exercise helps to explain where the AIDS pandemic is moving and how quickly—we begin to see why similar stories are legion in sub-Saharan Africa and India, why they are fast becoming commonplace in Thailand and other parts of Asia. The experiences recounted here may be textbook cases of vulnerability, but their moral is deciphered only if we clearly understand that these women have been rendered vulnerable to AIDS through *social* processes—that is, through the economic, political, and cultural forces that can be shown to shape the dynamics of HIV transmission. The anthropologist Brooke Schoepf, writing from Zaïre, explains how AIDS has "transformed many women's survival strategies into death strategies":

> Women, who often lack access to cash, credit, land or jobs, engage in "off-the-books" activities in the informal sector. Some exchange sex for the means of subsistence. Others enter sex work at the behest of their families, to obtain cash to purchase land or building materials, to pay a brother's school fees, or to settle a debt. Still others supplement meager incomes with occasional resort to sex with multiple partners. [Whether

these women are] married or not, the deepening economic crisis propels many to seek "spare tires" or "shock absorbers" to make ends meet.[32]

Taken together, the dynamics of HIV infection among women and the responses to its advance reveal much about the complex relationship between power/powerlessness and sexuality. But many questions remain unanswered. For example, by what mechanisms, precisely, do social forces (such as poverty, sexism, and other forms of discrimination) become embodied as personal risk? What role does inequality per se play in promoting HIV transmission?

Although many would agree that forces such as poverty and gender inequality are the strongest enhancers of risk for exposure to HIV, this subject has been neglected in both the biomedical and the social science literature on HIV infection. Let us take, as an example, an investigation of heterosexually transmitted HIV infection in "rural" Florida, conducted by Ellerbrock and co-workers. The study, published in 1992 in the *New England Journal of Medicine*, revealed that fully 5.1 percent of 1082 asymptomatic women attending a public prenatal clinic in Palm Beach County had antibodies to HIV. What risk factors might account for such high rates of infection? The researchers reported a statistically significant association between HIV infection and having used crack cocaine, having more than five sexual partners in a lifetime, or having more than two sexual partners per year of sexual activity. Also associated with seropositivity to HIV was a history of exchanging sex for money or for drugs or of having sexual intercourse with a "high-risk partner."

These associations are not surprising. How are they interpreted? The study concludes that "in communities with a high seroprevalence of HIV, like this Florida community, a sizable proportion of *all women of reproductive age* are at risk for infection through heterosexual transmission."[33] Is this in fact the most significant (or the most pragmatically valuable) conclusion to be drawn from such a study? In settings with an even higher seroprevalence of HIV, such as parts of New York City, it is clear that not *all* women of reproductive age are at increased risk of HIV infection; rather, *poor women*, who in the United States are often women of color, are at high risk.

A conclusion such as that drawn by the researchers is possible only if we place the "community" being studied under a Bell jar, so that both the glittering towers of West Palm Beach and the vast fields of sugarcane—and their owners—are outside the field of analysis. But if these parts of the "community" are invisible, so too is the political economy of AIDS, for many of the women studied, like their partners, have worked in these wealthy communities or in the nearby fields. Thus, *arbitrarily constricting the social field generates the illusion of equally shared risk.* It obscures inequalities central to the advance of HIV. An equivalent exercise would be to recount Darlene's story as if Central Harlem were an island nation rather than a rich city's ghetto. Guylène's narrative would make no reference to the wealthy households in which she was forced to work. Lata's social field would be bordered by the margins of the Kamathipura district, into which no wealthy clients entered.

A closer look at the language in which Ellerbrock and co-workers couched their conclusions suggests that a meaningful discussion of risk cannot be limited to medical issues, narrowly construed. Nowhere in their article does the word "poverty" appear, even though the authors mention that over 90 percent of the women who knew the amount of their income belonged to households earning less than $10,000 per year.[34] Nowhere in the article do we see the word "racism," even though in Florida, as elsewhere, the African American and Latino communities are those most affected by the epidemic. The terms "sexism," "despair," and "powerlessness" are also absent from the discussion, even though many of the women studied were pulled into the region by the possibility of jobs as servants or farmworkers. One might as easily conclude that, in Palm Beach County, it is the women who are "at risk" of attending a public prenatal clinic who are at higher risk of acquiring HIV—unemployed women of color, that is, who are more likely to have unstable sexual unions or to exchange sex for drugs or money.[35]

Like all societies characterized by extreme inequality or structural violence, the linked societies of Darlene, Guylène, and Lata require other kinds of violence in order to maintain the status quo, which is so unbearable for the majority. In the United States, the enormous number of African Americans in prisons reflects this violence, as do death squads in Haiti and police brutality in Bombay. Other forms of violence are more strikingly gendered. HIV and direct violence against women are intimately linked. Among sex workers, risk of assault and risk of HIV are both highest among the poorest prostitutes.[36] Many of the estimated four million U.S. women who are assaulted by their male partners are also those at heightened risk for HIV. As Sally Zierler observes, "This figure, awful as it is, obscures the fact that some women are more at risk than others. For like HIV's distribution, partner violence against women follows social divisions marked by class position, and race/ethnicity, creating strata of extreme vulnerability to violence victimization."[37]

In an era of widespread and instantaneous communication, *symbolic violence* is also used to accomplish these ends: structural violence requires its apologists, witting or unwitting. We now turn to the role played by researchers and other opinion shapers in buttressing the myths and mystifications related to the topic of women and AIDS.

WOMEN AND AIDS: MYTHS AND MYSTIFICATIONS

Throughout the world, the majority of women with HIV infection are poor. They are denied access not merely to resources and services but also to symbolic capital. In her thoughtful examination of the gendering of American AIDS discourse, Paula Treichler asks, "Why were women so unprepared? And why do they continue to take it so quietly?"[38] She responds to her own question with a candor that is all too rare:

> As evidence of AIDS in women mounted, speculations linked the disease to prostitutes, intravenous drug users, and women in the Third World (primarily Haiti and countries in central Africa). It was not that these three groups were synonymous but, rather, that their *differentness of race, class, or national origin* made speculation about transmission possible—unlike middle-class American feminists, for example. American feminists also by this point had considerable access to public forums from which to protest ways in which they were represented, while these other groups of women were, for all practical purposes, silenced categorically so far as public or biomedical discourse was concerned.[39]

This silencing refers to the absence of the voices of poor women in public forums ranging from conferences to published material. In truth, however, these women have not been silent; they have simply been unheard. In rural Haiti, for example, a group of poor women committed to preventing AIDS worked together in 1991 to generate a list of common myths about women and AIDS.[40] The document prepared by the group referred to the following myths:

AIDS Is a Disease of Men

The data are overwhelming: AIDS was never a disease of men. Given transmission dynamics, AIDS may in fact become a disease *predominantly* afflicting women.

"Heterosexual AIDS" Won't Happen

Heterosexual AIDS has already happened. Indeed, in many parts of the world, AIDS is the leading cause of death among young women.

Women's Promiscuity Causes AIDS

Most women with AIDS do not have multiple sexual partners; they have never used i.v. drugs; they have not received tainted blood transfusions. Their major risk factor is being poor. For others, the risk is being married and unable to control not only their husbands but also what jobs their husbands have to perform to make a living.

Women Are AIDS Vectors

Women are too often perceived as agents of transmission who infect men and "innocent babies." Prostitutes have been particularly hard hit by such propaganda, but prostitutes are far more vulnerable to infection than to infecting: AIDS is an "occupational risk" of commercial sex work, especially in settings in which sex workers cannot safely demand that clients use condoms.[41]

Condoms Are Panaceas

Gender inequality calls into question the utility of condoms in settings in which women's ability to insist on "safe sex" is undermined by a host of less easily confronted forces. Furthermore, many HIV-positive women *choose* to conceive children, which means that barrier methods that prevent conception are not the answer for many. Woman-controlled viricidal preventive strategies are necessary, if women's wishes are to be respected.

While these were the myths deemed salient in Haiti, other, related mystifications flourish in every setting in which poor women must now add HIV to a long list of quotidian threats. In the United States, Martha Ward complains of "urban folklore" about mothers with AIDS: "'Those women have food stamps. They buy alcohol or luxury items. They have infected their innocent babies. They should use birth control, get abortions, get a job, finish school, use condoms, and say "no" to drugs.' "[42]

What many of the dominant myths and mystifications have in common is an *exaggeration of personal agency*, often through highlighting certain psychological or cultural attributes, even though it is not at all clear that these attributes are in any way related to women's risk for HIV infection. Condoms are a classic case in point. Most U.S. women at high risk of HIV infection are already aware that condoms can prevent transmission, but many of these women are unable to insist that condoms be used because their precarious situations often force poor women to rely on men. For example, a study conducted among African American women in Los Angeles showed that couples in which the woman depended on her male partner for rent money were less likely to use condoms than couples in which the woman had no such dependence.[43]

There is nothing wrong with underlining personal agency, but there is something unfair about using personal responsibility as a basis for assigning blame while simultaneously denying those who are being blamed the opportunity to exert agency in their lives. "A patronage that simultaneously grants 'victims' powerlessness and then assigns them blame for that powerlessness is nothing new," observes Jan Grover. "It is therefore important to make connections between the construction of AIDS victimhood and similar constructions of the poor, who also suffer the triple curse of objectification, institutionalized powerlessness, and blame for their condition."[44]

Although most acknowledge the link between poverty and low rates of condom use, few studies have carefully explored the association. The objectification of "the poor," as noted, is a risk run by anyone who uses the term, but striving to understand a person's material constraints does not imply a refusal to recognize the salience of personal experience. Recognizing a commonality of constraint—in addition to, say, a commonality of psychology or of culture—is an important part of unraveling the nature of risk. Indeed, failure to embed personal experience in the larger social and economic matrices in which it takes on meaning is often synonymous with intense focus on personal psychology or "deviant subcultures."

Among the myriad mystifications that obscure the nature of women's risk, three are recurrent and important. One is the *focus on local factors and*

local actors to the exclusion of broader analyses that would implicate powerful forces and powerful actors outside the field of view. A second is the
conflation of structural violence and cultural difference. A third, centrally related to the others, is the *absence of serious consideration of social class.*[45]
These are not infrequently the mechanisms by which personal agency is
exaggerated in both scholarly and popular commentary. To cite Brooke
Schoepf again: "The structure of the wider political economy establishes
the situations and restricts the options that people can choose as a means
of survival. A focus on 'sub-cultures,' as on individual behaviors, tends
to obscure the underlying causes of social interaction."[46]

These expedient erasures and exaggerations are buttressed, rather
than challenged or exposed, by research published in a host of key journals. For example, a review of the ever-enlarging epidemiologic literature
reveals that although racism, sexism, and powerlessness go unmen-
tioned, we usually *do* find mention of culture.[47]

An example is a study conducted by Nyamathi and co-workers in the
Los Angeles area among 1173 women ages 18 to 75. Half were African
Americans; half were called "Latinas" and described as either "high-
acculturated" or "low-acculturated." Recruited through homeless shelters or drug-treatment programs, all of these women had histories of
using drugs, being the sexual partner of an injecting drug user, being
homeless, or having a sexually transmitted disease. Some had histories of
sex work; some had multiple sexual partners. A survey administered to
these women revealed that "African-American and Latina women were
equally knowledgeable about AIDS symptomatology; the etiologic agent
of AIDS; and behaviors known to reduce risk of HIV infection, such as
using condoms and cleaning works used by intravenous drug users."[48]
Greater differences existed in how much the women knew about modes
of transmission, but the women tended to *overestimate* transmissibility,
not to underestimate it.

In a sense, then, what the researchers found was that ignorance about
HIV was not really the issue for these women. What put them at risk was
something other than cognitive deficits. But the researchers' interpretation of their findings, published in the influential *American Journal of Public Health,* was not in keeping with the data: "These findings suggest the
need for culturally sensitive education programs that cover common

problems relating to drug use and unprotected sex and, in addition, offer sessions for women of different ethnic groups to address problematic areas of concern."[49] Was this truly a key implication of the research? By the researchers' own standards, these women were by and large *fully aware* of transmission of HIV through injection drug use and unprotected sex. Moreover, the more a woman had used drugs or had multiple sexual partners, the more likely she was to perceive herself, correctly, as being at increased risk of HIV infection.

By insisting that "culturally sensitive education programs" have a large role to play in protecting poor women from AIDS, the authors are suggesting, all evidence to the contrary, that ignorance of the facts is centrally related to high HIV risk and that, consequently, the way to diminish risk is to increase knowledge. Through this cognitivist legerdemain, we have expediently moved the locus of the problem—and thus the focus of the interventions—away from certain features of an inegalitarian society and toward the women deemed "at risk." The problem is with the women; thus the interventions should change the women.

The cost of all this desocialization might well be significant, for cognitivist, behaviorist, or culturist assumptions often privilege effects over cause. Immodest claims of causality, and even undue focus on the psychological or cultural peculiarities of those with AIDS, are not only intellectual errors; they also serve to deflect attention away from the real engines of the AIDS pandemic. Thus, when the *éminences grises* of sexually transmitted disease control examine the possibilities for effective AIDS control in developing countries, their list of suggested interventions ranges from public lectures to "long-term psychotherapy for HIV-positive individuals" and "group therapy for commercial sex workers."[50]

Similar themes are widely echoed in a society known for its obsession with individualism. It is not surprising, then, to hear the same exaggerations of agency even from those most committed to preventing AIDS. Often we hear about a certain community's "denial" of risk or about the epidemic of "low self-esteem" among those living with HIV infection. These cultural and psychological factors are then granted etiologic power: they are construed as the *source* of increased risk rather than the *effects* of structural violence.

Sadly, if predictably, the same calculus of causality occurs in the comments of those afflicted by AIDS. The founder of one group for women living with HIV infection put it this way: "Low self-esteem is a significant 'co-factor' that led many women to be at risk of acquiring HIV."[51] Surely there exist important co-factors for "low self-esteem"—and poverty (otherwise known in post-welfare America as hunger, joblessness, and homelessness) is the obvious leader among them. Other variations on this theme of inequality, including racism and sexism, are also high on the list.

Such immodest claims of psychological and moral causality expediently divert attention away from structural violence. No wonder, then, that U.S. Republicans and their friends among the Democrats are so eager to advance the same hypotheses. In the recently promulgated "Personal Responsibility Act," AFDC recipients are called to work a minimum of thirty-five hours per week in a designated "work slot." Since these women have, apparently unlike the authors of the act, more than a passing knowledge of math, they know that, with a median disbursement of $366 per month and an hourly wage in such "slots" of well under $3, they will be unable to assemble the funds necessary to provide day care—let alone health care and safe housing—for their children. Even in cities with a modest cost of living, a single mother of two children would need an hourly wage of $10 in order to cross the poverty line.[52] We are left to surmise that these women's infants and toddlers will buy and prepare their own formula and meals. As Valerie Polakow, who recently interviewed scores of single American mothers, bitterly notes, this experience should give these babies an early lesson in the importance of personal responsibility. "As their rhetoric against won't-work mothers and promiscuous teens escalates," concludes Polakow, "it advances the pernicious idea that poverty is a private affair, that destitution and homelessness are simply products of bad personal choices."[53]

From typhoid to tuberculosis and AIDS, blaming the victim is a recurrent theme in the history of epidemic disease.[54] In case after case, analysis can lead researchers to focus either on the patients' shortcomings (failure to drink pure water, failure to use condoms, ignorance about public health and hygiene) or on the conditions that structure people's risk (lack of access to potable water, lack of economic opportunities for women, unfair distribution of the world's resources). The results are not indifferent. One of the chief benefits of choosing to see illness in global-systemic terms is that it encourages physicians (and others concerned to protect or promote health) to make common cause with people who are both poor and sick. In addition, analyses that resolutely embed personal experience in the larger social fields in which experience takes on meaning have far more explanatory power in examining epidemics of infectious disease—particularly those that, like AIDS, move along the fault lines of our interlinked societies.

The most frequently encountered and easily circulated theories about women and AIDS are far more likely to include punitive images of women as purveyors of infection—prostitutes, for example, or mothers who "contaminate" their innocent offspring—than to include images of homelessness, barriers to medical care, a social service network that doesn't work, and an absence of jobs and housing. Dominant readings are likely to suggest that women with AIDS have had large numbers of sexual partners, but are less likely to show how girls like Lata are abducted into the flesh trade, and even less likely to reveal how political and structural violence—for example, the increasing landlessness among the rural poor and the gearing of economies to favor exports—come to be important in the AIDS pandemic today.

For women most at risk of HIV infection, life choices are limited by racism, sexism, political violence, and grinding poverty. It is a wonder, then, that discussions of AIDS so rarely focus on these issues. Complex indeed are the mechanisms by which such structural violence can be effaced and the apparent significance of personal choice (or cultural difference) inflated. But when dominant myths about women and AIDS are contrasted with the experiences of Darlene and Guylène and Lata, we are forced to call into question many of these understandings.

WHAT IS TO BE DONE?

As I described earlier, a group of poor women in rural Haiti, some of them living with HIV, met in 1991 to consider AIDS and its effects on their communities. They agreed that, although many were infected with HIV through means well beyond their own control, not enough had been done to educate the people in the region. How could they join forces to make up for this deficiency?

Written materials would have limited utility in a setting of nearly universal illiteracy, and the military government had just taken control of many of the area's radio stations. In the end, these women—who had never had electricity in their homes and had never owned televisions—decided to produce a videotape that told a story very similar to Guylène's. They then worked with a community-based organization to acquire a portable generator, a video projector, and a screen. Condom demonstrations and community discussion accompanied each showing of the video.

Proud of their success, the women subsequently spoke of their experience at a number of meetings and conferences held in rural Haiti. At one of these conferences, a Haitian physician (herself not unsympathetic to the trials of the women who'd made the video) listened to a presentation by one of the women and saw the video. During the discussion, the doctor faced the project participant, who had proudly introduced herself as a *malerez*, a "poor woman," and asked, "So what? In other words, if we are manifestly failing to prevent HIV transmission in this region, what is the significance of your project?"

The *malerez* did not hesitate in answering: "Doctor, when all around you liars are the only cocks crowing, telling the truth is a victory." Telling the truth about the nature of women's risk would be no mean feat in the current climate.

A second, and related, set of tasks concerns prevention. Making condoms readily available is an altogether insufficient response. Getting the right message across remains a priority and always will, as HIV is unlikely to be eradicated soon. Adolescents everywhere in the world simply must learn about sexually transmitted diseases before becoming sexually active. Universal HIV education needs to become part of growing up, which might also help to attenuate AIDS-related stigma. Clearly such efforts will need to be different in different settings, but the universal finality (and obstinacy) of AIDS has changed the way we think about sexuality and sexism. Teenagers throughout the world need to learn about the relationship between HIV transmission and social forces such as poverty and gender inequality.

A third set of activities might target specific groups of those at risk for HIV infection. In northern Tanzania, for example, improving the quality and accessibility of treatment for sexually transmitted infections reduced the incidence of HIV by 42 percent.[55] Injecting drug users need ready access to drug-treatment programs, but we also know that needle-exchange efforts can decrease the incidence of new infections even in the absence of adequate drug treatment.[56]

Stopping exploitative prostitution would require addressing poverty, gender inequality, and racism, but in the absence of serious societal programs with such aims, public health authorities can make a priority of protecting, rather than punishing, sex workers.[57] Commercial sex workers benefit from high-quality medical care, especially when it is provided with the well-being of the prostitutes—rather than that of their clients—in mind. "It is important," notes one advocate, "that a full range of health care services, including health care for their children and not just STD services, be made more accessible—and more acceptable—to prostitutes."[58] Attacking AIDS-related stigma will require an attack against the scapegoating of sex workers, gays, and other groups.

For women already living with HIV disease, improved clinical services are critical. This means, among other things, educating health care professionals about women and AIDS.[59] HIV infection is underrecognized in women, with many cases diagnosed during pregnancy—or at autopsy. When AIDS case definitions were changed to include, among other conditions, invasive cervical cancer, the number of AIDS diagnoses in U.S. women doubled in a single year.[60]

Further improving services implies removing the barriers that currently prevent poor women, regardless of their HIV status, from obtaining much-needed resources. These resources range from access to certain medications to safe housing. Although we lack extensive data, research currently under way in the urban United States suggests that, in one large cohort of women, the majority of patients with advanced HIV disease were not receiving prophylaxis to prevent the most common opportunistic infections, to say nothing of antiretroviral therapy. In the same cohort, most women did not have secure housing; almost 20 percent stated that they had "no safe place to live."[61] Attention to matters such as these could, in principle, prolong the lives of millions of women already infected, in both rich and poor countries.[62]

Finally, it is important to recall that women are also affected by AIDS in indirect ways, for it is women who bear the brunt of caring for the sick, regardless of age or gender.[63] For this reason, improving the quality of care for *all people* living with AIDS will improve the lives of the women who care for them.

Through these three sets of tasks alone—that is, setting the record straight, rethinking prevention activities, and improving the array of services available to women and to all persons with AIDS—we can do much to strengthen the hand of women living in poverty. With perseverance and commitment, such measures might eventually result in slowing the rate of HIV transmission to poor women. Indeed, evidence suggests that the recently registered drop in AIDS deaths is attributable to more effective therapy.[64] Patients receiving highly active antiretroviral therapy often have undetectable viral loads; transmission is much less likely when viral burden is low.[65]

As important as these AIDS-focused activities are, they largely address only the symptoms of a deeper ill. Endeavors focused on AIDS, though crucial, must be linked to efforts to empower poor women. The much-abused term "empower" is not meant vaguely here; empowerment is not a matter of self-esteem or even of parliamentary representation. Those choosing to make common cause with poor women must help them gain control over their own lives. Control of lives is related to control of land, systems of production, and the formal political and legal structures in which lives are enmeshed. In each of these arenas, poor people overall are already laboring at a vast disadvantage; the voices of poor women in particular are almost unheard.

The occurrence of HIV in the wealthy countries, where even those living in poverty control more resources than women like Guylène and Lata, reminds us that *HIV tracks along steep gradients of power.* In many settings, HIV risks are enhanced not so much by poverty in and of itself but by inequality. Increasingly, what people with AIDS share are not personal or psychological attributes. They do not share culture or language or a certain racial identity. They do not share sexual preference or an absolute income bracket. What they share, rather, is a *social position*—the bottom rung of the ladder in inegalitarian societies. Writing from Bombay, Sarthak Das underlines similarities in the experiences of the untouchable

castes of India and poor people of color in U.S. cities: "We need only re-
place the categories of 'Black' and 'Hispanic' with the low-caste, untouchable titles of *Harijan* and *Sudra* in order to observe a parallel epidemiological pattern on the subcontinent."[66]

The trials of women like Guylène and Lata pose challenges to
women—and, of course, to all people of good will—in the rich countries.
Can we somehow lessen the huge and growing disparities that characterize our world? Within rich countries, the struggles of women like Darlene Johnson are even more of a rebuke, challenging facile notions of
sisterhood and solidarity. Unlike Guylène and Lata, Darlene lives within
a mile of a world-class medical center. At key points in her experience,
however, that center might as well have been half a world away. Without
insurance, Darlene did not have ready access to it.

The rapidly growing literature on women and AIDS is well stocked
with pieties about solidarity, but the progress of the disease among
women seems to take particular advantage of the lack of solidarity
among the members of an AIDS-affected society. When solidarity fails,
the reasons are often less about color and more about class. A working-
class lesbian writes that "HIV makes a mockery of pretend unity and sisterhood." Those most affected, she notes, are women of color and poor
white women, many of whom are "struggling with long histories of
shooting drugs or fucking men for the money to get those drugs. These
are not the women usually identified as the women the feminist movement or the lesbian movement most value and try to organize to create a
progressive political agenda."[67] One of the contributors to *Listen Up*, a recently published collection of feminist essays, concurs: "Many feminists
seem to find the issues of class the most difficult to address; we are always faced with the fundamental inequalities inherent in late-twentieth-
century multinational capitalism and our unavoidable implication in its
structures."[68]

This is why efforts to promote pragmatic solidarity—that is, a solidarity that acknowledges and responds to the material needs of the destitute
sick—must engage not only local inequalities but also global ones. The
medical and social analysts whose work I prize most highly aim to link a
deep concern for pragmatic interventions—projects designed to prevent
or better treat complications of HIV infection—with more utopian aspi-

rations. If indeed inequality is an important co-factor in this pandemic, then stopping AIDS will require a more ambitious agenda, one that calls for the fundamental transformation of our world. What is at stake in these tasks is well expressed by anthropologist and activist Brooke Schoepf: "Unless the underlying struggles of millions to survive in the midst of poverty, powerlessness, and hopelessness are addressed, and the meanings of AIDS understood in the context of gender relations, HIV will continue to spread."[69]

In embracing a pessimism of the intellect, a certain optimism of the spirit is permitted. To paraphrase Patricia Hill Collins: as surely as HIV may be linked to oppression, so too are the conditions of oppression inherently unstable.[70]

4 The Exotic and the Mundane

HUMAN IMMUNODEFICIENCY VIRUS
IN THE CARIBBEAN

Typhoid, typhus, smallpox,

measles, cholera and

influenza . . . each disease in its

turn sweeps across the map,

moving through time and over

space to give every epidemic a

history and a geography.

PETER GOULD, *1993*

For any understanding of the

relationship between culture and

science, the problem of causation

is critically important because it

reflects directly on the

fundamental moral issue of

responsibility for disease.

ALLAN BRANDT, *1997*

Statistics, goes the old saying, are a lot like prisoners: they'll say anything if you torture them long enough. Although most of this book is based on research conducted in Haiti and Peru, some of it derives from a critical rereading of others' work, with an eye toward elucidating the role of social inequalities in the distribution of disease and poor outcomes. My first real turn at such a rereading came fifteen years ago, shortly after the first cases of AIDS were identified in Haiti. It was then, I believe, that I set out on a new path, at least as far as scholarship is concerned. By "new path," I mean new for me; the trail was blazed by many others. And it was not a path that led away from a life-long fascination with the natural sciences but rather one that led toward social theory and, particularly, anthropology. Like so many students, I'd been exposed to the great decentering paradigms of modern thought. But it was the insistent, questioning stance of anthropology—the "uncomfortable science"—that helped me to understand my deepening intimacy with what seemed, fifteen years ago, a very exotic place.

Mind you, anthropology also tripped me up, leading me down many interpretive dead ends. I've already mentioned how ill prepared I was to understand the effects of political economy on both the health and the health care of the Haitian poor: training in anthropology had induced me to "misdiagnose" structural violence as cultural difference. But the discipline also led me, ultimately, both to a deep appreciation for the remarkable cultural institutions of a remarkable people and to a better understanding of just why it is that so many of us who "study down" are likely to conflate social inequality and cultural difference.

This conflation was a staple of early AIDS-related commentary, and this proved to be as true of professional discourses as popular ones. In May of 1983, I found myself sitting in a crowded amphitheater in a middle-class neighborhood in Port-au-Prince. It was hot, I remember, though many of the people in the room were wearing coats, as physicians do when they convene. The participants were sodden, but the atmosphere was electric, since the topic that day was AIDS, a newly described affliction in which Haiti seemed to play a curious and ill-defined role.

It took me a while to identify the prevailing emotion. The stuffy air was thick with *accusation*—not at all what I'd expected from the Association Médicale Haïtienne (AMH, the Haitian Medical Association), which had convened the meeting. I saw one U.S. physician taken to task for his "racist speculations" about Haitians per se being a risk group for AIDS. I saw him repent meekly, even though he, like so many others, would later publish even more outlandish speculations purporting to explain AIDS in Haiti, including the assertion that "magic ritual provides a means for transfer of blood and secretions from person to person. Women have been known to introduce menstrual blood into the food and drink of their partners to prevent them from 'straying.' Worshippers of Erzulie, a benign deity, engage in rituals during which the *houngan*, or priest, may engage in intercourse with other male worshippers."[1] The thought flickered across my mind that perhaps Haitians who believed that AIDS was a U.S. biological experiment gone wrong were not as paranoid as they might seem—or at least that their vivid imaginations were of a kind with accredited U.S. experts.

No wonder the Haitians were irritated. I sat in the back of the auditorium, spellbound, delighted, a little appalled. Here, clearly, was a topic worthy of attention. Green as I was, I could recognize exoticism when I saw it, and the raggedy epidemiology seemed "off" in a somehow predictable way. I sensed that powerful templates helped to generate certain discourses, even if I could not, at that time, identify either the boundaries of these discourses or the templates that generated them. I knew that this was a battle, that there were sides, lines drawn in the sand. I knew that science, cultures, and transnational inequalities were coming together in a volatile mix. And I had a sense that I was in the middle of it, although I said not a word from my seat.

Looking back, I think of this as the beginning of my commitment to critical scholarship. Quests for personal efficacy are silly in the midst of settings like Haiti, but there's probably something to be said for discovering one's own hobby horse, even if it is in no way different from other voices. Working through the problem of AIDS in Haiti, combing a diverse body of literature (epidemiology, clinical medicine, virology, social theory, the popular press, even fiction) for clues and confirmations, I found a perspective—which might be termed "biosocial" rather than the fuzzy, now New Age term "holistic"—that has since served me well. When linked to properly ethnographic work, which was to come next, critical epidemiology had the power to reveal a great deal about a novel infectious disease.

This critique is not just the editorial clean-up of the seminar room; rather, it has practical effects on preventive strategies and treatment efforts.

Living in a village in rural Haiti at the time that both AIDS and political violence arrived on the scene can't be called serendipitous, in the sense of a lucky coincidence, but it certainly was instructive. Primed by my experience among Port-au-Prince professionals, I once again found accusation to be the dominant theme. Local interpretations of AIDS often hinged on allegations of sorcery; from earlier ethnographies, I learned to regard them as a sign of dread and hatred and a mark of social inequality. But what, precisely, was the cause of all this acrimony? Ethnographic fieldwork helped to illuminate both the curiously accusatory tenor of public discussions of AIDS and the forces that structured them.

Then too, the disciplinary focus of anthropology on patterns of human community proved well suited to address a number of questions that perennially vex epidemiologists. Why, for example, was HIV so quick to penetrate the city, and by what routes would it reach the countryside? Anthropology provided a great deal of help in seeking to answer these questions. Fieldwork confirmed what I had learned from my teachers: as Arthur and Joan Kleinman point out, "Local cultural worlds stand between the force of large-scale social changes—for example, economic and political transformations—and their outcomes in survival, mortality, morbidity, suffering, and coping."[2] Social responses to the new disease, like the disease itself, linked Haiti's rural Central Plateau to the city of Port-au-Prince and, beyond that, to the United States. This was not simply a matter of physical geography or of political geography, but of moral geography: a "geography of blame."

In the United States, too, it was clear that AIDS was embedded in the framework of blame and accusation. As in Haiti, observers were concerned to assess guilt, what historian Allan Brandt terms "the moral valence of individual risk."[3] In both settings, this condition was tightly linked to social inequalities.

The AIDS pandemic's complicated "geography of blame" became the leitmotiv—and subtitle—of my first book. Years later, when Françoise Héritier was kind enough to write an introduction to the French translation of *AIDS and Accusation*, she remarked that, following Marcel Mauss, I had used accusation as a *fait social total*—a "total social fact."[4] That result was not really because my methods were particularly subtle. It just happened that blame was everywhere, and any particular act of blaming networked indefinitely, connecting village-level enmities with the international financial and political order. In a sense different from Mauss's, the totality of the social fact was given, not something toward which one had to work painstakingly. It is this organizing principle of condemnation that has defined the world's conceptual definition of AIDS, the clinical responses to it, and the mobilization of political and material resources to address it. When the skin of accusation is peeled away, a "global" structure is laid bare, entire.

The text that follows is based on an essay I began a decade ago. It has an additional relevance here, as a means of highlighting what has happened in the ensuing years. The social fault lines that I limned ten years ago guaranteed that HIV would spread rapidly from men to women, and from city to countryside. As the next chapters show, this has tragically all come to pass.

.   .   .   .   .

At about 6 A.M. on 26 June 1982, Solange Éliodor died in Miami's Jackson Memorial Hospital. The twenty-six-year-old Haitian refugee had spent her final year first on a rickety boat, which had reached the shores of Florida the previous July, and then in prison, as the reluctant ward of the U.S. Immigration and Naturalization Service (INS).

Although the INS had initially maintained otherwise, the Dade County medical examiner later denied that the young woman had shown any signs of tuberculosis—"She didn't have it. Period." Responding to an allegation raised by the director of the Haitian Refugee Center, the medical examiner also asserted that "there was no sign the woman suffered a blow to the head." Other Haitians interned in the Krome Avenue INS detention facility may have been dealt blows to the head, but Solange Éliodor was apparently not one of them.[5] Instead, the medical examiner's verdict was toxoplasmosis of the brain, a common parasitic infection that is usually held in check by immune defenses. The woman's death merited a headline in the 30 June edition of the *Miami Herald:* "Krome Camp Detainee Died from Infection Transmitted by Cats."

Her story—flight by boat from Haiti, INS detention, newspaper headlines, mistaken diagnoses of tuberculosis and official violence—is of a piece with a single, if complicated, narrative. Early in the AIDS pandemic, a number of Haitians, including Solange Éliodor, fell ill with opportunistic infections characteristic of the new syndrome. Some of the affected Haitians lived in urban Haiti; some had emigrated to the United States or Canada. Unlike most other patients then being diagnosed with AIDS in the United States, the Haitian immigrants denied homosexual activity or intravenous drug use. Most had never had a blood transfusion. AIDS among Haitians seemed to be, in the words of North American researchers, "a complete mystery."

In 1982, U.S. public health officials inferred that Haitians qua Haitians were in some way at risk for AIDS and suggested that unraveling "the Haiti connection" would lead researchers to the culprit. Typifying the melodramatic prose that came to characterize American commentary about Haiti and AIDS, one reporter termed the disease's incidence in Haitians "a clue from the grave, as though a zombie, leaving a trail of unwinding gauze bandages and rotting flesh, had come to the hospital's Grand Rounds to pronounce a curse."[6]

The Haitian cases and the subsequent risk-grouping spurred a wide range of theories purporting to explain the epidemiology and origins of AIDS. In December 1982, for example, a physician with the U.S. National Cancer Institute was widely quoted expressing officialdom's suspicion that "this may be an epidemic Haitian virus that was brought back to the homosexual population in the United States."[7] This theory, unbolstered by research, was echoed by other physicians and scientists investigating (or merely commenting on) AIDS.

In North America and Europe, other pundits linked AIDS in Haiti to "voodoo practices." Something that went on around ritual fires, went the supposition, triggered AIDS in cult adherents—a category presumed to include the quasi-totality of Haitians. In the October 1983 edition of the *Annals of Internal Medicine*, for example, physicians affiliated with the Massachusetts Institute of Technology related the details of a brief visit to Haiti and wrote, "It seems reasonable to consider voodoo practices a cause of the syndrome."[8]

Did existing knowledge of AIDS in Haiti make such a hypothesis reasonable? Had voodoo been associated previously with the transmission of other illnesses? Careful review of the scholarly literature on AIDS and on voodoo would have made it clear that the answer to both questions was no. The persistence of these theories represents, in fact, a systematic misreading of existing epidemiologic and ethnographic data. But the appeal of such a reading had been predicted long before AIDS was described: "Certain exotic words are charged with evocative power," wrote Alfred Métraux in 1959. "Voodoo is one. It usually conjures up visions of mysterious deaths, secret rites—or dark saturnalia celebrated by 'blood-maddened, sex-maddened, god-maddened' negroes."[9]

What gradually became known about the new syndrome in Haiti seemed to have far less impact on popular and professional AIDS discourse than did preexisting conceptions of the place. In other words, the link between AIDS and Haiti seemed to resonate with a North American folk model of Haitians. The outlines of such a model are suggested by a study of Haitians living in New York, which recalls the image Haitian immigrants found waiting for them in the United States of the 1970s: "Haitians were portrayed as ragged, wretched, and pathetic and were said to be illiterate, superstitious, disease-ridden and backward peasants."[10]

Haiti has long been depicted as a strange and hopelessly diseased polity remarkable chiefly for its extreme isolation from the rest of the civilized world. This erroneous depiction fuels the parallel process of "exoticization" by which Haiti is rendered weird.[11] A journalist writing in 1989 in *Vanity Fair*, for example, claimed that "Haiti is to this hemisphere what black holes are to outer space"; a U.S. news magazine described the country as "a bazaar of the bizarre."[12] Over the past fifteen years, the AIDS association has been incorporated into that folk model as another necessary referent.[13]

Although both the folk model about Haitians and the nature of AIDS-related discrimination against them could best be studied in North America, my interest in AIDS in Haiti mandated research on the island: HIV affected Haiti not only indirectly, through the prejudices of North American scientists, employers, landlords, and tourists, but also directly, through the ravages of a fatal malady. In 1983, when I first traveled to Haiti, the country was in the first years of its own substantial AIDS epidemic.

Although it cannot be shown that HIV was present in Haiti before the close of the 1970s, the country is now among those most gravely affected by AIDS. Haitian researchers have concluded (in the absence of uniform data gathering) that HIV-related disorders have become the leading cause of death among adults between the ages of 20 and 49. Indeed, the disease has spread beyond any neatly defined "risk groups" and now constitutes what epidemiologists call a "generalized epidemic," in which infection is prevalent from mother to child. At this writing, Haiti, Guyana, and Brazil stand alone among this hemisphere's nations as countries afflicted with generalized epidemics.[14]

How did HIV come to cause such devastation in such a short amount of time? In Chapter 2, I argued that models of disease emergence need to be dynamic, systemic, and critical, uncovering connections and patterns that are often obscured by conventional epidemiology and examining the role of social forces and inequalities. Such an approach is essential to understanding the emergence of AIDS in Haiti and throughout the Caribbean.

A CHRONOLOGY OF
THE AIDS/HIV EPIDEMIC IN HAITI

Most chroniclers of the AIDS pandemic agree that awareness of the new syndrome began to emerge in California in 1981. Alerted to the possibility of an epidemic, U.S. public health specialists reviewed available documentation and observed that unexpected clusterings of Kaposi's sarcoma and opportunistic infections had first been noted early in 1977. Shortly thereafter, Haitian physicians began to see similarly puzzling cases of immunosuppression.

What was likely the first AIDS-related case of Kaposi's sarcoma in Haiti was detected in June 1979, when dermatologist Bernard Liautaud diagnosed the disorder in a twenty-eight-year-old woman from a city in the western part of the country. She had been referred to the nation's university hospital for worsening lower-extremity edema and arrived with nodular and papular lesions covering her face, trunk, and extremities. Neither her demographic background nor her clinical presentation fit the standard description of patients with the sarcoma: before AIDS, Kaposi's was considered a rare and indolent malignancy seen largely in elderly men of Eastern European and Mediterranean descent. The cancer behaved quite differently in Dr. Liautaud's patient, in whom it was aggressive and fatal.

After diagnosing Kaposi's in a young Haitian man later that year, Liautaud posed the following question: was the cancer of long-standing and unappreciated importance in Haiti, or was it new to the country? A survey of colleagues and an examination of pathologic specimens from other institutions led him to conclude that Kaposi's sarcoma had been virtually unknown in Haiti. Liautaud and his co-workers reported their findings to an international medical conference held in Haiti in April 1982.[15]

Concurrent outbreaks of Kaposi's reported in California and New York, as well as an increasing incidence of unexplained opportunistic infections, lent force to the idea that these illnesses might somehow be related to an epidemic infectious agent.[16] Several such unexplained infections, first noted in February 1980, were also described at the 1982 conference. This evidence of immunosuppression was strikingly similar to what the North American medical literature now termed "AIDS." The conviction that something new and significant was afoot led to the formation of the Haitian Study Group on Kaposi's Sarcoma and Opportunistic Infections (GHESKIO) in May 1982. The study group included thirteen physicians and scientists, who would eventually treat hundreds of AIDS patients while conducting important clinical and epidemiologic research.

In May 1983, the AMH dedicated its annual conference to the subject of AIDS. Research presented there left little doubt that in urban Haiti, at least, a new state of immunodeficiency was striking increasing numbers of young adults, especially men. It was clear from the presentations of the Haitian physicians that they were convinced their patients were ill with AIDS as it had recently been defined by the CDC. During the period from 1979 to the 1983 AMH conference, twenty cases of Kaposi's sarcoma had been diagnosed, along with more than sixty otherwise unexplained opportunistic infections. Using CDC criteria, Haitian researchers and clinicians had diagnosed a total of sixty-one cases of AIDS between June 1979 and October 1982.[17]

Despite the obvious parallels suggesting a new, acquired, and epidemic immunosuppression in both Haiti and the United States, there were important disparities between the two epidemics. Researchers noted early on that a smaller proportion of Haitian AIDS patients had *Pneumocystis carinii* pneumonia, the most common opportunistic infection in North Americans with AIDS. *M. avium-intracellulare*, an infection common in North American AIDS patients, was rare in Haiti; although the Haitian patients did have mycobacterial infections, these infections were almost exclusively tuberculosis. In fact, tuberculosis was soon documented to be the most common presenting illness among Haitians with AIDS.[18] Disparities in time of survival after diagnosis also existed: whereas mean survival after diagnosis was usually greater than a year in the United States at that time, survival was less than six months in the majority of Haitian patients, and none had lived more than twenty-four months after diagnosis. Despite these differences, most of those attending the AMH conference were confident that the Haitian and North American epidemics were caused by the same organism.

The research presented in 1983 offered important epidemiologic clues to Haiti's "role" in the larger pandemic. Although the Haitian researchers had initially concluded that "no segment of Haitian society appears to be free of opportunistic infections or Kaposi's sarcoma,"[19] AIDS did not strike randomly. Pape and co-workers found that 74 percent of all men with opportunistic infections lived in greater Port-au-Prince, home to approximately 20 percent of all Haitians. Curiously, 33 percent of all AIDS patients lived in a single suburb, Carrefour. This finding was underlined because several of the patients interviewed by Pape and other researchers reported that they had been remunerated for sex: "The prevalence rate of men with opportunistic infections in Carrefour was significantly higher than that of men in Port-au-Prince ($p < 0.001$ by the chi-square test). This is of interest since Carrefour, a suburb of Port-au-Prince, is recognized as the principal center of male and female prostitution in Haiti."[20]

These investigations also revealed that only 13 percent of the remaining men with opportunistic infections were from elsewhere in the country. An equal number had been living outside Haiti: two patients in New York, one in Miami, one in Belgium, and one in the Bahamas. Five of twenty-one men interviewed by a GHESKIO clinician stated that they were bisexual, as did two patients referred by other Haitian physicians.[21] Of these seven men, all had lived in either Carrefour (four) or the United States (three). Three of them admitted having sexual contact with North American men in both Haiti and the United States, and two others had had sexual contact with Haitian men known to have opportunistic infections.[22]

Furthermore, fully half of the allegedly heterosexual men had either lived or traveled outside Haiti. Although the U.S. popular press was hastily concocting a "history" of AIDS that emphasized supposed connections between Africa and Haiti, none of the Haitians ill with the new syndrome had ever been to Africa.[23] All denied sexual contact with persons from that continent; most, in fact, had never met an African. But 10–15 percent of these patients *had* traveled to North America or Europe in the five years preceding the onset of their illness, and several more admitted sexual contact with tourists.[24] The GHESKIO team offered other important demographic data: 71 percent of these patients also suffered from a sexually transmitted disease, and 20 percent had histories of blood transfusion.

Also in 1983, members of the GHESKIO team surveyed the twenty-one dermatologists and pathologists known to be practicing in Haiti, questioning them about their experiences in diagnosing and treating Kaposi's sarcoma. A simultaneous review of more than one thousand biopsy specimens from the Hôpital Albert Schweitzer revealed that only one case of the disease had been diagnosed in Haiti before the recent outbreak—in 1972—and that one had afflicted an older man, arousing no suspicions of immunodeficiency. GHESKIO concluded, as had Liautaud, that the new cases of Kaposi's represented an epidemic of recent onset.

Thus, given the latest research, those who attended the AMH conference could draw several important conclusions:

Haitians with AIDS were then largely men, though increasing numbers of women were reporting to the GHESKIO clinic.

The epicenter of the Haitian epidemic was in the city of Carrefour, home to Haiti's largest red-light district.

A large percentage of the early cases were linked to homosexual contact, some of it with North Americans and involving the exchange of money.

The association with a history of blood transfusions seemed to be greater in Haiti than in the United States.

Although the opportunistic infections often differed from those seen in North Americans with AIDS, the Haitian epidemic was strikingly similar to that in the United States.

The microbial agent that led to AIDS was probably new to Haiti, as no one could report cases predating the much larger North American epidemic.

Subsequent research, based on the development of assays for antibodies to the newly discovered HIV, also suggested that the virus was new to Haiti. Blood samples drawn from adults during a 1977–79 outbreak of dengue fever were later tested for antibodies to HIV; none of the 191 samples tested contained these antibodies.[25] The sole suggestion that AIDS existed in Haiti prior to 1979, when Dr. Liautaud noted two cases of Kaposi's sarcoma, were the autopsy records of a previously healthy twenty-year-old man who had died in 1978, two weeks after the sudden onset of generalized seizures. Postmortem studies at the Hôpital Albert Schweitzer revealed cerebral toxoplasmosis, an opportunistic infection common in persons with AIDS. "These data and studies from Africa," concluded Johnson and Pape, "are consistent with the hypothesis that HIV most likely originated in that continent, came to the United States and Europe, and subsequently was introduced into Haiti by either tourists or returning Haitians."[26]

The research conducted in the first years of the Haitian epidemic spoke to many of the questions raised as speculations by North American researchers and journalists. Was AIDS caused by "an epidemic Haitian virus"? Had overworked or undertrained Haitian physicians merely overlooked the disease, as some seemed to imply?[27] Was AIDS caused by an African virus brought to the United States by Haitians?[28] Was the disease caused by an organism endemic among isolated, superstitious peasants who transmitted it through some bizarre voodoo practice? Some of the Haitian researchers felt, understandably, that their research, which had been published in refereed, international journals, had answered these questions. And yet their contributions—in wide circulation by 1983—did little to dampen the apparently self-sustaining "exotic theories" that continued to influence popular opinion in the United States and elsewhere.

In 1986, for example, the *Journal of the American Medical Association* published a consideration of these theories under the fey title "Night of the Living Dead." Its author asks, "Do necromantic zombiists transmit

HTLV-III/LAV during voodooistic rituals?" Tellingly, he cites as his source not the (by then) substantial scientific literature on AIDS in Haiti, but the U.S. daily press:

> Even now, many Haitians are voodoo *serviteurs* and partake in its rituals (*New York Times*, May 15, 1985, pp. 1, 6). (Some are also members of secret societies such as Bizango or "impure" sects, called "cabrit thomazo," which are suspected to use human blood itself in sacrificial worship.) As the HTLV-III/LAV virus is known to be stable in aqueous solution at room temperature for at least a week, lay Haitian voodooists may be unsuspectingly infected with AIDS by ingestion, inhalation, or dermal contact with contaminated ritual substances, as well as by sexual activity.[29]

Social scientists were also seduced by the call of the wild. In a heroic effort to accommodate all of the exotic furbelows available in the American folk model of Haitians, Moore and LeBaron depict the following scene: "In frenzied trance, the priest lets blood: mammal's [*sic*] throats are cut; typically, chicken's [*sic*] heads are torn off their necks. The priest bites out the chicken's tongue with his teeth and may suck on the bloody stump of the neck." These sacrificial offerings, "infected with one of the Type C oncogenic retroviruses, which is [*sic*] closely related to HTLV," are "repeatedly [*sic*] sacrificed in voodoo ceremonies, and their blood is directly ingested by priests and their assistants." They complete the model with the assertion that "many voodoo priests are homosexual men" who are "certainly in a position to satisfy their sexual desires, especially in urban areas."[30]

Similarly lurid scenarios were promoted in the popular press, which offered images of voodoo, animal (and even human) sacrifice, and boatloads of disease-ridden refugees. Such articles had a considerable impact on Haiti, which once counted tourism as an important source of foreign currency. "Already suffering from an image problem, Haiti has been made an international pariah by AIDS," concluded one 1983 report. "Boycotted by tourists and investors, it has lost millions of dollars and hundreds of jobs at a time when half the work force is jobless. Even exports are being shunned by some."[31]

The AIDS association affected Haitians everywhere, especially those living in the United States and Canada. Many of the million or so Haitians living in North America complained that speculation about a

Haitian origin of AIDS had led to a wave of anti-Haitian discrimination. Gilman was not exaggerating when he suggested in 1988 that "to be a Haitian and living in New York City meant that you were perceived as an AIDS 'carrier.'"[32]

HIV IN HAITI:
THE DIMENSIONS OF THE PROBLEM

How far has HIV spread in Haiti? Given the natural history of HIV infection, this question is best answered not by the epidemiology of AIDS but through the study of HIV seroprevalence in asymptomatic populations. During 1986 and 1987, blood samples from several cohorts of healthy adults were analyzed for antibodies to HIV; Table 1 summarizes the results. In a group of individuals who worked in hotels catering to tourists, for example, HIV seroprevalence was 12 percent. Among urban factory workers, the rate was 5 percent. In both series, rates were comparable for men and women, which suggested that the high attack rate in Haitian men would slowly give way to a pattern like that seen in parts of Central Africa, where men and women are equally affected.

In a group of 502 mothers of children hospitalized with diarrhea and in a group of 190 urban adults with a comparable socioeconomic background, seroprevalence rates were 12 percent and 13 percent, respectively. All of 57 medical workers involved in the care of AIDS patients were seronegative, corroborating claims that HIV was not easily spread by nonsexual contact. Overall, GHESKIO researchers found that approximately 9 percent of 912 healthy urban adults (in the categories listed in Table 1, excluding pregnant women) were HIV-seropositive.[33]

The highest seroprevalence rates during these years were reported among female Haitian sex workers (reaching 41.9 percent by 1989),[34] underlining for some their role in the transmission of HIV. But few observed that such high rates among sex workers might simply reflect occupational risk—an increased likelihood of coming into contact with a seropositive man—and proved little about their role in propagating the virus.

Other investigations, focusing on Cité Soleil (the vast slum north of Port-au-Prince) and Gonaïves, Haiti's third largest city, confirmed the

Table 1.   HIV Seroprevalence Among Healthy Adults in Haiti, 1986–87

	N	Mean Age (Years)	% HIV+
Urban Haiti (Port-au-Prince area)			
Hotel workers	25	45	12.0
Factory workers	84	30	5.0
Mothers of sick infants	502	29	12.0
Medical workers	57	40	0.0
Other adults:			
High socioeconomic status	54	35	0.0
Low socioeconomic status	190	33	13.0
Pregnant women (1986)	1,240	29	8.4
Total	2,152	27	9.0
Rural Haiti (outside Port-au-Prince)			
Mothers of sick infants	97	25	3.0
Pregnant women	117	27	3.0
Blood donors	245	32	4.0
Other adults (rural village)	191	29	1.0
Total	650	30	3.0

SOURCE: Pape and Johnson 1988.

impression of high rates of HIV infection in Haiti's urban areas, especially among the poor.[35] In compiling available data from these early seroprevalence studies of ostensibly healthy urban adults, one is led to conclude that, by the late eighties, a substantial fraction of urban Haitians had been infected with HIV. By contrast, the situation in rural areas was considerably less acute. As of 1986, seroprevalence averaged 2 percent in unspecified "rural areas." Five years later, that figure was 5 percent—half that of the cities.[36]

What of seroprevalence among children? The GHESKIO team studied three groups of children: the offspring of a parent with AIDS; children hospitalized for diarrheal disease in Port-au-Prince's public hospital; and healthy, age-matched controls from the same neighborhoods as the hospitalized children. Their findings (summarized in Table 2) suggest that pediatric infection with HIV was perinatal: rates are highest in the children of parents with AIDS—especially in children less than one year old, when maternal antibodies may give false-positive antibody tests. Furthermore, the children of a seropositive father and a seronegative mother were all seronegative, which also strongly suggests vertical (mother-to-infant) transmission.

Disturbingly, the overall rates of seropositivity were identical for the children of parents with AIDS and the children hospitalized with diarrhea: 6.5 percent in both groups—three times greater than in controls. This finding suggests that by the late eighties, in Port-au-Prince at least, pediatric infection with HIV was leading to significant morbidity (through diarrheal disease and other infections) well before HIV infection was diagnosed. The relative contribution of HIV to mortality versus that of other pathogens was of course difficult to assess, since infant death due to diarrheal disease has long been commonplace in Haiti. Nevertheless, one recent study estimates that AIDS is responsible for as many as 20 percent of Haiti's infant deaths.[37]

In summary, then, large numbers of urban Haitians, particularly those living in poverty, had already been infected with HIV by the time the first studies were conducted. The speed of spread has been great indeed: sera stored in 1977–79 were found to be free of HIV. Since then, the only tested groups without a single seropositive adult have involved small cohorts

Table 2. Prevalence of HIV Antibodies Among Haitian Children, 1985–86

AGE (YEARS)	Children of a Parent with AIDS		Children Hospitalized with Diarrhea		Age-Matched Controls	
	N	% HIV+	N	% HIV+	N	% HIV+
Younger than 1	96	28	260	8	119	3
1–4	252	3	52	2	41	2
4–10	218	2	5	0	7	0
Older than 10	43	0	0	—	0	—
Total	609	6.5	317	6.5	167	2

SOURCE: Pape and Johnson 1988.

of rural Haitians. The exceptions have been a group of health care workers and a series of adults from relatively privileged backgrounds, which leads us to question the assertion, made early in the epidemic, that Haitians from all economic backgrounds were equally vulnerable to AIDS. As Pape and Johnson came to conclude, "Collectively, these data indicate that HIV infection is widespread and more prevalent in urban areas and in lower socioeconomic groups."[38]

Studies of disease prevalence are merely descriptive. Taken alone, such surveys can never really explain why an epidemic takes the shape it does. Taken alone, conventional epidemiology is often unable to discern either the path along which an outbreak will move or the rate at which it will progress. Epidemiology is also ill placed to interpret social responses to epidemic disease, even though these responses can profoundly affect the force of an epidemic. Nor can conventional anthropology provide illumination. It may ask what features of Haitian culture were responsible for the rapid progress made by AIDS, but it too often ignores the overarching context, the global structures of power and meaning.

To understand the questions to be asked, broader perspectives are necessary: we must cast the analytic net much more widely than either discipline is typically prepared to do. Since AIDS in the Caribbean is a transnational pandemic shaped by conditions and structures long in place, a critical epidemiology will necessarily be historically deep and geographically broad. It is to such an effort that we now turn.

THE "AMERICAN PHASE" OF THE URBAN EPIDEMIC

In Haiti, the epidemiologic questions were the same as those posed in other settings facing the AIDS epidemic: Who is at risk for acquiring HIV infection? How is the virus transmitted? What specific behaviors or preexisting conditions are associated with seropositivity or HIV disease? How extensively has the virus spread among groups engaging in high-risk behaviors or facing high-risk conditions? Preliminary research conducted among Haitian Americans with AIDS had identified none of the "accepted risk factors"—that is, homosexuality, bisexuality, injection drug use, blood transfusion, or hemophilia—in the vast majority of Haitians living with AIDS in the United States. ("Accepted risk factors" were those identified by the CDC in research among North Americans with AIDS.) In Haiti, however, risk factors often were identified, although the specific factors deemed important have changed over the years.

Responding to calls for careful research that would answer questions raised at the 1983 AMH conference, the GHESKIO investigators began to gather more information from new patients in an effort to identify activities or events that could have led to HIV exposure. Unfortunately, questions pertaining to sexual history were not standardized, and little effort was made to gather ethnographic data that might complement information garnered in the clinic. Nevertheless, with a standardized questionnaire, the GHESKIO physicians were able to identify "accepted risk factors" in a majority of cases. Table 3 presents data from an initial group of thirty-four patients interviewed by the researchers.

The most striking revelation, in light of reports about Haitians with AIDS in the United States, was that fully half of the male patients interviewed in Port-au-Prince had a history of sexual relations with men. None of them, however, was exclusively homosexual: "The fact that all the male AIDS patients who have had sex with men are bisexual would also provide greater opportunity for heterosexual transmission of AIDS in Haiti. This also may contribute to the finding that 21 percent of our

Table 3. Risk Factors for HIV Infection in Thirty-Four Patients

	Males (N = 26)	Females (N = 8)
Bisexual contact	13 (50%)	0
Blood transfusion	3 (11%)	4 (50%)
IV drug use	1 (4%)	0
Spouse with AIDS	0	1 (12%)
None apparent	9 (35%)	3 (38%)

SOURCE: Pape, Liautaud, Thomas, Mathurin, St Amand, Boncy, Péan, Pamphile, Laroche, and Johnson 1986.

Haitian AIDS patients are women, as compared with only 7 percent in the United States."[39] Pape and his team further reported that half of the female patients had received a blood transfusion in the five years prior to the onset of symptoms, observing that Haitian women are more likely to receive blood—often in the course of childbirth—than are Haitian men.

Did these data, which clearly demonstrated "accepted risk factors" in a majority of those studied, suggest that transmission in Haiti was occurring through the same mechanisms as those elucidated in the United States? To determine the significance of presumed risk factors, the researchers initiated a case-control study with an ambitious research design: "Each of the most recent 36 AIDS patients was asked to provide three 'healthy' persons to serve as controls. The controls included a sibling of the same sex closest in age to the patient, a friend of the same sex who shared social activities, and a current or recent sexual partner."[40]

Pape's patients complied by recruiting twenty siblings, twenty friends, and twenty sexual partners. Interestingly, all the patients—including the men who had histories of homosexual contact—provided "current or recent sexual partners" of the opposite sex. Among the risk factors studied were transfusion, the use of parenteral medications (intramuscular injections of, for instance, vitamins or antibiotics), and frequency of "heterosexual promiscuity" (arbitrarily defined as greater than twelve different partners during the six months preceding onset of their illness).

Based on this case-control study, the GHESKIO team initially concluded that "accepted risk factors" were present in more than two-thirds of the Haitians diagnosed with AIDS. The fact that risk profiles among the first Haitian AIDS patients were similar to those reported in the United States reflects the U.S. origins of the Haitian epidemic. In fact, the initial phase of the Haitian epidemic might best be thought of as the "American phase." Given these similar risk profiles, why did only 6 percent of Haitians with AIDS in the United States report histories of bisexuality and only 1 percent report histories of injection drug use?[41] As Pape and co-workers later observed, "The disparity in the data from the United States and Haiti may be attributable, in part, to a greater willingness of Haitians to provide reliable responses to personal questions in their native country and language."[42]

With homosexual contact already a documented risk factor, researchers hypothesized that an additional factor might be the number of opposite-sex partners. The female siblings and friends in the case-control study had a mean of one sex partner per year during the five years preceding the study and an HIV seroprevalence rate of 9 percent. Male siblings and friends, in contrast, had six or seven opposite-sex partners annually and a seroprevalence rate of 22 percent. Although the numbers are small and the sample not random, these figures corroborate the initial impressions of those studying the epidemic: urban Haitian men were noted to have significantly more sexual partners than did urban women, suggesting a greater role for men in the spread of HIV.

THE FEMINIZATION OF THE URBAN EPIDEMIC

Biology and sociology come together to further accentuate men's role in the propagation of HIV when a sexually transmitted pathogen is more readily passed from male to female.[43] There are several reasons to believe that HIV is more efficiently transmitted from men to women than vice versa. Some are intuitive: HIV is concentrated in seminal fluid but often difficult to isolate in vaginal secretions. In addition, in comparing male ejaculate to vaginal secretions, inoculum size of course differs by several orders of magnitude. Data from the United States also suggest that HIV is inefficiently transmitted from women to men: in two studies of women whose date of transfusion-associated HIV infection could be ascertained, from 0 to 7 percent of their spouses or regular sexual partners showed evidence of HIV infection.[44]

Although rates of HIV transmission from women to men in Haiti were higher than those documented in the United States, the most efficient female transmitters had concurrent sexually transmitted infections.[45] The data from Haiti do not offer strong support for efficient female-to-male transmission in the absence of ulcerative lesions caused by a concurrent sexually transmitted disease. Lorna McBarnett has rightly termed HIV a "biologically sexist" microbe.[46] Still, female-to-male transmission is by no means trivial: if bisexuality is decreasingly common and yet HIV seropositivity continues to increase among men, women are necessarily a source as well as a "sink" for infection.[47]

By the mid-1980s, the patterns that had emerged in GHESKIO's first case-control cohort seemed to be shifting, and these shifts in the Haitian epidemic were tied in important ways both to gender inequality and to an intrinsically sexist pathogen. In addition to reports of changing clinical features,[48] researchers noted striking shifts in the sex distribution of persons with AIDS. An overwhelming majority of the early patients had been men, but the percentage of women among the GHESKIO patients was increasing with each passing year (see Table 4).

As sex differences in the incidence of AIDS continued to diminish, more and more patients were also denying that their histories included "accepted risk factors." Such risk factors had been found in only 20 percent of the first Haitian cohort (before 1983) because, it was hypothesized, researchers had not used a standardized approach to these questions. In a second cohort (1983–84), risk factors could be identified in a majority of patients. In contrast, only 11 percent of the 170 male and female AIDS patients who presented in or after 1986 reported bisexuality, blood transfusions, or injection drug use. AIDS was becoming "generalized."

With the passage of time, then, it became increasingly clear that HIV was heterosexually transmitted, especially from men to women. By 1988, heterosexual transmission was presumed for the 16 percent of patients who were female sex workers as well as for those who had a spouse with AIDS. It was the probable source of infection in the patients who denied all other "accepted risk factors"; by 1986, as Table 5 suggests, these patients represented more than 70 percent of Haitian AIDS cases. Cases associated with perinatal transmission were also increasing at a rate greater

Table 4.   Sex Distribution of Patients
with AIDS in Urban Haiti

	N (Female/All)	% Females
1979–82	10/65	15
1983–85	86/319	27
1986–88	144/458	31
1989–91	329/764	43

SOURCE: Marie-Marcelle Deschamps, personal communication to the author.

Table 5. Risk Factors in 559 Haitian AIDS Patients

	1983	1984	1985	1986	1987	All
	(N = 38)	(N = 104)	(N = 132)	(N = 185)	(N = 100)	(N = 559)
Bisexual contact	50%	27%	8%	4%	1%	13%
Blood transfusion	23%	12%	8%	7%	10%	10%
IV drug use	1%	1%	1%	0	1%	1%
Heterosexual contact	5%	6%	14%	16%	15%	13%
Undetermined	21%	54%	69%	73%	73%	64%

SOURCE: Pape and Johnson 1988.

than that of the epidemic in general. Additional evidence for heterosexual transmission of HIV was the rising seroprevalence among a cohort of 139 commercial sex workers: 49 percent in 1985, and 66 percent in 1986.[49] In Haiti, AIDS was afflicting increasing numbers of women, and especially poor women.

How, then, did the Haitian AIDS epidemic change in the course of its first decade? We can discern an "American phase" of the Haitian epidemic, in which risk factors for HIV seemed to reflect those identified in the United States. A second phase of feminization followed, as HIV disease became, in urban Haiti, "just another STD." The GHESKIO clinic has seen a marked decrease in the relative number of Haitians with AIDS who report a history of transfusion or same-sex contact.[50] There have been no recent cases with histories of sexual contact with North Americans. A third phase of the Haitian epidemic is now under way, as complex webs of commerce and kinship move HIV into rural Haiti; this ruralization is the subject of the next chapter. First, however, it is necessary to define the broader social forces that placed Haiti and other Caribbean nations at risk for a transnational epidemic.

AIDS IN THE CARIBBEAN: THE "WEST ATLANTIC PANDEMIC"

The history of the Haitian AIDS epidemic is brief and devastating. Less than three decades ago, HIV may not have been present in the country. Now, complications of HIV infection are among the leading causes of death in urban and rural Haiti. How have other Caribbean islands been affected? Is Haiti, as some believe, an AIDS-ridden pocket in an otherwise low-prevalence region?[51] Answering these questions is no mean task, as Pape and Johnson suggest:

> First, in many countries there is no registry system for AIDS and it was only in 1984 that most nations started reporting cases to [the Pan American Health Organization]. Secondly, the widely used CDC case definition for AIDS is inappropriate for defining tropical AIDS and requires sophisticated laboratory support that is not readily available in most countries.

In our experience in Haiti, the new [1987] CDC case definition for AIDS, which relies more on HIV testing and clinical presentation, should increase the actual number of reported cases by at least 30 per cent.[52]

Given these caveats, what do we know about the nature of the Caribbean pandemic? All of what are known as the "Caribbean basin countries" have reported AIDS cases to the Pan American Health Organization (PAHO). Among the islands, Haiti, the Dominican Republic, Trinidad and Tobago, and the Bahamas together accounted for 82 percent of all cases reported to PAHO between the recognized onset of the epidemic and September 1987. As of that date, Haiti had reported the largest number of cases in the Caribbean region—which apparently lent credence to the widely shared belief that Haitians were somehow uniquely susceptible to AIDS. When the number of cases was standardized to reflect per capita caseload, however, the uniqueness of Haiti disappeared: Haiti's attack rate was then actually lower than that of several of its regional neighbors.[53]

During the twelve months preceding September 1987, the number of reported Caribbean cases doubled. The largest rates of increase were in Barbados, Jamaica, Martinique, Guadeloupe, French Guyana, the U.S. Virgin Islands, and Grenada. In the Dominican Republic, the epidemic continued to spread: although no cases were reported before 1983, health workers documented 62 in the subsequent two years. From there, rates of infection rose rapidly, more than doubling between 1987 and 1989.[54] By the end of 1989, 1202 AIDS cases had been reported to the Ministry of Health, 43 percent of them during that year alone.[55]

What was the nature of HIV transmission in these countries? Using World Health Organization terminology, many public health specialists spoke of the entire Caribbean basin as demonstrating "Pattern II" transmission, which differs from Pattern I "in that heterosexual intercourse has been the dominant mode of HIV transmission *from the start*. . . . Homosexuality generally plays a minor role in this pattern."[56]

Reviewing the data from Haiti, however, suggests that the WHO terminology obscured more than it illuminated about the spread of HIV in that country. First, although "the start" was never fully documented, it seems clear that same-sex relations between men played a crucial role in the Haitian epidemic. Second, the WHO scheme underlines similarities between Haiti and Africa, a comparison that tends to draw attention away from the history of the Caribbean pandemic, which is, causally speaking, much more intimately related to the North American epidemic. Third, the WHO scheme is static, whereas the Haitian epidemic has been rapidly changing. Data from other Caribbean countries indicate that the WHO terminology is equally inappropriate there and that the patterns seen in Haiti are suggestive of what has occurred in other countries in the region.[57]

Table 6 suggests that transnational homosexual contact has also played an important role in other Caribbean islands. But even here, finer distinctions may be drawn. "For these homosexuals," note Pape and Johnson in reference to gay men in Jamaica, the Dominican Republic, and Trinidad, "sexual contact with American homosexuals rather than promiscuity per se appeared to be associated with increased risk of infection."[58]

What research allows such a conclusion? In an important study of Trinidad, which has one of the highest attack rates in the Americas, Bartholemew and co-workers compared the epidemiologic correlates of infection with two retroviruses, HTLV-1 and HIV.[59] Infection with the former virus, thought to be long endemic in the Caribbean, was significantly associated with age, African descent, number of lifetime sexual partners, and "duration of homosexuality"—that is, length of time as a sexually ac-

Table 6. HIV Seroprevalence in Caribbean Homosexuals and Bisexuals

	Jamaica, 1986		Dominican Republic, 1985		Trinidad[a]	
	N	% HIV+	N	% HIV+	N	% HIV+
Homosexual/						
Bisexual	125	10	46	17	106	40
Controls	4,000	0	306	2.6	983	0.2

SOURCE: Pape and Johnson 1988.

[a]For Trinidad, information about the control group was gathered in 1982; figures for the homosexual/bisexual group are from 1983–84.

tive gay man. In sharp contrast, "age and race were not associated with HIV seropositivity. The major risk factor for HIV seropositivity was homosexual contact with a partner from a foreign country, primarily the United States. Duration of homosexuality and number of lifetime partners were not significantly associated with HIV seropositivity."[60]

The same risk factor was documented in Colombia, also a Caribbean basin country. In Bogota, Merino and co-workers observed that "significant behavioral risk factors for HIV-1 seropositivity among this sample of Colombian homosexual men included receptive anal intercourse and, for the subgroup reporting receptive roles, contact with foreign visitors."[61] The Haitian experience suggested that Trinidad and Colombia could expect the relative significance of sexual contact with a North American gay man to decrease, as other risk factors—most notably, high numbers of partners—became preeminent. This has, in fact, come to pass.

A similar risk factor was also hypothesized for the Dominican Republic, where Haitians, long despised in this neighboring country, have come under even heavier fire as "AIDS carriers." And yet studies revealed high seroprevalence rates among homosexual/bisexual male prostitutes living in the tourist areas of the country—in 1986, 10 percent in Santiago and 19 percent in Puerto Plata—strongly suggesting that "tourists, and not Haitians, were the most likely source of virus transmission to Dominicans, because contact occurs frequently between tourists (e.g., male homosexuals) and Dominicans but rarely between Haitians and Dominicans."[62]

Further, it seems that the epidemiology of HIV in the Dominican Republic may resemble that in Haiti to an even greater extent than did the Trinidadian epidemiology. Koenig and co-workers underline the role of economically driven prostitution among young Dominican men who identify themselves as heterosexual: "Persons who engage in homosexual acts only to earn money usually consider themselves heterosexual. This situation, public health workers have indicated, is particularly prevalent in the tourist areas with young adolescents. It could explain our finding of three positive serum samples in schoolchildren from Santo Domingo."[63]

Later research in the Puerta Plata area suggests that, although homosexual prostitution has diminished, another form of sexual exchange fostered by economic inequity continues to flourish. García and co-workers have studied the "beach boys" who work the area's tourist hotels:

> Beach boys are charming, friendly young heterosexual males who provide escort service to women tourists, most of whom are 30 years old or more. The beach boys are known locally as "Sanky Panky"—a corruption of the term "hanky panky." Because these men have contact with tourists from different countries and continents, they are often skilled, if not fluent, in English, French, German, and Italian.[64]

Although these contacts are termed "brief holiday romances," the escort service typically involves monetary compensation. Qualitative research allows García to conclude that "beach boys have multiple sexual partners and ply their trade in an area where the prevalence of AIDS is among the highest in the country."[65]

Epidemiologic reports from other parts of the Caribbean suggest a similar history for other growing island epidemics. Composite data from Surinam and what has been termed the "English-speaking Caribbean," which includes twenty island nations, show that while 100 percent of those diagnosed with AIDS in 1983 were homosexual or bisexual, the relative significance of same-sex contact as a risk factor for AIDS plunged to 30 percent over the next five years. The number of AIDS cases related to blood transfusions remained low, at less than 5 percent, and pediatric AIDS continued to account for less than 10 percent of diagnosed cases. Cases among those claiming to be exclusively heterosexual and without a history of transfusion or intravenous drug use soared, from less than 10 percent before 1985 to 60 percent in 1988. The male-to-female ratio has declined each year, as more and more women fall ill with AIDS.[66] These trends imply that the percentage of pediatric cases will also climb.[67]

Taken together, Caribbean-wide data suggest that many of the forces that helped to shape the Haitian epidemic have been important throughout the region. The most important of these forces have been economically driven and historically given: sufficient data now exist to support the assertion that economically driven male prostitution, catering to a North American clientele, played a major role in the introduction of HIV to Haiti. Why might Haiti have been particularly vulnerable to such commodification of sexuality? It is almost a cliché, now, to note that Haiti is "the poorest country in the hemisphere." In a country as poor as Haiti, AIDS might be thought of as an occupational hazard for workers in the tourist industry. A similar observation could be made concerning several other Caribbean nations.

Tourists' attitudes toward Haiti throughout the earlier half of this century are nicely summarized by Carpenter, whose Anglo-American guidebook to the Caribbean describes Haiti as "a deplorable and almost unbelievable mixture of barbaric customs and African traditions."[68] Later, in a slightly different era, Haiti's "exoticism" could be peddled as an attraction.[69] Tourism truly began in 1949, when Port-au-Prince celebrated its two hundredth birthday with the inauguration of the "Cité de l'Exposition," a long stretch of modern buildings built on the reclaimed swampy waterfront of the capital. The country counted some 20,000 visitors that year, and slightly fewer in 1950 and 1951. During the next few years, however, approximately 250,000 tourists would spend an average of three days and $105 in Haiti—in the aggregate, bringing in approximately 25 percent of Haiti's foreign currency.[70]

There was every sign that the gains in tourism would be steady, but political instability in 1957, followed by the tyrannical rule of François Duvalier, led North American tourists to avoid Haiti for several years.[71] This was the case even though a number of casinos relocated to Haiti from Cuba after the overthrow of the Batista dictatorship. After he had silenced domestic opposition, Duvalier attempted to court tourists and their dollars in the late 1960s. In the same speech in which he welcomed U.S. Vice President Nelson Rockefeller to Haiti and promoted the country as an ideal site for U.S. assembly plants, Duvalier père suggested that "Haiti could be a great land of relaxation for the American middle class—it is close, beautiful, and politically stable."[72]

By 1970, the annual number of visitors was close to 100,000; not counting brief layovers and "afternoon dockings," the annual tally had risen to 143,538 by 1979. Club Méditerranée opened its doors the following year.[73] Tourism, it was predicted, would soon supplant coffee and the offshore assembly plants as the capital's chief source of foreign exchange. But the effects of the "AIDS scare" were dramatic and prompt: the Haitian Bureau of Tourism estimated that tourism declined from 75,000 visitors in the winter of 1981–82 to under 10,000 the following year. In 1983–84, during the season following the risk-grouping and spate of articles in the popular press, even fewer tourists came to Haiti. Six hotels folded, and as many more declared themselves on the edge of bankruptcy. Several hotel owners were rumored to be planning a lawsuit against the CDC.

Although the lawsuit seemed ridiculous to most non-Haitian commentators, the probable effects of the CDC classification were likely to have been apparent to some in the agency before the March 1983 announcement of the risk-grouping. Requesting anonymity, one public health officer made the following observations, cited in a front-page story in the *New York Times*: "It's a working definition. If there turned out to be a large national or ethnic group, you would single that group out. But when you translate a working definition to a small, poverty-struck [*sic*] country like Haiti, it is devastating. It destroys one of their main cash industries—tourism."[74] Of course, fluctuations in tourism and trade may be attributed to many factors, but there was little doubt in Haiti as to the cause of the collapse: Haiti had been accused of "starting the AIDS epidemic." As Abbott observed, "AIDS stamped Haiti's international image as political repression and intense poverty never had."[75]

Those earlier years in which tourism and poverty were both on the rise had brought something of lasting significance to Haiti, however: institutionalized prostitution. As one Haitian physician put it, "This country had—as far as promiscuity was concerned—replaced Cuba after 1959."[76] And as Haiti became poorer, both men's and women's bodies became cheaper. Although there were no quantitative studies of Haitian urban prostitution, it was clear that a substantial sector of the trade catered to tourists, and especially to North Americans. And some portion of the tourist industry catered specifically to a gay clientele, as Greco described in 1983:

> During the past five years Haiti, especially Port-au-Prince, has become a very popular holiday resort for Americans who are homosexual. There are also Haitians who are homosexual, and homosexual prostitution is becoming increasingly common. . . . For the young Haitian male between the ages of 15 and 30 there is no likelihood of escaping the despair that abounds in Port-au-Prince. As elsewhere, those with money can purchase whatever they want.[77]

Although not all gay sex was prostitution, the deepening poverty of Haiti helped to ensure that social inequalities played an inordinate role even in "voluntary" same-sex relations: "With the help of money," writes d'Adesky, "what existed as gay life in Haiti in the '60s and '70s flowed like a dream." In a report recently published in *The Advocate*, d'Adesky writes of "hotels that catered to a gay clientele," of "discreet fucking rooms" in tourist hotels, and of slum houses that "would be emptied for a price and arrangements made." She cites a North American participant in Haiti's "once-flourishing gay subculture":

> "There was a gay life that was very gala and that involved various sectors of society," said AIDS activist Stephen Machon, a former resident of Haiti who saw the tail end of what some call Haiti's gay golden period. "There would be the gay guys and the working boys and the tourists, of course, and the parties would be just fabulous. Some of it took place in the streets, but a lot went on behind the courtyard walls. You could lead a very flamboyant life-style within certain limitations, and it was wonderful."[78]

During the AMH-sponsored conference in 1983, one Haitian American researcher read aloud from the pages of the 1983 *Spartacus International Gay Guide*, in which Haiti was enthusiastically recommended to the gay tourist: handsome men with "a great ability to satisfy" are readily available, the publication claimed, but "there is no free sex in Haiti, except with other gay tourists you may come across. Your partners will expect to be paid for their services but the charges are nominal." Another advertisement, which ran in *The Advocate*, assured the prospective tourist that Haiti is "a place where all your fantasies come true."[79]

Murray and Payne have questioned the relevance of gay tourism in the Haitian AIDS epidemic: "Insofar as gay travel can be estimated from gay guidebooks, Haiti was one of the least-favored destinations in the Caribbean for gay travelers during the 1970s and the less-favored half of the island of Hispaniola."[80] But an assessment based only on frequency of listings in gay guidebooks is surely a less significant indicator of the relevance of such tourism than were the cluster studies that revealed direct sexual contact between Haitian men and North American gay tourists. In a key paper published in 1984, Guérin and co-workers from Haiti, North America, and Canada stated that "17 percent of our patients had sexual contact with [North] American tourists."[81] As this study demonstrates, the introduction of an epidemic of sexually transmitted disease need not involve some critical mass of sexual contact but requires only that the infectious agent be introduced into a sexually active population (in this case, Haitian men).[82]

Of course, the existence of sexual tourism, some of it gay, does not prove that such commerce was "the cause" of the Haitian AIDS epidemic, nor is it my intention to argue that it does. Such commerce does, however, throw into relief the ties between Haiti and nearby North America—ties not mentioned in early discussions of AIDS among Haitians, which often posited "isolated Haiti" as the source of the pandemic. In fact, a review of even the scholarly literature on Haiti leaves the impression that the country is the most "isolated" or "insular" of Caribbean countries. In an assessment resonant with the U.S. medical community's AIDS-related speculations, the author of one standard text remarks that "Haiti in 1950 was in general what it had been in 1900: a pre-industrial society inhabited by ignorant, diseased peasants oblivious to the outside world."[83]

More attentive study of Haiti's economy, however, reveals that the nation has long shared close ties with the United States. In fact, Haiti plays an interesting role in what Orlando Patterson has termed the "West Atlantic system," an economic network encompassing much of the Caribbean basin and centered in the United States:

> Originally a region of diverse cultures and economies operating within the framework of several imperial systems, the West Atlantic region has emerged over the centuries as a single environment in which the dualistic United States center is asymmetrically linked to dualistic peripheral units. Unlike other peripheral systems of states—those of the Pacific, for example—the West Atlantic periphery has become more and more uniform, under the direct and immediate influence of its powerful northern neighbors, in cultural, political and economic terms. Further, unlike other peripheral zones in their relation to their centers, the West Atlantic system has a physical nexus in the metropolis at the tip of Florida.[84]

The Caribbean nations with high attack rates of AIDS are all part of the West Atlantic system. A relation between the degree of involvement in this network and the prevalence of AIDS is suggested by the following exercise. Excluding Puerto Rico, which is not an independent country, the five Caribbean basin nations with the largest number of cases by 1986 were the Dominican Republic, the Bahamas, Trinidad/Tobago, Mexico, and Haiti. In terms of trade, which are the five Caribbean basin countries most dependent on the United States? Export indices offer a convenient marker of involvement in the West Atlantic system. The five countries linked most closely to the United States in 1977 and 1983 (the years for which such data are available) are precisely those with the largest number of AIDS cases.[85] The country with the largest number of cases, Haiti, was also the country most fully dependent on U.S. exports. In all the Caribbean basin, only Puerto Rico is more economically dependent on the United States. And only Puerto Rico has reported more cases of AIDS to the Pan American Health Organization.

To understand the West Atlantic AIDS pandemic, a historical understanding of the worldwide spread of HIV is crucial. The thesis that evolving economic forces run parallel to the lineaments of the American epidemics is confirmed by comparing Haiti with a neighboring island, the sole country in the region not enmeshed in the West Atlantic system. In Haiti, as we have seen, several epidemiological studies of asymptomatic city dwellers revealed HIV seroprevalence rates of approximately 9 percent in the late 1980s. Meanwhile, in Cuba, only 0.01 percent of 1,000,000 persons tested in 1986 were found to have antibodies to HIV.[86] Had the pandemic begun a few decades earlier, the epidemiology of HIV infection in the Caribbean might well be different. Havana, once the "tropical playground of the Americas," might have been as much an epicenter of the pandemic as Carrefour.

The challenge of this reanalysis is daunting, for the questions raised here bear on the frame of reference and scope of analysis appropriate to a subject such as AIDS in Haiti. The anthropologic literature on Haiti has tended toward the exotic, with lurid treatises on ritual sacrifice and possession, potent poisons and zombiism. AIDS fits all too neatly into this symbolic network, in the self-confirming way of stereotypes. The Haitians may be exotic to "us" (as that symbolic structure defines "us"), but "we" are not in the least exotic to Haitians such as the inhabitants of the Central Plateau who are introduced in the next two chapters. We should pose Eric Wolf's pointed query again: "If there are connections everywhere, why do we persist in turning dynamic, interconnected phenomena into static, disconnected things?"[87]

AIDS in Haiti is all about proximity, not distance. AIDS in Haiti is a tale of ties to the United States rather than to Africa; it is a story of unemployment rates greater than 70 percent and tax-advantaged "free-trade" zones. AIDS in Haiti is about steep grades of inequality, both local and transnational. AIDS in Haiti has far more to do with the pursuit of trade and tourism in a dirt-poor country than with "dark saturnalia celebrated by 'blood-maddened, sex-maddened, god-maddened' negroes."

5 Culture, Poverty, and HIV Transmission

THE CASE OF RURAL HAITI

Violent deaths are natural deaths
here. He died of his environment.

DR. MAGIOT, IN GRAHAM
GREENE'S *The Comedians, 1966*

The preceding chapter describes some of the important work regarding HIV transmission that has been conducted in urban Haiti over the course of the past fifteen years. Haiti, however, a country of well over seven million inhabitants, is generally considered to be a substantially rural nation,[1] and it is significant that few studies of HIV transmission have been conducted in rural parts of the country. As the ties that link rural and urban Haiti are economically and affectively strong, an understanding of the urban epidemic is a necessary prologue to an investigation of HIV transmission in rural areas, the subject of this chapter.

Early reports by Pape and Johnson, based on small studies conducted in 1986–87, noted that the seroprevalence rate for HIV averaged 3 percent "in rural areas."[2] The seroprevalence in 97 mothers of children hospitalized with dehydration was 3 percent; of 245 unscreened rural blood donors, 4 percent had antibodies to HIV. In an area even more distant from urban centers, only 1 percent of 191 adults who came for immunizations were seropositive. Unfortunately, we know little about the individuals bled for these studies. Just how rural were they? What was the nature of their ties to Port-au-Prince and other high-prevalence cities? How did the seropositive individuals come to be at risk for HIV? How did they differ from seronegative controls? How rapidly was HIV making inroads into the rural population? What, in short, are the dynamics of HIV transmission in rural Haiti?

To understand the rural Haitian AIDS epidemic, we must move beyond the concept of "risk groups" to consider the interplay between human agency and the powerful forces that constrain it, focusing especially on those activities that promote or retard the spread of HIV. In Haiti, the most powerful of these forces have been inequality, deepening poverty, and political dislocations, which have together conspired to hasten the spread of HIV. This chapter details research on HIV transmission in a rural area of Haiti—and also recounts some of the ways such large-scale social forces become manifest in the lives of particular individuals.

AIDS IN A HAITIAN VILLAGE

The setting for the research described here is the Péligre basin of Haiti's Central Plateau, home to several hundred thousand mostly rural people. Although all parts of Haiti are poor, the Péligre basin region and its villages may be especially so.

Before 1956, the village of Kay was situated in a deep and fertile valley in this area, near the banks of the Rivière Artibonite. For generations, the villagers farmed the broad and gently sloping banks of the river, selling rice, bananas, millet, corn, and sugarcane in regional markets. Harvests were, by all reports, bountiful; life then is now recalled as idyllic. With the construction of Haiti's largest hydroelectric dam in 1956, however, thousands of families living in this region were flooded out. The displaced persons were largely peasant farmers, and they received little or no compensation for their lost land.

The hilltop village of Do Kay was founded by refugees from the rising water. The flooding of the valley forced most villagers up into the hills on either side of the new reservoir. Kay became divided into "Do" (those who settled on the stony backs of the hills) and "Ba" (those who remained down near the new waterline). By all standard measures, both parts of Kay are now very poor; its older inhabitants often blame their poverty on the massive buttress dam a few miles away and note bitterly that it brought them neither electricity nor water.

Though initially a dusty squatter settlement of fewer than two hundred persons, Do Kay has grown rapidly in the past decade and now counts about two thousand inhabitants. In spite of the hostile conditions, most families continue to rely to some extent on small-scale agriculture. But many villagers are involved in a series of development projects designed to improve the health of the area's inhabitants. Since 1984, for example, a series of outreach initiatives have complemented the work of our growing team of clinicians, based in Do Kay at the Clinique Bon Sauveur. The most significant efforts were undertaken under the aegis of Proje Veye Sante, the "health surveillance project." Proje Veye Sante, conducted in large part by village-based community health workers from about thirty nearby communities, provides preventive and primary care to close to fifty thousand rural people.

Through Proje Veye Sante, AIDS surveillance began well before the epidemic was manifest in the region. It is thus possible to date the index, or first, case of AIDS to 1986, when a young schoolteacher, Manno Surpris, fell ill with recurrent superficial fungal infections, chronic diarrhea, and pulmonary tuberculosis. Seropositive for HIV, he died a year later. (His experience is examined in Chapter 6.)[3]

Although Manno Surpris was from another part of the Central Plateau, it was not long before we began to diagnose the syndrome among natives of Do Kay. The sections that follow offer brief case histories of the first three villagers known to have died of AIDS. None had a history of transfusion with blood or blood products; none had a history of homosexual contact or other "risk factors" as designated by the CDC. They did, however, share two important, if poorly understood, risk factors: poverty and inequality.

Anita

Anita Joseph was born in approximately 1966 to a family that had lost its land to the Péligre dam. One of six children, she briefly attended school until her mother, weakened by the malnutrition then rampant in the Kay area, died of tuberculosis. Anita was then thirteen. Her father became depressed and abusive, and she resolved to run away: "I'd had it with his yelling. . . . When I saw how poor I was, and how hungry, and saw that it would never get any better, I had to go to the city. Back then I was so skinny—I was saving my life, I thought, by getting out of here."

Anita left for Port-au-Prince with less than $3 and no clear plan of action. She worked briefly as a *restavèk*, or live-in maid, for $10 a month but lost this position when her employer was herself fired from a factory job.

Cast into the street, Anita eventually found a relative who took her in. The kinswoman, who lived in a notorious slum north of the capital, introduced her to Vincent, a young man who worked unloading luggage at the airport. Anita was not yet fifteen when she entered her first and only sexual union. "What could I do, really?" she sighed as she recounted the story much later. "He had a good job. My aunt thought I should go with him."

Vincent, who had at least one other sexual partner at the time, became ill less than two years after they began sharing a room. The young man, whom Anita cared for throughout his illness, died after repeated infections, including tuberculosis. Not long after his death, Anita herself fell ill with tuberculosis.

Upon returning to Do Kay in 1987, she quickly responded to antituberculous therapy. When she relapsed some months later, we performed an HIV test, which revealed the true cause of her immunosuppression. Following a slow but ineluctable decline, Anita died in February 1988.

Dieudonné

Dieudonné Gracia, born in Do Kay in 1963, was also the child of two "water refugees." One of seven children, he attended primary school in his home village and, briefly, secondary school in a nearby town. It was there, at the age of nineteen, that he had his first sexual contact. Dieudonné remarked that his girlfriend had had "two, maybe three partners" before they met; he was sure that one of her partners had been a truck driver from a city in central Haiti.

When a series of setbacks further immiserated his family, Dieudonné was forced to drop out of secondary school and also to drop his relationship with the young woman. He returned to Do Kay to work with his father, a carpenter. In 1983, however, the young man decided to "try my luck in Port-au-Prince." Through a friend from Do Kay, Dieudonné found a position as a domestic for a well-to-do family in a suburb of the capital.

While in the city, Dieudonné's sexual experience broadened considerably. He had five partners in little more than two years, all of them close to his own age. Asked about the brevity of these liaisons, Dieudonné favored an economic explanation: "A couple of them let go of me because they saw that I couldn't do anything for them. They saw that I couldn't give them anything for any children."

In 1985, Dieudonné became ill and was dismissed from his job in Port-au-Prince. He returned to Do Kay and began seeing his former lover again. She soon became pregnant and moved to Do Kay as the young man's *plase,* a term designating a partner in a more or less stable conjugal union.[4]

During this interlude, Dieudonné was seen at the Do Kay clinic for a number of problems that suggested immunodeficiency: herpes zoster and genital herpes, recurrent diarrhea, and weight loss. In the months following the birth of their baby, the young mother fell ill with a febrile illness, thought by her physician to be malaria, and quickly succumbed. Less than a year later, Dieudonné, much reduced by chronic diarrhea, was diagnosed with tuberculosis. Although he initially responded to antituberculous agents, Dieudonné died of AIDS in October 1988.

Acéphie

Acéphie Joseph was born in 1965 on a small knoll protruding into the reservoir that had drowned her parents' land. Acéphie attended primary school somewhat irregularly; by the age of nineteen, she had not yet graduated and decided that it was time to help generate income for her family, which was sinking deeper and deeper into poverty. Hunger was a near-daily occurrence for the Joseph family; the times were as bad as those right after the flooding of the valley. Acéphie began to help her mother, a market woman, by carrying produce to a local market on Friday mornings.

It was there that she met a soldier, formerly stationed in Port-au-Prince, who began to make overtures to the striking young woman from Do Kay. Although the soldier had a wife and children and was known to have more than one regular partner, Acéphie did not spurn him. "What would you have me do? I could tell that the old people were uncomfortable, worried—but they didn't say no. They didn't tell me to stay away from him. I wish they had, but how could they have known? . . . I looked around and saw how poor we all were, how the old people were finished. . . . It was a way out, that's how I saw it."

Within a short time, the soldier fell ill and was diagnosed in the Do Kay clinic with AIDS. A few months after he and Acéphie parted, he was dead.

Shaken, Acéphie went to a nearby town and began a course in what she euphemistically termed a "cooking school," which prepared poor girls for work as servants. In 1987, twenty-two years old, Acéphie went to Port-au-Prince, where she found a $30-per-month job as a housekeeper for a middle-class Haitian woman who worked for the U.S. embassy. She began to see a man, also from the Kay region, who chauffeured a small bus between the Central Plateau and Port-au-Prince.

Acéphie worked in the city until late in 1989, when she discovered that she was pregnant. This displeased both her partner and her employer. Sans job and sans boyfriend, Acéphie returned to Do Kay in her third trimester.

Following the birth of her daughter, Acéphie was sapped by repeated opportunistic infections, each one caught in time by the staff of the clinic in Do Kay. Throughout 1991, however, she continued to lose weight; by January 1992, she weighed less than ninety pounds, and her intermittent fevers did not respond to broad-spectrum antibiotics.

Acéphie died in April 1992. Her daughter, the first "AIDS orphan" in Do Kay, is now in the care of Acéphie's mother. The child is also infected. A few months after Acéphie's death, her father hanged himself.

Sadly, however, this is not simply the story of Acéphie and her family. The soldier's wife, who is much thinner than last year, has already had a case of herpes zoster. Two of her children are also HIV-positive. This woman, who is well known to the clinic staff, is no longer a widow; once again, she is the partner of a military man. Her late husband had at least two other partners, both of them poor peasant women, in the Central

Plateau. One is HIV-positive and has two sickly children. The father of Acéphie's child, apparently in good health, is still plying the roads from Mirebalais to Port-au-Prince. His serostatus is unknown.

Individual Experience in Context

When compared to age-matched North Americans with AIDS, Anita, Dieudonné, and Acéphie have sparse sexual histories: Anita had only one partner; Dieudonné had six; Acéphie had two. Although a case-control study by Pape and Johnson suggested that HIV-infected urban men, at least, had larger numbers of partners than our patients did,[5] research conducted in Anita's neighborhood in Port-au-Prince suggests that her case is not as unique as it would seem:

> The high seropositivity rate (8%) found in pregnant women 14 to 19 years of age suggests that women [in Cité Soleil] appear to acquire HIV infection soon after becoming sexually active. Moreover, this age group is the only one in which a higher seropositivity rate is not associated with a greater number of sexual partners. Women with only one sexual partner in the year prior to pregnancy actually have a slightly higher prevalence rate (although not significantly so) than the others. This suggests that they were infected by their first and only partner.[6]

The stories of Anita, Dieudonné, and Acéphie are ones that reveal the push-and-pull forces of contemporary Haiti. In all three cases, the declining fortunes of the rural poor pushed young adults to try their chances in the city. Once there, all three became entangled in unions that the women, at least, characterized as attempts to emerge from poverty. Each worked as a domestic, but none managed to fulfill the expectation of saving and sending home desperately needed cash. What they brought home, instead, was AIDS.

How representative are these case histories? Over the past several years, the medical staff of the Clinique Bon Sauveur has diagnosed dozens more cases of AIDS and other forms of HIV infection in women who arrive at the clinic with a broad range of complaints. In fact, the majority of our patients have been women—a pattern rarely described in the AIDS literature, as noted in Chapter 3. With surprisingly few exceptions, those so diagnosed shared a number of risk factors, as our modest case-control study suggests.

We conducted this study by interviewing the first twenty-five women we diagnosed with symptomatic HIV infection who were residents of Do Kay or its two neighboring villages. Their responses to questions posed during a series of open-ended interviews were compared with those of twenty-five age-matched, seronegative controls. In both groups, ages ranged from 16 to 44, with a mean age of about 27 years. Table 7 presents our findings.

None of these fifty women had a history of prostitution, and none had used illicit drugs. Only two, both members of the control group, had received blood transfusions. None of the women in either group had had more than five sexual partners in the course of their lives; in fact, seven of the afflicted women had had only one. Although women in the study group had on average more sexual partners than the controls, the difference is not striking. Similarly, we found no clear difference between the two groups in the number of intramuscular injections they had received or their years of education.

The chief risk factors in this small cohort seem to involve not number of partners but rather the professions of these partners. Fully nineteen of the women with HIV disease had histories of sexual contact with soldiers

Table 7.   Case-Control Study of AIDS in Rural Haitian Women

Patient Characteristics	Patients with AIDS (N = 25)	Control Group (N = 25)
Average number of sexual partners	2.7	2.4
Sexual partner of a truck driver	12	2
Sexual partner of a soldier	9	0
Sexual partner of a peasant only	0	23
Ever lived in Port-au-Prince	20	4
Worked as a servant	18	1
Average number of years of formal schooling	4.5	4.0
Ever received a blood transfusion	0	2
Ever used illicit drugs	0	0
Ever received more than ten intramuscular injections	17	19

or truck drivers. Three of these women reported having only two sexual partners: one a soldier, one a truck driver. Of the women diagnosed with AIDS, none had a history of sexual contact exclusively with peasants (although one had as sole partner a construction worker from Do Kay). Among the control group, only two women had a regular partner who was a truck driver; none reported contact with soldiers, and most had had sexual relations only with peasants from the region. Histories of extended residence in Port-au-Prince and work as a domestic were also strongly associated with a diagnosis of HIV disease.

How can we make sense of these surprising results? In the sociographically "flat" region around the dam—after all, most area residents share a single socioeconomic status, poverty—conjugal unions with nonpeasants (salaried soldiers and truck drivers who are paid on a daily basis) reflect women's quest for some measure of economic security. In the setting of a worsening economic crisis, the gap between the hungry peasant class and the relatively well-off soldiers and truck drivers became the salient local inequality. In this manner, truck drivers and soldiers have served as a "bridge" from the city to the rural population, just as North American tourists seemed to have served as a bridge to the urban Haitian population.

But just as North Americans are no longer important in the transmission of HIV in Haiti, truck drivers and soldiers will soon no longer be necessary components of the rural epidemic. Once introduced into a sexually active population, HIV will work its way to those with no history of residence in the city, no history of contact with soldiers or truck drivers, no history of work as a domestic. But these risk factors—all of which reflect a desperate attempt to escape rural poverty—are emblematic of the lot of the rural Haitian poor, and perhaps especially of poor women.

HIV in a Haitian Village

Extended residence in Port-au-Prince, work as a servant, and sexual contact with nonpeasants—although these risk factors were far different from those described for North Americans with AIDS, they characterized the majority of our male and female patients afflicted with AIDS. The majority of the residents of the area served by Proje Veye Sante shared none of these attributes, however. Did this suggest that few would prove to be infected with HIV? Although a good deal of ethnographic research into the nature of AIDS had already been conducted in the region, no research had addressed the question of HIV prevalence among asymptomatic adults.

Troubled by this lacuna, the staff of the clinic and of Proje Veye Sante established the Groupe d'étude du SIDA dans la Classe Paysanne.[7] GESCAP has a mandate to research the mechanisms by which poverty puts young adults, and especially young women, at risk of HIV infection.[8] With community approval, GESCAP is attempting to illuminate case histories with serologic surveys, an expanded case-control study, and cluster studies (such as those that revealed how a single HIV-positive soldier came to infect at least eleven natives of the region, one of whom was Acéphie).

After considerable discussion, the members of GESCAP decided to undertake a study of all asymptomatic adults living in Do Kay. The study was to include all members of the community who might plausibly be sexually active (fifteen years and older) and who were free of any suggestion of immunodeficiency; patients with active tuberculosis were excluded from this study. Anyone who was the regular sexual partner of a person with known HIV infection was also excluded.

Of the first one hundred villagers enrolling in the program, ninety-nine were seronegative for HIV.[9] The one young woman with HIV infection, Alourdes, had a history of extended residence in Port-au-Prince and also in 1985 of regular sexual contact with a salaried employee of the national electric company. This man, who had several sexual partners during his tenure in central Haiti, was rumored to have died of AIDS. In 1986, Alourdes had been the partner of a young man from her home village, a construction worker. He later developed tuberculosis, initially attributed to respiratory contact with his wife, who had pulmonary tuberculosis. Both were later found to be infected with HIV; neither had ever had sexual contact outside the Do Kay area. The discovery of HIV infection in Alourdes, who was known to have risk factors as defined in the case-control study, helped to identify the routes of exposure of the couple who had HIV-related tuberculosis.

Such discrete studies do not, however, fully define the nature of the large-scale social forces at work. The discussion in the following sections summarizes the factors that seem to be most significant in the ultimate rate of progression of HIV in rural Haiti. Perhaps an examination of these forces can serve to inform understandings of the dynamics of HIV transmission in other parts of Latin America and also in areas of Asia and Africa where prevalence rates in rural regions are currently low. It is a cautionary tale that argues for aggressive preventive measures:

> If a disaster is to be prevented in rural Haiti, vigorous and effective prevention campaigns must be initiated at once. And although such efforts must begin, the prospects of stopping the steady march of HIV are slim. AIDS is far more likely to join a host of other sexually transmitted diseases—including gonorrhea, syphilis, genital herpes, chlamydia, hepatitis B, lymphogranuloma venereum, and even cervical cancer—that have already become entrenched among the poor.[10]

Only massive and coordinated efforts may yet avert the ongoing disaster that has befallen urban Haiti, Puerto Rico, inner-city North America, Thailand, Brazil, and many nations in sub-Saharan Africa.

THE DYNAMICS OF
HIV TRANSMISSION IN RURAL HAITI

Wherever HIV infection is a sexually transmitted disease, social forces necessarily determine its distribution. Cultural, political, and economic factors, while each inevitably important, cannot be of equal significance in all settings. In rural Haiti, we can identify a number of differentially weighted, synergistic forces that promote HIV transmission.

Population Pressures

Haiti, which covers 27,700 square kilometers, is one of the most crowded societies in the hemisphere. In 1980, only 8,000 square kilometers were under cultivation, giving an effective population density of 626 persons per square kilometer. Unfortunately, Haiti's topsoil is now prey to runaway forces that further compound the overcrowding: "The land suffers from deforestation, soil erosion and exhaustion; the country is periodically ravaged by hurricanes which cause enormous damage."[11] As the land becomes increasingly exhausted, more and more peasants abandon agriculture for the lure of wage-labor in cities and towns.

Indeed, one of the most striking recent demographic changes has been the rapid growth of Port-au-Prince. More than 20 percent of the Haitian population now lives in the capital, a city of over 1.5 million. Although this concentration is not impressive by Caribbean standards (more than 30 percent of Puerto Ricans live in San Juan), the rate of growth in Port-au-Prince has been striking: "The urban population was 12.2% of the total in 1950, 20.4% in 1971 and an estimated 27.5% in 1980."[12] Haitian demographers estimate that by the year 2000 urban dwellers will constitute 37 percent of the total population.

As is the case with so many Third World countries, internal migration has played the most significant role in the growth of the capital. Locher estimates that "between 1950 and 1971 rural-urban migration accounted for 59% of Haitian urban growth, while natural population increase accounted for only 8%."[13] Neptune-Anglade has observed that the growth of Port-au-Prince is substantially the result of a "feminine rural exodus," leaving the city approximately 60 percent female.[14] Younger women of rural origin—women like Anita and Acéphie—are most commonly employed as servants.[15] Migrants of both sexes maintain strong ties with their regions of origin. In these respects, the three index cases of AIDS from Do Kay are illustrative of the trends documented by demographers and others who speak of Port-au-Prince as "a city of peasants."

Economic Pressures

Rural Haiti, always poor, has become palpably poorer in recent decades. A per capita annual income of $315 in 1983 masked the fact that income hovered around $100 in the countryside; in the late 1990s the average annual per capita income is down to around $175.[16] Accompanying the population growth and a loss of arable land to erosion and alkalinization has been an inevitable growth in landlessness. All of these factors have inevitably had a devastating effect on agricultural production. For example, Girault typifies the decade preceding 1984 as marked chiefly "by the slowdown of agricultural production and by a decrease in productivity."[17]

This decline has been further compounded by striking rural-urban disparities in every imaginable type of goods and service. In 1984, Girault was able to complain that "Port-au-Prince with 17–18% of the national population consumes as much as 30% of all the food produced in the country and a larger share of imported food."[18] Government statistics reveal that the "Port-au-Prince agglomeration" consumed 93 percent of all electricity produced in the country in 1979. As Trouillot notes, the city "houses 20% of the national population, but consumes 80% of all State expenditures."[19]

In short, current economic conditions push people out of the countryside and into the city or, often enough, out of the country altogether. The Haitian people have long since left behind a peasant standard of living (which did not necessarily mean an exceptionally low one). Whereas Haiti was once a nation with an extremely high percentage of landholders, late-twentieth-century Haiti is increasingly a country of unemployed and landless paupers. When the Population Crisis Committee published its "international index of human suffering" in 1992, based on a variety of measures of human welfare, Haiti had the dubious distinction of heading the list of all countries in this hemisphere. Of the 141 countries studied, only three were deemed to have living conditions worse than those in Haiti—and all three of these countries were at the time being consumed by civil war.[20]

Patterns of Sexual Union

In the numerous studies of conjugal unions in rural Haiti, most have underlined the classic division between couples who are *marye* (joined by civil or religious marriage) and those who are *plase* (joined in a conjugal union that incurs significant and enduring obligations to both partners). *Plasaj* (from French, *plaçage*) has generally been the most common form of conjugal union in rural Haiti, outnumbering marriages by two or three to one.

Early studies usually considered *plasaj* to be polygamous, with one man having more than one *plase* partner. This is often no longer the case, as Moral suggested over three decades ago: "It is 'plaçage honnête'—that is, monogamy—that best characterizes matrimonial status in today's rural society."[21] The reason for this shift toward monogamy, he believed, was the same one that leads many rural people to avoid marriage in the first place: formal unions are costly. "If the considerable growth of *plaçage* is to be explained in part by economic factors," continued Moral, "the form that *plaçage* now takes is greatly influenced by the poverty spreading throughout the countryside."

Allman's review suggests that contemporary sexual unions are considerably more complex than the bipolar model just described. In a survey in which women who had sexual relations with the same partner for a minimum of three months were considered to be "in union," interviews revealed an emic typology with five major categories: three of these—*rinmin, fiyanse,* and *viv avèk*—did not usually involve cohabitation and engendered only slight economic support; two others—*plase* and *marye*—were deemed much stronger unions, generally involving cohabitation as well as economic support.[22]

In addition, a number of other sexual practices have often been loosely termed "prostitution," in Haiti a largely urban phenomenon and much understudied.[23] It is clear, however, that unemployed women from rural areas may become involved in occasional and often clandestine sex work (variously described by terms such as *ti degaje, woulman*) when other options are exhausted. There are few avenues of escape for those caught in the web of urban migration, greater than 60 percent unemployment, and extreme poverty.[24]

How are these forms of sexual union related to the dynamics of HIV transmission? To those working in rural clinics, *plasaj* is often implicated in the spread or persistence of sexually transmitted diseases such as gonorrhea and chlamydial disease. Treatment of one or two members of a network is of course inadequate, as even women who have but one sexual partner are indirectly in regular sexual contact with any other *plase* partners of their mate. Regarding HIV, polygamous *plasaj* may be considered a preexisting sociocultural institution that serves to speed the spread of HIV and that constitutes a risk in and of itself, particularly for monogamous women. Women throughout the world bear similar risks—which are compounded wherever gender inequality erodes women's power over condom use.

The unremitting immiseration of Haiti has clearly undermined stable patterns of union such as marriage and *plasaj* by creating economic pressures to which women with dependents are particularly vulnerable. In the wake of these pressures, new patterns have emerged: "serial monogamy" might describe the monogamous but weak unions that lead to one child but last little longer than a year or two. After such unions have dissolved, the woman finds herself with a new dependent and even more in need of a reliable partner.

Equally dangerous, as we have seen, is the quest for a union with a financially "secure" partner. In rural Haiti, men of this description once included a substantial fraction of all peasant landholders. In recent decades, however, financial security has become elusive for all but a handful of truck drivers, representatives of the state (such as soldiers and petty officials), and landholders (grandòn). As noted, truck drivers and soldiers are clearly groups with above average rates of HIV infection.

Gender Inequality

"The ability of young women to protect themselves from [HIV] infection becomes a direct function of power relations between men and women."[25] As Chapter 3 discussed, gender inequality has weakened women's ability to negotiate safe sexual encounters, and this sapping of agency is especially amplified by poverty. The Haitian economy counts a higher proportion of economically active women—most of them traders—than any other developing society, with the exception of Lesotho.[26] It is not surprising, then, that the machismo that has so marked other Latin American societies is less pronounced in Haiti.[27] (Even the head of the Duvaliers' dreaded paramilitary force was a woman.) But gender inequality is certainly a force in political, economic, and domestic life. It would be difficult to argue with Neptune-Anglade when she states that, in all regards, rural women "endure a discrimination and a pauperization that is worse than that affecting [rural] men."[28]

Preliminary ethnographic research in the Do Kay area suggests that many rural women do not wield sufficient authority to demand that plase partners (or husbands) use condoms. A growing literature documents similar patterns throughout the developing world and in the inner cities of the United States.[29] These considerations lead us to agree with those calling for preventive efforts that are "women-centered." "In societies where the female has a weaker hand," Desvarieux and Pape argue, "effective methods of prevention have a better chance of working if the woman does not have to rely on either the consent or the willingness of her partner."[30]

Other "Cultural" Considerations

Practices such as the widespread and unregulated use of syringes by "folk" practitioners unschooled in aseptic techniques received a fair amount of attention as possible sources of HIV transmission. But far more frequently invoked were "voodoo practices," which played a peculiarly central role in early speculations about the nature of the AIDS epidemic, as Chapter 4 describes. These speculations, which sparked waves of anti-Haitian sentiment, had the added disadvantage of being incorrect; none of these leads, when investigated, panned out. In urban Haiti, GHESKIO did not even consider these hypotheses worthy of serious investigation.

In our small-scale but in-depth study of AIDS in the Central Plateau, we did not find any strong implication of nonsexual transmission of HIV.[31] Similarly, the Collaborative Study Group of AIDS in Haitian-Americans initiated the first and (so far) only controlled study of risk factors for AIDS among Haitians living in the United States. Compiling data from several North American research centers, the investigators reached the following conclusion: "Folklore rituals have been suggested as potential risk factors for [HIV] transmission in Haiti. Our data do not support this hypothesis."[32] Such hypotheses reflect less an accurate reading of existing data and more a series of North American folk theories about Haitians.[33]

There have been few ethnographic studies of Haitian understandings of AIDS, and most of these have been conducted in Montreal, New York, or Miami. To my knowledge, the only such study conducted in rural Haiti (reviewed in Chapter 6) demonstrated that such understandings were in fact changing, at first quite rapidly. Over time, however, a stable illness representation of *sida*—as AIDS is termed—seemed to evolve.[34]

In the Do Kay region, serial interviews with the same group of villagers permitted us to delineate a complex model of illness causation, one linked fairly closely to understandings of tuberculosis. As Chapter 6 explains, villagers often, but not always, cited sorcery in discussions about *sida*, which nonetheless came to be seen as a fatal illness that could be transmitted by sexual contact. Local understandings of *sida* did not seem to affect disease distribution, but certainly they may hamper preventive efforts if not taken into account when designing interventions. Far more disabling, however, has been the nation's political situation.

Political Disruption

It is unfortunate indeed that HIV arrived in Haiti shortly before a period of massive and prolonged social upheaval. Political unrest has clearly undermined preventive efforts and may have helped, through other mechanisms, to spread HIV. Although many commentators observed that political struggles served to divert the public's interest away from AIDS, this was not the case in the Do Kay region. In fact, periods of increased strife were associated with increased public discourse about the new sickness.

But the same political disruptions that may have stimulated commentary about AIDS also served to paralyze coordinated efforts to prevent HIV transmission. For example, although the Haitian Ministry of Health has identified AIDS prevention as one of its top priorities, the office charged with coordinating preventive efforts has been hamstrung by six coups d'état, which have led, inevitably, to personnel changes—and to more significant disruptions. At the time GESCAP was founded, in 1991, *there had been no comprehensive effort to prevent HIV transmission in rural Haiti.* Even in Port au Prince, what has been accomplished thus far has often been marred by messages that are either culturally inappropriate or designed for a small fraction of the population (for example, Haitians who are francophone, literate, and television-owning). These messages are especially unsuccessful in rural areas, where even well-funded "social marketing" schemes have had little cultural currency.

A sense of hopefulness, rare in Haiti, returned to the public health community in 1991, when the country's first democratic elections brought to office a social-justice government headed by a progressive priest. A new Ministry of Health promised to make AIDS, tuberculosis, and other infectious pathogens its top priority. But in September of that year, a violent military coup brought a swift end to Haiti's democratic experiment. The impact on the population's health was incalculable.[35]

Political upheaval did not simply hobble coordinated responses to the AIDS epidemic. It has had far more direct effects. One of the most epidemiologically significant events of recent years may prove to be the coup d'état of September 1991. As noted earlier, surveys of asymptomatic adults living in Cité Soleil revealed seroprevalence rates of approximately 10 percent, whereas surveys of asymptomatic rural people were likely to find rates an order of magnitude lower. Following the coup, the army targeted urban slums for brutal repression. A number of journalists and health care professionals estimated that fully half of the adult residents of Cité Soleil fled to rural areas following the army's lethal incursions. It takes little imagination to see that such flux substantially changes the equations describing the dynamics of HIV transmission in rural areas sheltering the refugees.[36] Similar patterns have been noted elsewhere, particularly in sub-Saharan Africa:

> Women living in areas plagued by civil unrest or war may be in a situation of higher risk. In many countries, relatively high percentages of male military and police personnel are infected and their unprotected (voluntary or forced) sexual encounters with local women provide an avenue for transmission. Patterns of female infection have been correlated with the movements of members of the military in parts of Central and Eastern Africa.[37]

Concurrent Disease

The progression of HIV disease depends on host variables such as age, sex, and nutritional status; viral load, CD4-cell number and function; and concurrent disease. Concurrent illness can alter this progression in at least three ways: first, any serious illness, including opportunistic infections (most notably, tuberculosis), may hasten the progression of HIV disease; second, various diseases can heighten an individual's "net state of immunosuppression," rendering him or her increasingly vulnerable to infection; and, third, certain infections seem to increase the risk of *acquiring* HIV—the point considered here.

Sexually transmitted diseases have been cited as AIDS co-factors in a number of studies, especially those conducted in tropical and subtropical regions.[38] Researchers view STDs as particularly important in the heterosexual spread of HIV, as the virus is less efficiently transmitted from women to men than vice versa. Thus vaginal and cervical diseases—even those as ostensibly minor as trichomoniasis—may increase the risk of HIV transmission through "microwounds" and even through mere inflammation (as certain lymphocytes are, after all, the target cells of HIV).[39]

Although researchers are now collecting important data about STDs in Port-au-Prince,[40] few studies have focused on rural areas.[41] But there is no evidence to suggest that villagers are more sexually active than their urban counterparts; there is even less evidence to suggest that rural Haitians are more sexually active than age-matched controls from North America. What is evident is that a majority of STDs go untreated—which certainly implies that sores, other lesions, and inflammation will persist far longer in rural Haiti than in most areas of the world.

Other diseases—including leprosy, yaws, endemic syphilis, and various viruses—have been suggested as possible co-factors in "tropical" AIDS, but their roles have not been clarified. It seems safe to add, however, that serious co-infections do enhance the net state of immunosuppression. Similarly, malnutrition clearly hastens the advent of advanced, symptomatic disease among the HIV-infected, although this dynamic may lessen the risk of transmission: the Haitian variant of "slim disease" is now popularly associated with AIDS, and visible cachexia is likely to drive away potential sexual partners.[42]

Access to Medical Services

Finally, in seeking to understand the Haitian AIDS epidemic, it is necessary to underline the contribution, or lack thereof, of a nonfunctioning public health system. Medical care in Haiti is something of an obstacle course, one that places innumerable barriers before poor people seeking care. Failure to have an STD treated leads to persistence of important co-factors for HIV infection; failure to treat active tuberculosis causes rapid progression of HIV disease and death—to say nothing of its impact on HIV-negative individuals, for HIV-infected patients with tuberculosis have been shown to be efficient transmitters of tuberculosis.[43] Contaminated blood transfusions alternate with no transfusions at all. Condoms are often not available even to those who want them. The cost of pharmaceuticals, always prohibitive, has skyrocketed in recent years. Antivirals are in essence unavailable to most Haitians: in February 1990, "local radio stations announced . . . that for the first time, the drug AZT is available in Haiti. It might as well have been on Mars. A bottle of 100 capsules costs $343—more than most Haitians make in a year."[44] Since that time, it has become possible to find newer, highly active antiretroviral agents in Haiti—but for a prince's ransom.

AIDS, ANALYSIS, ACCOUNTABILITY

Identifying and weighting the various social forces that shape the HIV epidemic is a perennial problem, but one too rarely addressed by medical anthropology, which is often asked to elucidate the "cultural component" of particular subepidemics. By combining social analysis with ethnographically informed epidemiology, however, we can identify the most significant of these forces. The factors listed here are differentially weighted, of course, but each demonstrably plays a role in determining HIV transmission in rural Haiti:

1. Deepening poverty
2. Gender inequality
3. Political upheaval
4. Traditional patterns of sexual union
5. Emerging patterns of sexual union
6. Prevalence of and lack of access to treatment for STDs
7. Lack of timely response by public health authorities
8. Lack of culturally appropriate prevention tools

Many of these factors are a far cry from the ones that anthropologists were exhorted to explore—for example, ritual scarification, animal sacrifice, sexual behavior in "exotic subcultures"—during the first decade of AIDS. But the forces underpinning the spread of HIV to rural Haiti are as economic and political as they are cultural, and poverty and inequality seem to underlie all of them. Although many working elsewhere would agree that poverty and social inequalities are the strongest enhancers of risk for exposure to HIV, international conferences on AIDS have repeatedly neglected this subject. Of the hundreds of epidemiology-track posters presented in 1992 in Amsterdam, for example, only three used "poverty" as a keyword; two of these were socioculturally naïve and did not seem to involve the collaboration of anthropologists.

What were anthropologists doing in the early years of AIDS? The mid- to late 1980s saw the formation of task forces and research groups as well as an increasing number of AIDS-related sessions at our professional meetings. The central themes of many of the early sessions focused on the "special understanding of sexuality" that was, suggested certain speakers, the province of anthropologists. The scenario most commonly evoked was one in which ethnographers, steeped in local lore after years of participant-observation, afforded epidemiologists and public health authorities detailed information about sexual behavior, childbearing, and beliefs about blood and blood contact. This knowledge transfer was deemed indispensable to determining which "behaviors" put individuals and communities at risk for HIV infection.

Fifteen years into the AIDS pandemic, after at least a decade of social science studies of AIDS, we must ask, How substantial were these claims? How many secret, AIDS-related "behaviors" have we unearthed in the course of our ethnography? Anthropologists deeply involved in AIDS prevention now know that many such claims were immodest. Everywhere, it seems, HIV spreads from host to host through a relatively restricted set of mechanisms. We've also learned that preventive efforts, even the most culturally appropriate ones, are least effective in precisely those settings in which they are most urgently needed. Africa, long a favored proving ground for anthropology, offers the most obvious and humbling example. Haiti offers another.

In the interest of enhancing the efficacy of interventions, it's important to pause and take stock of the situation. How might anthropology best contribute to efforts to prevent HIV transmission or to alleviate AIDS-related suffering? One major contribution would be to help show where the pandemic is going, which leads us back to analytic challenges such as these:

Identifying and differentially weighting the major factors promoting or retarding HIV transmission

Linking the sexual choices made by individual actors to the various shifting conditions that restrict choice, especially among the poor

Understanding the contribution of the culturally specific—not only local sexualities but also kinship structures and shifting representations of disease—without losing sight of the large-scale economic forces shaping the AIDS pandemic

Investigating the precise mechanisms by which such forces as racism, gender inequality, poverty, war, migration, colonial heritage, coups d'état, and even structural-adjustment programs become embodied as increased risk

Anthropology, the most radically contextualizing of the social sciences, is well suited to meeting these analytic challenges, but we will not succeed by merely "filling in the cultural blanks" left by epidemiologists, physicians, scientists, and policy makers. Nor will we succeed without a new vigilance toward the analytic traps that have hobbled our understanding of the AIDS pandemic.[45]

First, we often find widespread, if sectarian, ascription to behaviorist, cognitivist, or culturalist reductionism. Just as many physicians regard social considerations as outside the realm of the central, so too have psychologists tended to reify individual psychology, while economists have reified the economic. Anthropologists writing of AIDS have of course tended to reify culture. We must avoid confusing our own desire for personal efficacy with sound analytic purchase on an ever-growing pandemic: HIV cares little for our theoretical stances or our disciplinary training. AIDS demands broad biosocial approaches. Jean Benoist and Alice Desclaux put it well:

The conditions limiting or promoting transmission, illness representations, therapeutic itineraries, and health care practices—none of these subjects are captured by disciplinary approaches. They evade even the distinction between biology and social sciences, so tightly are biological realities tied to behaviors and representations, revealing links that have not yet been fully explored.[46]

Second, much anthropologic analysis focuses overmuch (or exclusively) on local factors and local actors, which risks exaggerating the agency of the poor and marginalized. Constraints on the agency of individual actors should be brought into stark relief so that prevention efforts do not come to grief, as they have to date. To explore the relation between personal agency and supraindividual structures—once the central problematic of social theory—we need to link our ethnography to systemic analyses that are informed by history, political economy, and a critical epidemiology. It is not possible to explain the strikingly patterned distribution of HIV by referring exclusively to attitude, cognition, or affect. Fine-grained psychological portraits and rich ethnography are never more than part of the AIDS story.

Third, the myths and mystifications that surround AIDS and slow AIDS research often serve powerful interests. If, in Haiti and in parts of Africa, economic policies (for example, structural-adjustment programs) and political upheaval are somehow related to HIV transmission, who benefits when attention is focused largely or solely on "unruly sexuality" or alleged "promiscuity"? The lasting influence of myths and immodest claims has helped to mask the effects of social inequalities on the distribution of HIV and on AIDS outcomes.

The recent advent of more effective antiviral therapy could have an enormous impact on what it means to have AIDS at the close of the twentieth century—if you don't happen to live in Africa or Haiti or Harlem. Protease inhibitors and other drugs raise the possibility of transforming AIDS into a chronic condition to be managed over decades, but they also remind us that there are two emerging syndromes: an AIDS of the North, and an AIDS of the South.

Perhaps this does not sound much like an anthropologist speaking. Why talk of latitude (North/South) and class (rich/poor) before speaking of culture? One answer to this question is that, for many of us, the view that AIDS is a culturally constructed phenomenon is not open to debate. AIDS, like sexuality, is inevitably embedded in local social context; representations and responses must necessarily vary along cultural lines. The contribution of cultural factors to the lived experience of AIDS is and will remain enormous. Indeed, the true and vast variation of HIV lies not, as we had been led to believe, in its modes of spread, nor is it found in the mechanisms by which the virus saps the host. The variation of HIV lies, rather, in its highly patterned distribution, in its variable clinical course among the infected, and in the ways in which we respond, socially, to a deadly pathogen.

Miracles and Misery

AN ETHNOGRAPHIC INTERLUDE

This wasn't the music of pain. Pain

has no music, pain is a story: it starts,

Eurydice was taken from the fields.

She did not sing—you cannot sing in

hell—but in that viscous dark she

heard the song flung like a rope into

the crater of hell.

ELLEN BRYANT VOIGT,
"Song and Story," 1993

The margin between social theory and

the ethnography of social suffering is

a space of vital liminality. It is a

threshold to something new, an

unoccupied no-man's-land open for

exploration. Such a liminal position

can animate a critically different

reflection on medicine and society, a

reflection that need not accept things

as they are.

ARTHUR KLEINMAN, *1995*

I have worked in the same village in Haiti's Central Plateau since 1983, and every year since has brought more of the misery and miracles that fuel me and my writing. The misery is everywhere; the miracles are discerned, often, by others. A pair of simple examples will suffice. One is from 1984 and the other from 1996. In the former instance, still a student, I was learning the ropes. I've told the story before, erasing myself from the scene in keeping with canonical trends in ethnographic writing:

In January 1984, Église Saint-André was commandeered as a clinic for residents of [Do] Kay and surrounding villages. Present were Dr. Pierre, the Haitian physician then working with Père Aléxis [the Episcopalian priest who directs the Haitian projects described throughout this book], and a few North American doctors and nurses. Early in the morning, the headmaster of the school (Maître Gérard) asked the visiting physicians to see Marie, an adolescent student who had collapsed while doing exercises on the new soccer field. When she regained consciousness, she complained of nausea and a severe headache. Her temperature was normal, and she stated that she had not "recently had a fever." The doctors found her to be quite anemic, but were unsure as to what had caused her collapse. She was given aspirin, a supply of vitamins, and tucked into the school sick bay, where she was to be seen later in the day. At noon it was discovered that Marie had declared herself "much better," and had walked home. With a long line of patients still waiting to see them, the physicians were perfectly satisfied with this response.

The next day, however, Marie slipped into a coma. Père Aléxis brought her and her mother to see Dr. Pierre at the clinic in Mirebalais. Dr. Pierre examined Marie, and said very little other than "malaria." Marie, it was then revealed, had been experiencing intermittent fevers in the preceding weeks. She now presented with the symptoms of cerebral or "pernicious" malaria, and her chances of survival were estimated by Dr. Pierre to be "one or two in ten." Marie was carried to the nearby house of a kinswoman, and Dr.

Pierre followed with injectable chloroquine and other requisite supplies. It was agreed that she would be watched very closely.

She was not watched closely for long—not, at least, in Mirebalais. As I learned from Mme. Aléxis the following day, Marie's father had "somehow rented a vehicle and driver, [come] in the middle of the night, and [taken] the girl." Mme. Aléxis had little else to add. But knowing Marie's family, the rest of the scenario was easy to piece together.

Marie was then eighteen years old, and lived with her parents and siblings in a house a few hundred yards down the road from the school in [Do] Kay. Though soft-spoken, she was one of Aléxis's "leaders," and was active in church activities. Her mother, too, was an Episcopalian, and a regular at Père Aléxis's services. Her father, however, was an irregular churchgoer, and had closer ties to Tonton Mèmè's place of worship (houmfor) in nearby Vieux Fonds. Tonton Mèmè was the Kay region's most well-known voodoo priest (houngan). Marie's father had arrived in the night, confident that doctors could not help his mysteriously felled daughter. Someone was trying to do her in, and he needed to find out who it was. As one of his friends later told me, Marie's father feared that "her illness was not simple. He thought it had an author." And he knew that only a houngan was going to be able to help him divine the author of her illness.

The reactions to this news ranged from dismay (on the part of the visiting physicians, who felt Marie's chances were nil without chloroquine), to weary resignation (evinced by Dr. Pierre, who also believed that Marie would not survive without chloroquine, but felt that there was nothing he could do about it), to angry anxiety (both Père and Mme. Aléxis). Upon hearing the news, Père Aléxis got into his pick-up truck and drove back to Do Kay, in an attempt to "wrest the girl from the clutches of a potentially fatal error." Her father refused to let anyone touch the still comatose Marie, and the priest left empty-handed and angry. A bargaining team then went to the house to ask if Marie could continue her chloroquine treatment there. A deal was struck, and Marie eventually emerged from her coma without any residual effects.

There were, however, residual effects on the community. These included a rift between Père Aléxis and Marie's mother ("as one of my parishioners, she should have prevailed upon her husband to leave their daughter in the care of the physicians"), and a great deal of speculation whether it was the chloroquine or the *houngan* that had saved Marie's life. I learned of these debates in a second-hand manner. Of the dozen or so villagers interviewed about Marie's illness, only one spoke as if there was even a chance that she had been the victim of maleficence. The woman, who was an elderly relative of Marie's mother, insinuated a push and pull between opposing forces:

> I'm not saying that the medicines did not help her. I'm saying that the way the thing happened suggests that it might not be God's illness (*maladi bondjè*) that she had. She is well and then one minute, plop!, she's on the ground. This happens to an old lady, yes, but not a child. . . . Did Marie go to communion on Sunday? I think not, even though she always goes to communion. Could they have been trying to eat her (*manje li*)? I'm not saying that the medicines did not help her, but I'm glad she works in the sacristy. I'm glad she works with Père Aléxis. A man his age should have high blood pressure, lower back pain, and problems with his eyes. But him—nothing.

The expression *manje li*, "to eat her," means to kill through magic, regardless of the specific mechanism (for example, illness, accident, even suicide). The insinuation was that Marie, weakened by her inhabitual abstention from communion, was laid open to attack by a jealous rival. The rival must have engaged the services of a *bokor*, a *houngan* specializing in sorcery, who initiated the train of events necessary to *manje moun nan*—"eat the person."[1]

That's the way I told the story years ago, replete with the requisite local color and references to sorcery. The absent part of the story, of course, is that I was the "bargaining team" who pleaded with Marie's father to let me treat her. To tell the truth, he readily assented—even though the version written years ago does not reveal just how easy it was to convince him. I injected the chloroquine into Marie's muscle, hung intravenous fluids from the rafters of her hut, and found myself on the horns of what I now see as a false dilemma.

The problem as I saw it at the time was this: what is the role of the outsider when confronted with alien cultural institutions, such as those manifest in the desire of Marie's father to counter the spell that laid low his daughter? It's not that I was given to the spineless relativism now native to our own culture. Having by then had malaria a couple of times, I knew first-hand that chloroquine worked. I believed in the power of modern biomedicine, and nothing about this experience changed my perspective. But where I then saw cultures in conflict—and Marie's father as acting to preserve his culture's integrity—I now see the symptoms of unequal access to effective remedies.

It's not that "culture" doesn't matter. Far from it: the father's conviction that his daughter was the victim of sorcery, a conviction grounded in properly Haitian understandings of illness, led to his decision to remove her from the clinic, a decision that the priest correctly identified as potentially fatal. The question is, What does Marie's close call mean at the end of the twentieth century?

Do these events speak to the power and integrity of Haitian cultural traditions? Or do they point instead to inequalities of access which mean that, in rural Haiti, understandings of acute infectious disease even now evolve largely in the absence of effective interventions that are readily available to nonpoor Haitians? Is Marie's a story about rural "beliefs" or rather a story about poverty and its effects on health outcomes among people who share her circumstances? I've spoken about "selective blindness." When an observer witnesses the effects of structural injustice and sees little more than cultural difference, is this not a conflation of cultural difference and structural violence?

The published version also left out the wave of gratitude from Marie and her family and the ambivalence it triggered in me. There were testimonies in church—a miracle!—letters of thanks, hugs and handshakes from everyone, even Marie's father. In fact, I later became the godfather of her first baby, a boy. I was proud and happy, but I remember hearing, even then, a nagging voice in my head.

Yes, said the voice, sarcastically. *It's almost as if she had some treatable infectious disease.*

Fourteen years later, having completed my training as an infectious disease specialist and anthropologist, I hear that voice ever more persistently. The power of biomedical interventions in the Clinique Bon Sauveur, of which I am now medical director, is at times nothing short of astonishing to the children and young adults who come in febrile and chattering and leave, often enough, cured of their infections. A visit, a shot, a pill, a cure—a miracle! But how often are these miracles really reflections of misery?

Take the case of Wilfrid. In Haiti, in the summer of 1996, I had the privilege of hosting one of my medical students from Harvard. During the course of a vaccination clinic in a small village two hours' walk from Do Kay, a community health worker asked us to visit a young man who was "paralyzed from the waist down." He had been to another clinic, we were told, but was later "sent home to die." Since tuberculosis of the spine is the leading cause of lower-extremity paralysis in young adults in rural Haiti, I immediately thought that there was surely something we could do.

A ten-minute walk brought us to the house of Wilfrid, a thirty-three-year-old man who was lying on a straw mat under the small granary near his hut. Wilfrid had a beautiful smile, but he was already wasted; his legs looked like knobby walking sticks. The story he told was straightforward and recounted in a matter-of-fact tone; his voice contained no self-pity. His wife and children stood by silently as he spoke.

Stricken by a fever, Wilfrid had gone to the nearest clinic. There he was given some antibiotics, and the fever fell, but he then developed terrible pain in his right hip. After two weeks, he said, the doctor taking care of him said that she could do nothing more. Because he was going to die, she needed to give his bed to someone else. "Then they put me on this little cot for people who are going to die. My wife said that this wasn't right and came to take me home." That had been three weeks before our meeting, and Wilfrid's fevers had since recurred.

As we looked at Wilfrid, it didn't take long to make a differential diagnosis. Upon examination, it became clear that he was not actually paralyzed; rather, the pain in his right hip was so extreme that he simply couldn't move. A month's immobility accounted for the atrophy and weight loss. Since his hip was affected, and not his spine, as we'd been told, tuberculous osteomyelitis seemed less likely. And his village, we knew, was in the midst of a typhoid epidemic. Because of the high number of treatment failures reported from the nearby clinic, we'd already concluded that the strain was resistant to chloramphenicol.

I will not forget the look on Wilfrid's face, or on that of my student, when I announced that he was not paralyzed, needed and would promptly receive treatment, and therefore would not die. He and his wife were amazed, not by the horrible injustices already meted out to him but by the fact that some of them might be remedied. We made arrangements with community health workers and family members to carry Wilfrid on a stretcher to the road, where we would pick him up and take him to the clinic.

Wilfrid weighed well under one hundred pounds when he reached the clinic. I drained his hip with the help of a spinal needle; finding pus there confirmed the diagnosis of septic arthritis, likely due to *Salmonella typhi*. He was treated for a couple of months with a single, powerful antibiotic, and he walked out of the clinic having regained thirty pounds. Within three months, with the help of the student's careful ministrations, Wilfrid ceased even to limp. A miracle, according to all concerned.

Yes, said the voice. *It's as if he had some treatable infectious disease.*

It would be very dishonest of me to suggest that I was not thrilled by this miraculous recovery. But this time the misery hit harder than the miracle. The conditions that made us look like heroes showed only how little we and our local allies had been able to accomplish. The misery of contaminated water—Wilfrid's wife and son were ill with typhoid, too—was a rebuke to all of us who had spent a decade arguing that educational strategies will not change rates of typhoid when basic sanitation does not exist. We had even started a water-protection project in Wilfrid's village, but it was one of many efforts abandoned during the difficult years after the 1991 coup d'état.

I've called this an ethnographic interlude, but it's really a prelude to the next chapter, which is a properly ethnographic exploration of the slow, painful arrival of AIDS in the village of Do Kay. I can write with some authority on the subject because, through accident of history rather than planning, I was there. Geertz has reminded us that "the ability of anthropologists to get us to take what they say seriously has less to do with either a factual look or an air of conceptual elegance than it has with their capacity to convince us that what they say is a result of their having actually penetrated (or, if you prefer, been penetrated by) another form of life, of having, one way or another, truly 'been there.'"[2]

In rereading my own prose—both in Marie's story, told earlier, and in the chapter to follow—I see numerous signs of this effort to establish authenticity: the insertion of "local color" (Creole words) and of the exotic (sorcery, naturally), with here and there the first-person pronouns of an eyewitness. Eyewitness testimony matters, of course: it isn't just a matter of claiming authenticity. An eyewitness account of the *introduction* of a new and fatal illness can never be written twice—it can be done only one time in any setting, because a plague of these dimensions arrives, and evokes initial reactions, only once. And, in the case of rural Haiti, there is usually no written record—no diary entries, no newspaper clippings, no recordings of radio programs—to consult later.

Infections and Inequalities is not ethnographic in any sense of the word, but it is underpinned by previous ethnographic study, and the complementary narratives and studies presented here build on the messy vagaries of having been there. Notes Kleinman: "The empirical result of this utterly human—because contextualized and uncertain— though professionally disciplined engagement is positioned knowledge; that is, a view from somewhere."[3] The "somewhere" in question has been a shifting locale. Fifteen years after beginning this fieldwork, fifteen years after being there at that fateful moment, I now know that ethnographic work is in a sense apodictic and unlikely to be contested. As the phrase goes, "You had to be there." In terms of people who'd be interested in conducting such research—well, nobody else was there. And this is another reason that I have not elected to write another ethnography, but have instead brought together patients' stories and, with a nod to the sociology of knowledge, critical reanalyses of pressing problems in infectious disease. These stories and analyses are intended to serve as correctives to the lurid exoticism that too often creeps into ethnographic writing about Haiti. At the same time, it is clear that careful ethnography—and perhaps careful ethnography alone—can reveal the strengths and limitations of epidemiologic categories. As the next chapter shows, the "accepted risk factors" for AIDS were even more invalid in rural Haiti than they were in the city. What's more, the advent of AIDS to a Haitian village evoked social responses with obvious implications for AIDS prevention and control. Ethnographic work revealed what was happening "on the ground" when other methodologies were stymied.

6 Sending Sickness

SORCERY, POLITICS, AND CHANGING CONCEPTS
OF AIDS IN RURAL HAITI

Deep in the lungs a cloudiness not clearing;

Vertigo, nausea, slowed heart, thick green catarrh,

Nosebleeds spewing blood across the room—

As if it had conscripted all disease.

Once, finding a jug of homemade corn

Beneath the bed where a whole fevered family

lay head to foot in their own and the others' filth,

I took a draft and split the rest among them,

Even the children, these very children named for me,

who had pulled them into this world—

it was the fourth day and my bag was empty,

small black bag I carried like a Bible.

ELLEN BRYANT VOIGT, *Kyrie*, 1995

Among the new challenges that AIDS presents to anthropology, some are theoretical and not substantially different from the challenges faced by other ethnographers who seek to study, comprehend, and describe new phenomena. Others involve the ethical dilemmas inherent both in the study of a terrible new affliction for which we have only limited therapeutic recourse and in the deeply vexed question of how anthropologists might best contribute to preventive efforts. What follows is a processual ethnography of the advent of AIDS in the small village of Do Kay. While Chapter 5 focused on the historical and practical dynamics of HIV transmission in rural Haiti, this chapter attempts to examine the problems inherent in studying cultural meaning—in this case, the meaning and description of a new illness—while it is taking shape.

The need for a more processual approach to the study of illness representations is most dramatically illustrated when one is witness to the advent of a disorder previously unknown to one's host community. Some of the steps in this process of growing awareness are easily intuited. Before the arrival of the new malady, there exists no collective representation of the disorder; then comes a period of exposure, either to the illness or to rumor of it. With time and experience, disagreement and uncertainty about the nature of the disease may give way to a cultural model shared by the majority of a community.[1]

In studies of illness representations, medical anthropologists have usually investigated the degree to which a model is shared. But when we study a truly novel disorder, a new set of questions pertains. How does cultural consensus emerge? How do illness representations, and the realities they organize and constitute, come into being? How are new representations related to existing structures? How does the suffering of particular human beings contribute to collective understandings, and how much of individual experience is not captured by cultural meaning?

Although this chapter is primarily a study of a cultural model, it is also the story of three individuals with AIDS, for their experience is what made AIDS matter in Do Kay. This account is distilled from a series of interviews dating from 1983–84 to 1990, which reveal not only the role of culture in structuring illness narratives—we already know a great deal about that— but also the ways in which those accounts are elaborated, how they change over time, how representations (also changing) are embedded in narratives, and how they are significant to the experience of illness.

As Chapter 5 described, the first case of AIDS was registered in Do Kay in 1986. For the inhabitants of the village, the advent of a new and fatal disorder was, in the words of one person who lives there, "the last thing"—the last thing, that is, in a long series of trials that have afflicted the rural poor of Haiti.

Because I had already begun to investigate local understandings of AIDS in Do Kay four years earlier, it became possible to document the subsequent elaboration of a fairly detailed and widely shared cultural model of AIDS. By conducting serial interviews with the same people, I was able to document the rate at which consensus was achieved and to discern the events leading to it.[2] Most of these events were of local salience. But important national events also occurred during the course of this study.[3] In 1986, Haiti's long-standing family dictatorship collapsed, which led to changes felt keenly in village Haiti. These changes profoundly affected the process of illness representation, for they substantially altered the ways in which illness and other kinds of misfortune were discussed.

1983-84: "A CITY SICKNESS"

In 1983, when my research began, the word "sida" was often heard in Port-au-Prince. The term had gained currency there following rampant speculation by the North American press that associated AIDS with Haiti. As Chapter 4 details, the CDC in the United States had inferred that Haitians as a group were in some way at risk for AIDS, and the popular press had begun to paint Haitians as the principal cause of the American epidemic.[4]

The effects on Haiti of this association with AIDS were quickly felt and far-reaching.[5] By 1980, tourism had become the country's second largest source of foreign currency, generating employment for thousands living in and around Port-au-Prince. In response to the AIDS scare, however, tourism begin to decline dramatically, forcing the closure of hotels, restaurants, and other businesses and throwing many Haitians out of work. Haitian government officials reacted to this crisis in a manner reflecting the deep contradictions of the Haitian ruling class. Within months one was hearing the classic mixture of antiracist nationalism followed by local repression of those held responsible for "spreading AIDS." These measures did nothing, of course, to counter the collapse of the nation's tourist industry.

As thousands of urban Haitians were left without jobs, the word "sida" took on specific connotations, many of which linked the disease to the media furor over its alleged Haitian origins. Few city dwellers were unaware of the syndrome, though most of them could not have known individuals with AIDS. But the word "sida" was not yet well established in the rural Haitian lexicon. In interviews in early 1984, only one of seventeen Do Kay informants mentioned *sida* as a possible cause of diarrhea. The term never came up during unprompted discourse about tuberculosis, the most common infection among Haitians with AIDS, nor did it figure in talk about diarrhea or other disorders. When I questioned them, fifteen out of twenty villagers said that they had heard of *sida*, and a dozen of them associated certain symptoms or stigmata with this label (although many of these attributes were not in fact commonly seen in Haitians with AIDS). Most of the villagers who spoke of *sida* had heard of the disorder on the radio or during trips to the capital.[6]

Villagers voiced considerable disagreement as to what the chief characteristics of *sida* might be. In the 1983–84 interviews, most mentioned at least one or two of these three aspects of *sida:* the novelty of the disorder, its relation to diarrhea, and its association with homosexuality. Only five noted that *sida* was lethal. Two others asserted that "*sida* is the same thing as tuberculosis." Three villagers believed that *sida* had originally been a disease of pigs. Three were also of the opinion that, despite claims to the contrary made by the foreign press, *sida* had been brought to Haiti by North Americans.

In early 1984, Mme. Sylvain, a thirty-six-year-old market woman, offered this commentary, which was fairly typical of other remarks heard in the village: "*Sida* is a sickness they have in Port-au-Prince and in the United States. It gives you a diarrhea that starts very slowly but never stops until you're completely dry. There's no water left in your body. . . . *Sida* is a sickness that you see in men who sleep with other men."

She had little else to say about the syndrome, although Mme. Sylvain was seldom at a loss for words when sickness was the topic.[7] These preliminary interviews demonstrated that in Do Kay, where illnesses were usually much discussed, *sida* was not. When I asked one villager whether he and his associates were reluctant to speak about *sida*, he responded, "Why should that be? There is no one who says we can't talk about *sida*. But it is nothing that we have seen here. It's a city sickness (*maladi lavil*)."

In the first year of my research, then, all talk about the disorder was prompted by questioning; no illness stories or "therapeutic narratives" about *sida* were forthcoming. The people of Do Kay, already bent under the unremitting burdens of poverty and sickness, had little at stake regarding AIDS. Despite the elaborate explanatory models propounded by several individuals, despite the savvy of market women like Mme. Sylvain, the lack of natural discourse about *sida* and the lack of agreement on its core characteristics suggest that, during the 1983–84 period, no cultural model of AIDS existed in the area around Do Kay.

1985–86: MÉLANGE ADULTÈRE DE TOUT

During the course of 1985–86, relative silence concerning *sida* gave way to discussion of the new illness in the Kay area, and a more widely held representation slowly began to emerge. Villagers began to recount illness stories, but they were invariably the tales of someone else, somewhere else—people who had died in Mirebalais, the nearest market town, or in Port-au-Prince. There was rumor, too, of the mistreatment of Haitians in far-off North America; one villager often spoke of a cousin in New York who had lost her job "because they said she was a Haitian and an AIDS carrier."

Fully eighteen of twenty informants interviewed during this period referred directly to "blood" in our discussions of *sida*, and for many other residents of Do Kay as well, *sida* was a sickness of the blood. Perhaps the most commonly heard observation was that *sida* "dirties your blood" (*li sal san w*). Villagers frequently alluded to "poor blood"—usually a gloss for anemia—as a prodrome of *sida*, and some referred to the dangers of blood transfusion. For example, when Ti Malou Joseph needed a unit of blood during an obstetrical intervention, several villagers observed that, given the "sickness going around" (*maladi deyò a*), a transfusion was tempting fate.[8] For some, it was a question of exposing the transfusion recipient to a microbe (*mikwòb*); for others, one of "mixing bloods that don't go together," causing reactions that eventually "degenerate into *sida*." Several informants began to speak of *sida* as a slow but irreversible process that was invariably fatal.

Others interviewed in the summer of 1985 stated that "bad blood" (*move san*), a somatosocial disorder widespread among Haitian women, put one at risk for *sida*.[9] As Mme. Mathieu put it, "You're very weak when you have *move san*, and you can more easily catch *sida*." Although two of the twenty villagers interviewed that year felt that the new illness was a "very severe form of *move san*," the rest of those who mentioned *move san* underlined the distinctions between it and *sida*. The observations of Mme. Kado, a fifty-one-year-old woman who worked with the activist priest in Do Kay, were typical of the opinions garnered in late 1985:

> [*Sida*] spoils your blood, makes you have so little blood that you become pale and dry. It first causes little blemishes (*bouton*) that rise all over your arms and legs. That tells you that the blood is bad, and makes you think of a simple case of *move san*. But *sida* has no treatment, it's not like *move san*. Anyone can get this, but it is most common in the city.

In much of Haiti, disvalued experiences—shocks, disappointments, anger, fright—may be embodied as disorders of the blood. The significance of this conceptual framework led Hazel Weidman and her co-workers to speak of the "blood paradigm" underlying the health-related beliefs of their Haitian informants in Miami.[10] Within this paradigm are found the causal links between the social field and alterations in the quality, consistency, and nature of blood. During much of 1985–86, preexisting beliefs about blood lent form to vague understandings of *sida*, which was coming to represent an irreversible pollution caused, depending on whom you asked, by blood transfusions, same-sex relations, weakness from overwork in the city, or travel to the United States. The contributions of this paradigm to the emerging representation waned with direct experience of the disorder, however, and the "tuberculosis paradigm" emerged as the more important of preexisting models.

The year 1985 also marked the debut of a preventive campaign conducted by the nation's health authorities. There were songs about *sida* and numerous radio programs, all in Creole and targeted toward the peasantry. Less influential were the many articles in the print media and the posters and billboards declaring *sida* to be a public menace to which all were vulnerable. Although villagers may have known more about the syndrome as a result of these public health efforts, it was not yet a compelling subject of everyday discourse—which was increasingly, if somewhat clandestinely, dedicated to discussion of national-level political events.

The Duvalier dictatorship, in place for almost thirty years, was beginning to totter, and more and more rural Haitians joined the chorus calling for Duvalier's removal. After years of silence, the people of Do Kay lent their voices to this chorus. Because peasants had long been excluded from direct participation in politics, the shift was significant and had an impact on the way that illness was discussed in rural Haiti.

At first, talk of *sida* was simply submerged in all-important discussions of national politics. When the syndrome was addressed, it often seemed that the speaker was invoking it to malign the regime or the United States. On New Year's Day of 1986, several of my friends from Mirebalais joked that Duvalier was a *masisi* (homosexual) who had contracted the syndrome from one of his *masisi* cabinet members. More common, however, were commentaries often dismissed as conspiracy theories. For example, shortly after Duvalier's departure, one market woman in her mid-fifties angrily denounced AIDS as part of "the American plan to enslave Haiti. . . . The United States has a traffic in Haitian blood. Duvalier used to sell them our blood for transfusions and experiments. One of these experiments was to make a new sickness."[11]

Later it became clear that the fall of the Duvalier dictatorship, in February 1986, had given a boost to stories about *sida*. To judge from trends observed in Do Kay and surrounding villages, rural Haitians began to feel that they could speak more candidly about misfortunes in general, and this alteration in the "rhetoric of complaint" may have had a determinant effect on what would prove to be enduring understandings of *sida*.[12]

One of the first slogans to become popular shortly after Duvalier's fall was *baboukèt la tonbe*. A literal English equivalent is "the bridle has fallen off," but the phrase would be better rendered as "the muzzle is off." Although few in Do Kay began openly talking about politics until March, and a full year had elapsed before the adventurous were wholeheartedly joined by a majority of the villagers, the transformation seemed complete by the spring of 1987. Do Kay and surrounding villages saw a sudden proliferation of transistor radios (or at least a sudden surfacing of them). Some persons—men especially—spent entire days cradling their radios, switching from one news program to another. Community councils, drastically overhauled in other villages, were strengthened in the area around Do Kay; meetings that once drew a score or so now often drew well over a hundred people. New groups were formed and set to civic activities such as repairing roads and planting trees. All this was worked into the daily round of gardening and marketing, but the changes stood out nonetheless.

The subject of *sida*, however, was only temporarily submerged in this sea of activity. In Port-au-Prince, many knew people who had died or were ill with the syndrome. Hospitals and sanatoriums were faced with large numbers of *moun sida*—as persons with AIDS were labeled. Haitian researchers continued to document a large and growing epidemic. Government health officials conceded that *sida* was not a public-relations issue but rather a major public health problem.

In the Do Kay area, too, *sida* was once again a regular topic of conversation. In the summer of 1986, questions I posed about the sickness triggered long and elaborate responses. Yet respondents expressed many discrepant ideas. In natural discourse about *sida*, the number of references to blood declined. In interviews conducted late in 1986, only eleven of nineteen informants used the term when speaking at length about the new sickness. Public health campaigns may have contributed to this shift: the more one heard about *sida* on the radio, the less it seemed to resemble other well-known disorders of the blood.

The declining significance of the blood paradigm is suggested by a comment from a 1986 interview with Tonton Sanon, a *doktè fey*, or herbalist. "I'm wondering if it is really a sickness of the blood," he said, "because we know how to put blood in its place. There's a part of it that is in the blood, yes, but it is not only in the blood, and it's not blood that is the principal problem. The problem is in other systems."

He was seconded by others who spoke as if the blood paradigm had been used to assess the nature of *sida* and found wanting. Interviews with other healers revealed a similar lack of accord about the new illness, although some allowed that *sida* was beyond their competence. "Truly it's a sickness that is slippery (*enpwenab*)," observed Mme. Victor, a midwife known for her efficacious herbal remedies. "To this day, they're struggling with it, but they haven't yet found an herbal treatment for it." Another *doktè fey* predicted that "the herbal remedy that will heal *sida* has not yet reached us, but when it does, we'll learn how to use it."[13]

Thus it seemed that, during 1985 and 1986, when mention of *sida* began to stimulate more interest, villagers made an effort to compare the disorder to other illnesses, especially those involving the blood. But *sida* failed to fit neatly into the existing blood paradigm. Lack of a perfect fit between the new disorder and the old framework posed no real problems, as clear and defensible understandings of *sida* were not yet a necessity: no one from Do Kay had fallen ill with the syndrome.

1987: PROTOTYPES AND PROTOMODELS

In many ways, 1987 was the decisive year in the process leading to a shared understanding of AIDS. During the course of that year, a protomodel of illness causation rose to prominence—a model that proved influential in the elaboration of a more stable collective representation of *sida*. By the fall of that year, narratives about *sida* were easily triggered, and it was clear that a consensus—albeit a tenuous one—had emerged.

Interviews conducted in 1987 and afterward revealed that the semantic network in which *sida* was embedded had changed substantially since 1983–84. In 1987, the syndrome was mentioned by over half of those asked to cite possible causes of diarrhea in an adult. The majority also associated *sida* with tuberculosis. Furthermore, ideas about how the new disorder became manifest in the afflicted were more widely shared.

Equally striking was the increasing frequency with which rural people mentioned the social and political origins of illness, including *sida*. There were perhaps two primary reasons for this: first, the unmuzzling of the rural poor had led to a new rhetoric of complaint; and second, and most important, the syndrome had come to matter locally. Someone in Do Kay had fallen ill with *sida*.

Comparing earlier interviews to these later ones reveals the increasing importance of the shift in styles of complaining, triggered by the large-scale political changes. Although I did not alter my interviewing style or methods, the narratives—whether relating a case of diarrhea or some other misfortune—became increasingly tinged with a new political sensibility. Yet "politicization of discourse" is an altogether unsatisfactory description of a far more complicated process. The stories told were superficially similar to those heard earlier, but how tellers gave shape and sense to their stories had changed. For example, in speaking of misfortune, informants' attributions of blame seemed to be changing subtly. Narrative shifts similar to those in the following interviews with Mme. Jolibois abound.

Mme. Jolibois, a young woman who supports her family by working a small patch of land, had traveled from the Kay area to a clinic in a nearby town in February 1984, when her infant son had a bad case of diarrhea. When I interviewed her that year and asked what had caused the diarrhea, she answered, "I don't know what causes it. Microbes, perhaps, or gas from milk. Microbes, especially—they're little bugs that can make children sick. Or it could be my milk. I think he must be getting too old for milk."

In May 1987, over three years after the first interview, she again went to the clinic—the new one in Do Kay. This time a nine-month-old daughter had severe diarrhea. When I asked the same question, "What caused the diarrhea?" she responded, "It's the bad water we have in [my village]. We have to drink it even when it's muddy and full of microbes. It gives the babies diarrhea, and they die, and the government does nothing about it. It's always promises without action (promèt san bay)."

The methodologically minded reader might ask a series of important questions. Were the differences related to the severity of the episode? The sex of the child? Are contextual or performative factors important? Did the ethnographer have closer rapport with the informant years later? Perhaps Mme. Jolibois was simply in a bad or accusatory mood? I slowly discovered that such questions were secondary, however, as similar trends emerged in the discourse of other villagers.

The collapse of the Duvalier regime also had a palpable effect on the way in which AIDS-related accusations were marshaled and used. Conspiracy theories abounded: the Duvalier regime had caused sida, asserted some. Others thought that no, the Duvaliers were too stupid to create a sickness, despite a talent for creating zombies. But the rulers had allowed the people of their nation to be used as guinea pigs in an American plan to stem migration. Referring to the North American suggestion that AIDS originated in Haiti, I heard more than one villager remark, "Of course they say it's from Haiti; whites say all bad diseases are from Haiti."[14] Indeed, accusations against the accusers were perhaps the most prevalent of these commentaries.

The illness of Manno Surpris was the second reason that the same villagers who were aware of, but generally uninterested in, sida in 1984 were universally interested in the syndrome less than three years later. In 1987, sida came to be a social drama that left few adults in Do Kay untouched.[15]

The observations of a young schoolteacher, himself a native of the village in which we worked, suggest the impact of this change. I interviewed him several times between 1983 and 1990. In a 1984 interview, he noted, "Yes, of course, I've heard of [*sida*]. It's caused by living in the city. It gives you diarrhea and can kill you. . . . We've never had any *sida* here. It's a city sickness." A long exchange recorded late in 1987 clearly showed that the man's understanding of *sida* had changed substantially. He could now hold forth at great length about the disorder, especially since he could now refer to the death of Manno Surpris, his fellow schoolteacher: "It was *sida* that killed him; that's what I'm trying to tell you. But they say it was a death sent to him. They sent a *sida* death to him. . . . *Sida* is caused by a tiny microbe. But not just anybody will catch the microbe that can cause *sida*."

Manno's illness and death made a lasting contribution to the cultural model of *sida* that took shape in these years, and this contribution was not substantially lessened by the subsequent deaths from AIDS of other villagers. Manno had moved to Do Kay in 1982, when he became a teacher at a large new school there. He was then twenty-five years old. An enthusiastic and hardworking man, Manno came to be held in high esteem by the school administrators. They entrusted him with a number of public—and remunerative—tasks, including taking care of the village's new water pump and the community pig project, both of which were administered by the priest who ran the school. That an outsider would be granted such favors was deeply resented by some of the villagers, as became clear after Manno fell ill.

In early 1986, Manno began to be bothered by intermittent diarrhea. Superficial skin infections recrudesced throughout the summer; the patches would clear up with treatment, only to appear again—usually on the scalp, neck, or face. Several of us began to worry that Manno might be ill with AIDS, but we felt reassured that an internist in Port-au-Prince did not leap to this conclusion. By December, Manno's decline was drastic, however, and he began to cough. In January 1987, Manno's physician in Port-au-Prince finally referred him to the public clinic for the serologic test used to diagnose HIV infection.

In the first week of February, while awaiting the test results, Manno revealed his fears about the disorder: "Most of all, I hope it's not tuberculosis. But I'm afraid that's what it is. I'm coughing. I've lost weight. . . . I'm afraid I have tuberculosis, and that I'll never get better, never be able to work again. . . . People don't want to be near you if you have tuberculosis."

Manno did indeed have tuberculosis and initially responded well to the appropriate treatment; by March, he no longer looked ill at all. However, he also had antibodies to HIV, which suggested to us that immune deficiency caused by the virus was at the root of his health problems. Although other villagers were not privy to the results of Manno's test, they had other reasons for believing that his tuberculosis was "not simple," as people often remarked. A rumor circulated around Do Kay, which was not dampened by Manno's rapid clinical improvement when his tuberculosis was treated. Manno was the victim, it was whispered, of sorcery. Some angry or jealous rival had consulted a voodoo priest in order to have a *mò*, a dead person, "sent" against Manno.[16] And, as Métraux observed years ago, "whoever has become the prey of one or more dead people sent against him begins to grow thin, spit blood and is soon dead."[17]

Manno's wife was among those I interviewed in 1984. She had then opined that *sida* was "a form of diarrhea seen in homosexuals." Informed in February 1987 by Manno's Port-au-Prince physician that her husband was infected with HIV, she accepted this diagnosis as correct. But Manno and she also knew that he was the victim of sorcery: "They did this to him because they were jealous that he had three jobs—teaching, the pigsty, and the water pump."

Because treatment of a "sent sickness" requires identifying the sorcerers, Manno and his family were increasingly obsessed not with the course of the disease but with its ultimate origin. They consulted a voodoo priest who revealed through divination the authors of the crime. One of those accused of killing Manno was his father-in-law's brother's daughter; another, a schoolteacher, was more distantly related to his wife. The third, the "master of the affair," was also a teacher at the school.

But divination and the indicated treatment could not save Manno. By the end of August, his breathing had become labored. Painkillers no longer relieved severe bone and joint pain, and he was unable to sleep. He vomited after most meals and again lost a great deal of weight. Manno succumbed in mid-September, and his death was the chief topic of "semi-private" conversation for months.

Although a few villagers subsequently cast their analysis in terms of the familiar dichotomy of voodoo versus Christianity, most spoke in less clear-cut terms. A series of oppositions, rather than one, came to guide many of our conversations: an illness might be caused by a "microbe" or by sorcery or by both. An intended victim might be "powerful" or "susceptible." For example, some spoke of the night, years ago, when Manno had been knocked out of bed by a bolt of lightning. The shock, they said, had left him susceptible to a disease caused by a microbe and "sent by someone." An illness as serious as *sida* might be treated by doctors, or voodoo priests, or herbalists, or prayer, or any combination of these.

Anita Joseph, whose story was introduced in Chapter 5, was the second villager to fall ill with *sida*. Anita once referred to herself as "a genuine resident of Kay," but her name did not surface in the census of 1984. The following year, however, a study of villagers' ties to Port-au-Prince and the United States revealed that Luc Joseph had a daughter in "the city." She was, he reported, "married to a man who works in the airport."

Less than two years later, Anita, gravely ill, was brought back to Do Kay by her father. Her husband had died some months previously of a slow, wasting illness. Shortly after Anita's return, I heard that she might have *sida*. The rumor was not surprising, as there was at that time a great deal of talk about Manno's illness. Anita, people remarked, looked the way Manno had earlier that year. Anita had been in the city, and was *sida* not a city sickness?

More than one villager asserted that Anita did not have *sida*, as she was "too innocent." The logic behind this statement was radically different, however, from that underpinning similar statements made in North America. "Innocence" had nothing to do with such things as sexual practices (though some villagers incorrectly believed that Anita had led a "free life"); rather, it underlined the fact that very often a string of bad luck signifies that one is the victim of *maji*, sorcery. Sorcery is never random; it is sent by enemies. Most people make enemies by inspiring jealousy (often through inordinate accumulation) or by their own malevolent magic. Dogged by bad luck, Anita had never inspired the envy of anyone, and she was widely regarded as unwise in the ways of *maji*. Two persons who had earlier explained the role of sorcery in Manno's illness queried rhetorically, "Who would send a *sida* death on this poor unfortunate child?" Since many believed that the sole case of *sida* known in the Kay area had been caused by sorcery, and since Anita was an unlikely victim of this form of malice, it stood to reason, some thought, that Anita could not possibly have *sida*.

Perhaps equally important to this interpretation was the course of Anita's illness. She did not have skin infections or other dermatologic manifestations, as had Manno. Furthermore, as Manno began his final descent, Anita was recovering her strength under a treatment regimen for tuberculosis. When Manno died, Anita was hard at work, as a servant in Mirebalais. That Manno had initially shown a striking response to antituberculous medications (or some other concurrent intervention) seemed irrelevant to the widely shared assessment of Anita's malady. To judge from the total absence of reference to Anita in interviews about *sida* in the autumn of 1987, people widely assumed that she was not in fact ill with the new disorder.

Six months after the initiation of the antituberculous regimen, however, Anita declined precipitously. Her employer in Mirebalais sent her back to Do Kay. Anita had bitter words for the woman, stating that "they just use you up and when they're finished with you, they throw you in the garbage." She also felt that she had made an error in returning to "the same kind of work that got me sick in the first place." By early December, she could no longer walk to the Do Kay clinic; she weighed less than ninety pounds and suffered from intermittent diarrhea. Convinced that she was indeed taking her medications, we were concerned about AIDS, especially when she recounted the story of her husband and his illness.[18]

Her deterioration clearly shook her father's faith in the clinic, as well as her own, and they began spending significant sums on herbal treatments. As her father later reported, "I had already sold a small piece of land in order to buy treatments. I was spending left and right, with no results." Since the treatment for tuberculosis was entirely free of charge, he was obviously spending his resources in the folk sector. Anita's father later informed me that he had consulted a voodoo priest but soon abandoned that tack as he came to agree that his daughter was an unlikely victim of sorcery.

By the close of 1987, many villagers came to believe that Anita was ill with *sida*, and this time the label stuck. The disorder again became a frequent topic of conversation, edged out of prominence only by national politics. Election-related violence in November 1987 had shocked villagers and led many to observe that "things simply can't continue like this." The unpleasant turn of national events was related in several ways to continued hard times for "the people." The advent of *sida* was simply one manifestation of these trials. Another would be the predicted return of the big *tonton makout*, the members of the Duvaliers' security forces who had fled Haiti after February 1986. Several people whispered that some of the cruelest of the *makout*, even those rumored dead, were bringing back new weapons. One twenty-three-year-old high school student from Do Kay informed me that one of the Duvaliers' most notorious henchmen was returning from South America with "newly acquired knowledge." In a manner revealing not his own cynicism but rather that of Duvalierism, the student continued:

> They say he went [to South America] to study the science of bacteriology. He learned how to create microbes and then traveled to [North] America to study germ warfare. . . . They can now put microbes into the water of troublesome places. They can "disappear" all the militant young men and at the same time attract more [international] aid in order to stop the epidemic.

1988: NEW DISORDER, OLD PARADIGMS

In Do Kay, an increased concern with *sida* fit neatly into the almost apocalyptic winter of 1987–88. A military dictatorship was declared. Manno was dead, and Anita was dying. Why was it, several villagers queried, that Do Kay alone of the villages in the area had people sick with *sida*? If the disorder was indeed novel, as most seemed to believe, why should it strike Do Kay first? Some cautioned that the mysterious deaths of two persons from nearby villages may not have been due to "sent" tuberculosis, as had been suspected: perhaps they had died, undiagnosed, from *sida*. Other questions were asked in more hushed tones: was it true that others, such as Dieudonné Gracia and Calhomme Viaud, were also ill with the disorder? Was it really caused by a simple microbe, or was someone at the bottom of it all?

Rumors flew. Some said that Acéphie, another young villager back from Port-au-Prince, had contracted the disorder by sharing clothes with Germaine, a kinswoman from another village in the plateau. A voodoo priest in a neighboring village was reported to have signed a contract with a North American manufacturing firm to "load tear-gas grenades with *mò sida*." Demonstrators who found themselves in a cloud of this brand of tear gas would later fall ill with a bona fide case of *sida*. One person with tuberculosis was cautioned not to cross any major paths, stand in a crossroads, or walk under a chicken roost, lest his malady "degenerate into *sida*."

At the same time, one noted the parallel activities of the village health workers. At the January 1988 meeting of the village health committee, there was talk of initiating a much-needed antituberculosis project—one that would also include the task of HIV education. The community health workers from Do Kay and surrounding villages also held a second conference on *sida*. But these attempts at activism were mired in a widely shared resignation that cast the new disorder as a ruthless killer against which "doctors' medication" could offer little comfort. Dispirited physicians and nurses seemed to feel that any assertions to the contrary were hollow ones, that there really was nothing they could do. The mood was grim and affected us all.

Anita's death in mid-February coincided with an obvious dampening of discussion about the political disorder. What had once seemed a sort of struggle for preeminence between politics and *sida*, with the former eclipsing the latter whenever the political situation was "hot," now appeared to be more like a symbiotic relationship between the two. When the muzzle was off, it was off for everything; when it was applied with new force, those with the most to lose simply spoke less. *Sida* was discussed less and less as villagers, increasingly cowed by the climate of insecurity, stopped discussing national politics.

During the months following Anita's death, the commentaries offered by the villagers seemed to contain a new confidence and clarity. It was widely agreed that she had died of *sida*, yet people noted that her sickness had been outwardly different from that of Manno. It was almost universally accepted that *sida* was a "sent sickness" (that is, the result of sorcery), and yet few believed that Anita had been the victim of sorcery. How did the nascent representation accommodate these disparities? As one of Anita's aunts put it, "We don't know whether or not they sent a *sida* death to [her husband], but we know that she did not have a death sent to her. She had it in her blood, she caught it from him." Her father's lack of success in his quest for magical therapy indicated the virulence of her "natural" illness, not the power of her enemies.

Anita's aunt was reflecting the view of many in Do Kay who had come to understand that a person can contract *sida* in two ways: "You catch it by sleeping with a person with *sida*. You might not see that the person is sick, but the person nonetheless has it in the blood. The other way is if someone sends a *mò sida*. When Manno died, he didn't have *sida* in the blood. They sent a *mò sida* to him, but it wasn't in his blood." The proof that Manno's *sida* was "not simple" was that his wife did not have the disorder. "If it was in his blood, his wife would have it, and she did not," observed one of Anita's aunts. "She had a test, and she did not have it."

By the end of Anita's illness, these distinctions between the causal mechanisms operating in the two cases became sharper and had a great influence on a rapidly evolving collective representation of *sida*. In the eyes of a majority of those interviewed in early 1988, Manno's sickness has been sent to him by a jealous rival or a group of rivals. Anita had contracted *sida* through sexual contact with a person who had the syndrome. She was not the victim of sorcery. Indeed, this would have been a very unlikely fate for Anita Joseph. As villagers repeated many times, Anita had lost her mother, run away at age fourteen, and been forced into a sexual union by poverty. Several people, including Anita's uncle, added that they were all the victims of the dam at Páligre.

Dieudonné Gracia, whose story was also introduced in Chapter 5, was the third villager to fall ill with *sida*. Once again, many features of the case were found to be compatible with the nascent model. He had spent two years in Port-au-Prince, where a relative from Do Kay had helped him find a position as "yard boy" for a well-to-do family. He worked opening gates, fetching heavy things from the car, and tending flowers in the cool heights of one of the city's ostentatious suburbs. Most villagers saw Dieudonné's subsequent illness as the result of an argument with a rival domestic, which had led him to return to Do Kay in 1985. Two informants felt that his *sida* was the result of poison: an invisible "powder" laid in his path. But most villagers, including his family, came to agree that Dieudonné's illness was another "sent sickness," a suspicion later confirmed by a voodoo priest consulted by Boss Yonèl, the young man's father.

Although Dieudonné had visited the clinic for recurrent diarrhea and weight loss in 1986 and early 1987, his cousin, a community health worker, felt that his illness had begun in August of 1987:

> His gums began to hurt him, to bleed easily. He was coughing, and he had diarrhea that went on and on, and fever and vomiting. This was when he was first ill, when he was working in Savanette [a neighboring village]. It was on the way home from Savanette; he got to [another community health worker's] house, and he thought it was a cold. He gave him cold medications, and I took care of him when he came home. He got better.

Dieudonné did seem to improve, which may explain why his illness was not attributed to sent *sida* until about the time of Anita's death, when he was again coughing and complaining of shortness of breath (*retoufman*). By April, his night sweats led us to suspect tuberculosis, and physicians from another clinic offered the same opinion. But Boss Yonèl was reluctant to believe that diagnosis.

During the last week of September 1988, Boss Yonèl took his son to see Tonton Mèmè, a well-known voodoo priest who lived in a neighboring village. Mèmè diagnosed *sida* and stated that it had been sent by "a man living in Port-au-Prince, but from somewhere else." This was seen as confirmation of the original reading of the illness. Tonton Mèmè later explained that *sida* "is both natural and supernatural, because they know how to send it, and you can also catch it from a person who already has *sida*." He spoke, too, of the protections he could offer against the sickness, of charms that could "protect you against any kind of sickness that a person would send to you."

In an interview shortly before his death, Dieudonné observed that "*sida* is a jealousy sickness." When I asked him to explain more fully what he intended by this observation, Dieudonné replied:

> What I see is that poor people catch it more easily. They say the rich get *sida*; I don't see that. But what I do see is that one poor person sends it to

another poor person. It's like the army, brothers shooting brothers. The little soldier (*ti solda*) is really one of us, one of the people. But he is made to do the bidding of the state, and so shoots his own brother when they yell, "Fire!" Perhaps they are at last coming to understand this.

Dieudonné based his optimism on the September 1988 coup d'état, which was initially seen as "deliverance" from a bloody and now universally detested regime, the most recent in a series of military governments. Indeed, a widespread, if ill-advised, optimism was registered among many. But Dieudonné's mood did not match his condition: his diarrhea and cough worsened; his open sores were compared to Manno's dermatologic problems.

Dieudonné died in October. His mother told me that she had been alerted well in advance: "A woman I know came to the clinic. . . . She was sitting with me and said, 'Oh! Look how death is near you! (*gade jan lamò a pre w!*)' So I knew the week before." Although one dissenting opinion held that "tuberculosis killed him because it circulated too long in his blood," most agreed with Dieudonné's cousin, who explained the relationship between tuberculosis and sent *sida*: "Tuberculosis and *sida* resemble each other greatly. They say that 'TB is *sida*'s little brother,' because you can see them together. But if it's a sent *sida*, then it's really [*sida*] that leaves you weak and susceptible to TB. You can treat it, but you'll die nonetheless. *Sida* is TB's older brother, and it's not easy to find treatment for it."

A decade has passed since Dieudonné's death. Villagers still talk about *sida*, and they still greatly fear it—as they do many other misfortunes.[19] Numerous other people, also natives of the region, have since died of AIDS. But it was the experience of the three individuals described here—Manno, Anita, and Dieudonné—that informed the emerging cultural model of *sida*. Based on statements such as that of Dieudonné's cousin and also on more structured interviews, we can summarize the shared understanding of AIDS in this Haitian village in 1989 as follows:

Sida is a "new disease."

Sida is strongly associated with "skin infections," "drying up," "diarrhea," and, especially, tuberculosis.

Sida may occur both "naturally" (*maladi bondjè*, "God's illness") and "unnaturally." Natural *sida* is caused by sexual contact with someone who "carries the germ." Unnatural *sida* is "sent" by someone who willfully inflicts death upon the afflicted. The mechanism of malice is through "expedition (sending) of the dead," in the same manner that tuberculosis may be sent.

Whether "God's illness" or "sent," *sida* may be caused by a "microbe."

Sida may be transmitted by contact with contaminated or "dirty" blood, but earlier associations with homosexuality and transfusion are rarely cited.

The term "*sida*" reverberates with associations, drawn from the larger political-economic context, to North American imperialism, a lack of class solidarity among the poor, and the corruption of the ruling Haitian elite.

For many living in Do Kay, then, two related but distinguishable entities exist: *sida* the infectious disease and *sida* caused by sorcery. One may take preventive measures against each. Condoms are helpful against the former, useless against the latter. Certain charms (*gad* and *arèt*) are widely believed to offer some protection against *sida*-caused-by-sorcery, and people are uncertain about whether the charms will work in the event of exposure to *sida*-the-infectious-disease.

Whether or not this uncertainty is supplanted by consensus remains to be seen, but the rapid rate of change in local understandings of *sida* appears to be a thing of the past. Although the current meanings will be contested and will change, the points just listed summarize a *cultural* model, in that a high level of agreement regarding the nature of the illness has evolved among the villagers. And although we find a significant "surface variation" in models elicited from individuals, even these discrepant versions seem to be generated by a schema that includes these points.[20] In the absence of dramatic group experience, collective accord tends to be more stable and to shift more slowly than individual models, which are often more vulnerable to disputation and subject to rapid revision.

AIDS AND THE STUDY OF ILLNESS REPRESENTATIONS

Tracing the emergence of *sida* as a collective representation illuminates our understanding of AIDS in rural Haiti. Recall that in 1984, when *sida* was a "city sickness," the most frequent comments about it concerned the novelty of the disorder, its relation to diarrhea, and its association with homosexuality. The absence of illness stories regarding the malady call into question the very notion of a cultural model of *sida* at that time. As of October 1988, however, there were many stories to tell. Manno's remained the prototypical case—the standard against which other illnesses could be judged. When two other villagers succumbed to *sida*, their illnesses—though quite different in several ways from Manno's—confirmed many of the tentatively held understandings that had been elaborated in 1987.

While many of the ideas and associations were indeed new, it was clear that *sida*—both the word and the syndrome—came to be embedded in a series of distinctly Haitian ideas about illness. This "adoption" of a new illness category into an older interpretive framework is well documented in the medical anthropology literature. "As new medical terms become known in a society," notes Byron Good, "they find their way into existing semantic networks. Thus while new explanatory models may be introduced, it is clear that changes in medical rationality seldom follow quickly."[21]

The causal language used in reference to *sida* is in many respects similar to that employed when speaking of tuberculosis. For example, the new illness became linked to other diseases that can be caused by malign magic. Just as it is possible to "send a tuberculous death" (*voye yon mò pwatrinè*), so too is it possible to expedite an AIDS death.

The relation of these ideas to voodoo is unclear. Certainly, some of my informants readily ascribed both the ideas and the practice of sorcery to the realm of voodoo. But most of those interviewed made no such Manichean distinctions. Instead of adherence to a neatly defined "belief system," we found almost universal acceptance of the possibility of "sending sickness." This was as true of virulently antivoodoo Protestants as it was of regulars of Tonton Mèmè's temple. In other words, the expedition of the dead is more correctly a *rural Haitian* model of disease causation, rather than one influential among only a particular group of rural Haitians.

It is in the scholarly literature on voodoo, however, that we read about this form of illness causation. Mátraux refers to the "sending of the dead" as "the most fearful practice in the black arts" and describes Haitian understandings of *expédition:* "Whoever has become the prey of one or more dead people sent against him begins to grow thin, spit blood and is soon dead. The laying on of this spell is always attended by fatal results unless it is diagnosed in time and a capable *hungan* succeeds in making the dead let go."[22]

In Haiti, a fatal disease that causes one to "grow thin, spit blood" is tuberculosis until proven otherwise. Once referred to as "little house illness," in reference to the afflicted person's separate sleeping quarters, tuberculosis remains—as the next chapters show—the leading cause of death among rural adults. It is greatly feared. Although some say that virtually any death can be sent, the people of Do Kay and surrounding villages agree that a *mò pwatrinè* (a tuberculous death) is the most commonly dispatched. In research concerning tuberculosis that was conducted before the advent of AIDS, a few informants asserted that only a *mò pwatrinè* can be sent. These same informants, when interviewed in 1988, all agreed that there was a new "expeditable" death to be feared.

These two major causal schemes—sorcery and germ theory—are elaborately intertwined and subject to revision. For example, one person who was widely believed to have been the victim of a *mò pwatrinè* was considered to have "simple" tuberculosis after antituberculous therapy led to her dramatic recovery. The introduction of an effective antituberculous program seems to have led to numerous such reclassifications, although many people continue to associate tuberculosis with sorcery. There is debate as to whether medications are effective against "sent" tuberculosis. As one individual with tuberculosis put it, "If they had sent a *mò pwatrinè* to me, your medicines wouldn't be able to touch it." For *sida,* conversely, some believe that the sent variant is the less virulent form of the disease, since at least magical intervention is possible. The "natural" form is universally fatal.

The term "*sida*" has also become a prominent part of everyday discourse about misfortune. It has been the subject of several nationally popular songs, all of which tend to affirm associations that are important to the Haitian cultural model of AIDS. This discourse reveals the semantic network in which the term is embedded—a network that has come to include such diverse associations as the endless suffering of the Haitian people, divine punishment, the corruption of the ruling class, and the ills of North American imperialism.

Shifts in the rhetoric of complaint became prominent during the political turmoil around the collapse of the Duvalier dictatorship. For example, when the military government organized a carefully policed forum on the mechanics of army-run elections, the gathering was widely termed a "forum *sida*"—a play on the official name "forum CEDHA," the acronym designating the army's proposed electoral machinery. Conspiracy theories, especially those linking AIDS to the machinations of racist "America," are still prominent. Although such expressions emanated from Port-au-Prince, at one time they had a greater effect on the elaboration of rural illness realities than did the virus itself. Some rural regions have to date registered no local cases of *sida*; travel in northern and southern Haiti suggests to me that inhabitants of these regions are nonetheless familiar with many of these expressions.

As an illness caused by sorcery, *sida* stands for local, rather than large-scale, dissatisfaction. Several villagers referred to *sida* as a "jealousy sickness," an illness visited on one poor person by another, even poorer person. As such, the disorder has come to connote an inability of poor Haitians to develop enduring class solidarity. Such observations often served as codas in the illness stories recounted in Do Kay, as when Dieudonné concluded a conversation with a deep sigh and the prediction that "Haiti will never change as long as poor people keep sending sickness on other poor people." These associations are also important in other parts of Haiti. The 1988 pre-Lenten carnival was marred by a widespread rumor of a group of people who planned to spread *sida* by injecting revelers with HIV-infected serum. Some urban Haitians observed that those with such plans must be "poor people hurting their own brothers and sisters."

We can delineate several factors important to the crafting of this illness representation. Most significant, of course, has been the advent of the illness itself, with the suffering and pain it introduces into the lives of individuals and their families. *Sida*'s debut in Do Kay prompted its residents to care about AIDS, to urgently need a means of talking about the new affliction among themselves. Thereafter, Manno's illness served as a prototypical case, which meant that although the presentation and course of subsequent cases were much different, they did not quickly alter ideas about the etiology, symptomatology, and experience of *sida*.

When Manno's affliction made *sida* matter to the people of Do Kay, what "organizing principles" did they use to make sense of a new kind of suffering? The flurry of information that followed the arrival of AIDS in Haiti was important. Billboards, posters, and T-shirts all proclaimed AIDS to be a menace. But it was the radio that ensured a largely non-literate population a certain exposure to biomedical understandings of the syndrome, shaping at least the outline of an emerging cultural model of AIDS. Although the radio did not immediately stimulate strong interest in the disease in rural Haiti, it seems to have provided a vague grid— associations with homosexuality, blood transfusions, "America"—upon which genuinely interested villagers would evaluate their consociates' illnesses. In this respect, the efforts of a local clinic to disseminate information about AIDS—in church, community council meetings, and at conferences for health workers, injectionists, and midwives—supplemented the national media.

These sources of information seem far less significant, however, than the three preexisting meaning structures into which *sida* so neatly fit. The blood paradigm—which posits causal links between the social field and alterations in the quality, consistency, and nature of blood— was invoked early on, before the virulence of *sida* became clear. Disorders of the blood are all considered dangerous and require intervention, but they are rarely refractory to treatment, unlike the new disorder. *Sida* also recalled tuberculosis in many ways. All three villagers who fell ill with *sida* eventually developed active tuberculosis, as do most Haitians with HIV disease. In addition, people soon learned that the new disorder was far more serious than "bad blood"; it evoked significant fear. It was not only disfiguring but also chronic, sapping the body's strength over months or years. Given certain similarities in presentation, it is not surprising that the tuberculosis paradigm has been invoked in reference to *sida*. This long-standing conceptual framework includes elaborate understandings of causality (most notably through sorcery), divination, and treatment. Finally, the microbe paradigm, which has the official blessing of the local representatives of cosmopolitan medicine, has long endured alongside the other explanatory frameworks. It is widely accepted, with provisos, throughout rural Haiti.

These three frameworks—in which are embedded understandings of blood, tuberculosis, and microbes—have been worked into a "master paradigm" that links sickness to moral concerns and social relations. Writing of North America, Taussig observes that "behind every reified disease theory in our society lurks an organizing realm of moral concerns."[23] This is no less true in the Do Kay area, where *sida* has come to represent a "jealousy sickness" and a disease of the poor—victims' moral readings of the sources of their suffering.

Medical anthropology has by and large followed its parent discipline in studying illness representations in cultural, political, and historical contexts. When the illness under consideration is a new one, it is clear that our ethnography must be not only alive to the importance of change but also accountable to history and political economy.[24] AIDS, an illness that "moves along the fault lines of society," demands nothing less.[25]

Such a mandate is no license to give short shrift to the lived experience of the afflicted, however. Indeed, by attending closely to the understandings of the ill and their families, we are led to precisely this conclusion. I think of the words of Manno, who said of his disorder: "They tell me there's no cure. But I'm not sure of that. If you can find a cause, you can find a cure." Manno's search for a cause was the search for the enemies who had ensorcelled him, and it was guided by an assessment of his relations with those around him. Who was jealous of his relative success in the village?

Anita, even younger than Manno and a native of the village, was not a victim of sorcery. In contrast to the etiologic theories advanced by Manno and his family, Anita felt that she had "caught it from a man in the city." The rest of her analysis was more sociological, however, as she added that the reason she had a lover at a young age was "because I had no mother." After the death of her mother, she explained, her family's poverty deepened, and she felt that the only way to avoid starvation was to leave the village and go to the city.

Anita was equally insistent regarding the cause of her family's poverty. "My parents lost their land to the water," she said, "and that is what makes us poor." If there had been no dam, insisted Anita, her mother would not have sickened and died; if her mother had lived, Anita would never have gone to the city; had she not gone to Port-au-Prince, she would not have "caught it from a man in the city."

Neither the dam nor the AIDS epidemic would have been as they are if Haiti had not been caught up in a network of relations that are political and economic as well as sexual. Dieudonné underlined this point on several occasions. Like Manno, he was a victim of sorcery; like Anita, he tended to cast things in sociological terms. Dieudonné voiced what have been called "conspiracy theories" regarding the origins of AIDS. On more than one occasion he wondered whether *sida* might not have been "sent to Haiti by the United States. That's why they were so quick to say that Haitians gave [the world] *sida*." When asked why the United States would wish a pestilence on Haitians, Dieudonné had a ready answer: "They say there are too many Haitians over there now. They needed us to work for them, but now there are too many over there." A history of Haiti's entanglement in this international network should inform any understanding of *sida* as "sent sickness." The spread of HIV across national borders has taken place within our lifetimes, but the conditions favoring the rapid, international spread of a predominantly sexually transmitted disorder were established long ago and further heighten the need to historicize any understanding of this pandemic.

7 The Consumption of the Poor

TUBERCULOSIS IN THE LATE TWENTIETH CENTURY

Like the philosopher's stone, a cure for

consumption will continue, we apprehend,

to be a desideratum for ages yet to come.

Boston Medical and Surgical
Journal, 1843

In 1995, more people died of TB than in any

other year in history. At least thirty million

people will die from tuberculosis in the next

ten years if current trends continue. Millions

more will watch helplessly as friends and

family members waste away, racked with

coughing and sweating with fever. They may

wish that medical science could cure this

terrible disease. The truth is, medical science

can. Since 1952, the world has had effective

and powerful drugs that could make every

single TB patient well again.

WORLD HEALTH
ORGANIZATION, *1996*

BACK WITH A VENGEANCE?

The World Health Organization recently announced that in 1996 alone some three million persons died of tuberculosis.[1] Not since the turn of the century, when tuberculosis was the leading cause of young adult deaths in most U.S. cities, has the disease claimed so many lives. Tuberculosis, we're told, has returned "with a vengeance."[2] In the language of the day, it's an "emerging infectious disease." In scientific publications and in the popular press, the refrain is the same: tuberculosis, once vanquished, is now emerging to trouble us once again.

According to many of the voices echoed in this book, tuberculosis has been with us all along; only from a highly particular point of view can it be seen as an emerging, or even a "reemerging," disease. "Thinking in terms of a returned tuberculosis," objects Katherine Ott, "obscures the unabated high incidence of tuberculosis worldwide over the decades."[3] Those who experience tuberculosis as an ongoing concern are the world's poor, whose voices have systematically been silenced. Yet they deserve a hearing, if for no other reason than that the poor infected with the tubercle bacillus are legion. Some estimate that as many as two billion persons—a third of the world's population—are currently infected with quiescent but viable *Mycobacterium tuberculosis*. This figure corroborates another: tuberculosis remains, at this writing, the world's leading infectious cause of preventable deaths in adults.[4]

Tuberculosis is thus two things at once: a completely curable disease and the leading cause of young adult deaths in much of the world. As we approach the end of the millennium, it's instructive to compare our circumstances to the situation that prevailed at the end of the previous century. At that time, Robert Koch had recently identified the tubercle bacillus, but no effective treatment existed. "Consumption" was the leading cause of death and the most feared of diseases. "During the late nineteenth century," notes Ryan, "there was a growing fear that the disease might destroy European civilization."[5]

Although TB's victims during the eighteenth and nineteenth centuries included members of all classes, it has always disproportionately affected the poor. In the 1830s, for example, English mortuary registers revealed that although tuberculosis deaths were common, they were increasingly so at the lower end of the social ladder: "the proportion of 'consumptive cases' in 'gentlemen, tradesmen, and laborers' was 16, 28, and 30 percent respectively."[6] The affluent could "take the cure" in a number of ways—they could travel to different climes or enjoy protein-rich diets—but case-fatality rates were high among all those with "galloping consumption."

With the advent of improved sanitary conditions and the development of food and trade surpluses, tuberculosis incidence declined in the industrializing nations, particularly in those communities and classes that enjoyed the greatest benefits of these transformations. Still, tuberculosis remained common and patterned in its distribution. In 1900, annual death rates from tuberculosis for white Americans approached 200 per 100,000 population. "Among black Americans," adds historian Barbara Rosenkrantz, "the figure was 400 deaths per 100,000, approximately the same level recorded in the middle of the nineteenth century for the population as a whole."[7] Black Americans were thus enjoying the fruits of medical progress with a fifty-year lag.

Technology has often been presented as the remedy for social ills, and the development of effective tuberculosis chemotherapy was hailed as the beginning of the end of the disease. But the poor remained much more likely to become infected and ill with M. tuberculosis. When they were sick with complications of tuberculosis, they were more likely to receive substandard therapy—or no therapy at all. In the years after World War II, those with access to the new antituberculous medications could expect to be cured of their disease. Who had access to streptomycin and PAS in the late 1940s? Fortunate citizens of the United States and a handful of European nations, all with well-established and encouraging trends in tuberculosis incidence that predated effective chemotherapy. Thus risk, though never evenly shared, became increasingly polarized.

By mid-century, tuberculosis was still acknowledged as a problem in certain quarters, but it was becoming less and less of a concern. One historian has argued that "TB had all but disappeared from public view by the 1960s."[8] The reasons for this invisibility stem in part from the decreasing absolute incidence in wealthy nations and in part from persistent patterns of differential susceptibility. Writing in 1952, René and Jean Dubos observed that "while the disease is now only a minor problem in certain parts of the United States, extremely high rates still prevail in the colored population." Nor were poor outcomes distributed merely by race. Within racial categories, differential risk remained the rule. The case-fatality rate in whites, noted these authors, was "almost seven times higher among unskilled laborers than among professional persons."[9] Ironically, then, the advent of effective therapy seems only to have further entrenched this striking variation in disease distribution and outcomes. Inequalities operated both locally and globally: the "TB-outcome gap" between rich and poor grew, and so too did the outcome gap between rich countries and poor countries.

In short, the "forgotten plague" was forgotten in large part because it ceased to bother the wealthy. In fact, if tuberculosis is reexamined from the point of view of those living in poverty, a radically different picture emerges. In this century, at least, tuberculosis has not really emerged so much as *reemerged from the ranks of the poor*.[10] One place for diseases like tuberculosis to "hide" is among poor people, especially when the poor are socially and medically segregated from those whose deaths might be considered more significant. Who are these throwaway people? We begin our process of rethinking by examining the life histories of some people afflicted by the disease.

JEAN

Jean Dubuisson, who has never been sure of his age, lives in a small village in Haiti's Central Plateau, where he farms a tiny plot of land. He shares a two-room hut with his wife, Marie, and their three surviving children. All his life, recounts Jean, he's "known nothing but trouble." His parents lost their land to the Péligre hydroelectric dam—a loss that plunged their large family into misery. Long before he became ill, Jean and Marie were having a hard time feeding their own children: two of them died before their fifth birthdays, and that was before the cost of living became so intolerable.

And so it was a bad day when, some time in 1990, Jean began coughing. For a couple of weeks, he simply ignored his persistent hack, which was followed by an intermittent fever. There was no clinic or dispensary in his home village, and the costs of going to the closest clinic (in a nearby town) are prohibitive enough to keep men like Jean shivering on the dirt floors of their huts. But then he began having night sweats. Night sweats are bad under any conditions, but they are particularly burdensome when you have only one sheet and often sleep in your clothes.

Marie insisted that it was time to seek professional treatment for Jean's illness. But it was already late September, Jean argued, and school would be starting soon. There would be tuition to pay, books and notebooks to buy, school uniforms to sew. Jean did not seek biomedical care; he instead drank herbal teas as empiric remedies for the *grip*, a term similar to "cold" in North American usage.

Jean's slow decline continued over the course of several months, during which he lost a good deal of weight. The next event, in the story told by Jean and Marie, was when he began to cough up blood, in late December of 1990. Hemoptysis is common in rural Haiti, and most people living there do not believe that the *grip* can cause it. Instead, Jean and his family concluded that he was *pwatrinè*—stricken with tuberculosis—and they knew that he had two options: to travel to a clinic or to seek care from a voodoo priest. These were not mutually exclusive options, but, as Jean had no enemies, he concluded that his tuberculosis was due to "natural causes" rather than to sorcery. Emaciated and anemic, he went to the clinic closest to his home village.

At the clinic, he paid $2 for multivitamins and the following advice: eat well, drink clean water, sleep in an open room and away from others, and go to a hospital. Jean and Marie recounted this counsel without a hint of sarcasm, but they nonetheless evinced a keen appreciation of its total lack of relevance. In order to follow these instructions, the family would have been forced to sell off its chickens and its pig, and perhaps even what little land they had left. They hesitated, understandably.

Two months later, however, a second, massive episode of hemoptysis sent them to a church-affiliated hospital not far from Port-au-Prince. There Jean, still coughing, was admitted to an open ward. We were unable to review his records, but we know that he stayed for a full two weeks before being referred to a sanatorium. During his stay, Jean was charged $4 per day for his bed; at the time, the per capita income in rural Haiti was about $200 a year. When the hospital's staff wrote prescriptions for him, he was required to pay for each medication before it was administered.

Thus, although Jean could not tell us exactly what therapies he received while an in-patient, he knew that he actually received less than half of the medicine prescribed. Furthermore, the only meals Jean ate in the hospital were those prepared by Marie; most Haitian hospitals do not serve food.

Jean continued to lose weight, and he simply discharged himself from the hospital when the family ran out of money and livestock. He did not go to the sanatorium. Needless to say, the cough persisted, as did the night sweats and fever. "We were lucky, though," added Jean. "I stopped coughing up blood."

After reaching home, Jean, bedridden, was visited by a cousin who lived in Bois Joli, a small village served by Proje Veye Sante, which was then sponsoring the comprehensive tuberculosis-treatment project described in the next chapter. The program, which included financial aid and regular visits from community health workers, had been designed for people like Jean Dubuisson and for a country like Haiti—that is, it was designed for poor and hungry people with tuberculosis who receive shabby treatment wherever they go. Unfortunately, the project then served the permanent residents of only sixteen villages and was based in a village over two hours from Jean's house. "Several [villagers] had benefited from it," recalled Jean's cousin, "so I suggested that he move to Bois Joli, as then he would be eligible for this assistance."

Marie Dubuisson "took down the house" and moved her husband and children to Bois Joli. "We didn't have a tin roof or good land," she added philosophically, "so it wasn't as bad as it might have been. And Jean needed the treatment." The skeletal man with sunken eyes and severe anemia began therapy in May of 1991. Jean gained eighteen pounds in his first three months of treatment. His oldest daughter was found to have tuberculosis of the lymph nodes, and she too was treated.

Jean was cured of his tuberculosis, but this cure, in many respects, came too late. Although he is now free of active disease, his left lung was almost completely destroyed. He is short of breath after only minimal exertion. Marie now does most of the manual labor, depending on her daughter (who was also cured) for assistance in carrying water and hoeing. "I have a hard time climbing hills," Jean reports, surveying the steep valley before him. "And that's a bad thing when you're trying to get by up in the hills."

CORINA

Corina Bayona was born in 1942 in Huánuco, in Peru's Central Sierra. Like most of the region's poorer peasants, her parents found it increasingly difficult to wrest a living from the unforgiving countryside. When Corina married Carlos Valdivia, both had dreams of escaping the harshness of rural life. A son, Jaime, was born before Corina was twenty.

In 1974, the three of them emigrated to Carabayllo, the new and sprawling slum north of Lima, one of Latin America's most rapidly growing cities. The edges of the settlement consisted of "*invasiones*"—dry and dusty slopes dotted with ramshackle shelters built first of straw and cardboard and plastic and then rebuilt in dun-colored brick only years later, when the squatters no longer feared that they would be removed by force. To settlers and to visitors alike, the steep and treeless fringes of Carabayllo looked like the surface of the moon.

Soon Corina, Carlos, and Jaime moved into a one-room house. During the 1970s and 1980s, Corina worked as a maid in a schoolteacher's house; Carlos worked as a night watchman in the industrial area south of Lima. Their house eventually had electricity, if no running water, and Corina and Carlos were able to send Jaime to high school. Carlos recalls this time as relatively secure, despite the political violence that often marked the city. Unemployment was high in Carabayllo, although not as high as it would later become, and they were lucky to have two jobs, especially since their son's new wife and baby precipitously added two more mouths to feed in the mid-1980s.

At some point in 1989, Corina began coughing. Initially, she attempted to treat herself with herbal remedies, primarily because she was unable to visit the clinic. Although a public health post was based nearby, it was closed during the hours that Corina was in Carabayllo. What Corina lacked most was time: it took her more than two hours on public buses to commute to work each day. When her cough worsened, she finally went to the post, where a doctor raised the possibility of tuberculosis. A smear of her sputum revealed the tubercle bacillus, and she began standard antituberculous therapy.

In August of 1990, shortly after Alberto Fujimori was elected president of Peru, the urban poor underwent what they later termed *fujishock*—the

rapid implementation of one of the most draconian structural-adjustment policies in the hemisphere. Inflation spiraled, and public services,
including health care, were trimmed back sharply.[11] Soon Carlos was out
of work.

In the midst of all these problems, Corina began coughing again. More
sputum was collected for a smear, which was positive, and for culture.
When Carlos later returned for the culture results, however, he was informed that the specimen had been misplaced. In April of 1991, after
more delays and worsening symptoms, Corina was formally diagnosed
with relapsed pulmonary tuberculosis. Given the health post's inconve-
nient hours and long waits—and also, as one of her doctors noted, the significant stigma associated with tuberculosis—she began receiving treatment at a private clinic.

What Corina gained in privacy and convenience she lost in increased
costs. As was not uncommon in those months after *fujishock*, the family's
meager savings were soon expended; Corina was unable to complete her
treatment. As her husband recalls it, they could afford to buy only two of
the four drugs prescribed.[12] Corina's condition worsened, and she became unable to work. When she next sought care, this time in a public
health center in Carabayllo, physicians there discovered that she did not
respond to standard therapy. When her condition worsened still further,
in April of 1991, she was advised to seek care in a hospital.

Corina first presented to a private university teaching hospital, but she
was unable to purchase the medications and supplies prescribed. She
was referred to the public facility not far away. At the private hospital,
Corina had been told that she would have to pay for supplies; at the public facility, where supplies were extremely scarce, she was told that she
must bring her own—including syringes, gloves, and gauze. Further, Corina had the ill fortune to arrive at this hospital just before the national
health workers' strike, which was called in response to the new government's massive cuts in public spending. During the strike, most ambulatory treatment was simply suspended; Corina received, in essence, no
care for her tuberculosis during this time.

In August of 1991, shortly after the strike ended, Corina returned for
her medications. A physician roundly upbraided her: "Señora, it's your
own fault that you did not complete your treatment. Why didn't you

come before?" Brusquely, he sent her to yet another facility on the grounds that she was not from that hospital's catchment area. This third hospital, though close to the Valdivia household, was not highly regarded, and Corina complained that there too she received a cool welcome. She was summarily referred back to the local health post for her care.

Dr. Raúl García, who directs Socios en Salud, the Peruvian community-based organization described in Chapter 1, had just initiated a health survey of Carabayllo. He met Corina in the course of inquiring about drug-resistant tuberculosis in the area. She was, he recalls, scarred by her interactions with the health care system. "Every time she went to the hospital, the physicians were mean or impolite to her. They had labeled her as noncompliant." Thus branded, Corina "felt attacked." "She was filled with fear," continued Dr. García. "She had resolved not to return to seek care at the health center."

Carlos Valdivia was troubled by this resolution, for Corina continued to worsen. She coughed incessantly and became short of breath, even at rest. Her son, still living at home, worried for his mother. "You should go back to the health center," he pleaded, "so that they will cure you." But soon Jaime began to cough as well. "He didn't want to go either," recalled Dr. García, "because he didn't want to be treated the way they had treated his mother." Eventually Jaime sought treatment at the local post, but he too failed to respond to standard therapy.

For the next three years, Corina and Jaime lived with active pulmonary tuberculosis. Their household, wracked by coughing, was increasingly tense. Jaime's wife left, leaving behind their two infants, and Carlos began to drink. Late in the summer of 1994, Corina began to cough up blood. When at last she sought care for this condition, physicians documented that her infecting strain had become resistant to all first-line anti-tuberculous drugs except ethambutol. For reasons that remain unclear, the doctors then prescribed those same ineffective medications for her again. Corina of course failed to respond to these agents—and, worse, she had a life-threatening reaction to one of them in November. Shortly thereafter, Corina was advised to give up completely on her "futile" efforts to treat her disease.

But Corina and her family were not so easily dissuaded. Upon inquiring, they learned that other drugs were available, although the public health system could not provide them free of charge. Among the drugs prescribed by a pulmonologist were two new agents, ciprofloxacin and ethionamide, with an estimated cost of 500 *soles* a month—eight times her husband's income when he'd been fortunate enough to have a job.

Carlos Valdivia, seeing his family dying before him, each month searched high and low for 500 *soles* for his wife and for his son, because by then it had become clear that Jaime also had drug-resistant tuberculosis. Sometimes Carlos succeeded; often he did not. "What unemployed person in Caraballyo could find 1000 *soles* a month?" reflected Carlos sadly. His son died in December of 1995, leaving behind two small children.

Corina, finding herself the primary caregiver for her grandchildren, found new reasons to fight for survival. Dr. García recalls her saying, "I thought that I'd lived long enough until I had these two children to take care of. All I ask is for God to let me live in order to take care of them." Through the efforts of a local community-based organization, Corina eventually received therapy with a multidrug regimen designed for resistant tuberculosis disease. The medications were free, but she soon had another adverse reaction: bruises erupted on her legs. A pulmonologist advised her to stop taking all of her medications and recommended another culture of her sputum.

In February 1996, one week before Corina died, Carlos went to the health post with yet another sputum sample. The plan, he knew, was to find other medications that his wife might be able to take. Suddenly, however, Corina became severely short of breath. Carlos took her to the clinic, and an auxiliary nurse subsequently tried to place her in two different hospitals. In the emergency room of the teaching hospital, the staff informed Corina: "We have nothing we can do for you; your case is too chronic." After that, Corina stated that she would not return to the local public hospital, to which she had been again referred. "I would rather wait for the end at home than go back there," she said. This time, she did not have long to wait.

CALVIN

Calvin Loach was born in New York City in 1951. His parents were both from the Carolinas. Shortly before Calvin's birth, they had emigrated to the city hoping to find steady work and respite from the racism that had so limited their economic opportunities in the South. New York, they found, was not much better. As Calvin and his two sisters were growing up, their father worked in a series of unrewarding and short-lived jobs; later, and for many years, their mother worked in the medical records department of a Brooklyn hospital.

Calvin attended public high school, where his academic performance was fairly unremarkable, and graduated in 1969. There was talk, at the time, of his attending a local community college, but Calvin never completed an application. In the second month of his second job, at age nineteen, Calvin was drafted into the U.S. Army.

Calvin rarely spoke about his tour of duty in Vietnam. He saw active combat in April 1971 and was part of a platoon that sustained heavy fire and loss of life. Calvin was not wounded by gunfire, but during a march in rough terrain he sustained a penetrating wound to the sole of his right foot. This injury soon became infected, eventually requiring surgery and intravenous antibiotics. It subsequently became the source of many problems for Calvin.

Another problem stemming from Calvin's tour of duty concerned heroin. In one telling, Calvin linked the use of opiates to the chronic pain that resulted from his injury; in another account, his regular use of heroin preceded this injury by several months. In any case, it was in Vietnam, and not in New York, that Calvin first used the drug, which was inexpensive, readily available, and (according to many) widely used by the increasingly demoralized U.S. soldiers.

In 1972, Calvin returned to New York, where he lived with his mother and one of his sisters; his father had returned to North Carolina. Although he did drink and smoke, sometimes heavily, Calvin initially did not use heroin in the United States; at that time, he knew no one else who was involved with the drug. It was during a visit to Boston, where his mother's cousins owned part of a convenience store, that Calvin was reintroduced to heroin and also to cocaine. From the late 1970s until 1992, Calvin used heroin, sometimes steadily and sometimes intermittently.

Most social histories obtained from his medical records suggest that Calvin never had a steady job after Vietnam, but a more thorough interview, by a social worker at a Boston-area Veterans' Administration hospital, documented more than three years of full-time employment in a furniture warehouse. At that time, Calvin was living with a woman who had previously worked for his cousins. His girlfriend told another social worker that Calvin had turned again to heroin after he lost this job in 1982. This girlfriend strongly discouraged his drug use, and it led her to leave him.

In 1991, Calvin was hospitalized for an episode of staphylococcal endocarditis, which permanently damaged one of his heart valves. During this hospitalization, Calvin's old foot injury became increasingly painful and began to drain pus. He was diagnosed with osteomyelitis and received two months of therapy for the infection.

It was during this hospital stay, which lasted almost a month, that Calvin developed a dislike for the hospital milieu; the feeling, it seems, was mutual. Medical records describe Calvin as "difficult" and, in one instance, "verbally abusive." The word "noncompliant" is found throughout his records, although it is not entirely clear why: Calvin was well on his way to completing difficult therapy for endocarditis and osteomyelitis, and in the previous year he had used an antihypertensive medication with regularity.

By the time Calvin was referred for expert management of his addiction, he had already spent a month withdrawing from narcotics, without the help of opiates or benzodiazepines. By his account, he did not use heroin again, although he later received methadone.

Some months later, in the spring of 1992, Calvin began to cough. A heavy smoker, he initially attributed the cough to bronchitis, which he'd had intermittently for years. He was reluctant to return to the VA clinic. When he began to experience fevers and drenching sweats, Calvin was sure that he had AIDS; this made him even less enthusiastic about seeking medical care. These symptoms eventually drove him to the emergency room, however, and there he was promptly diagnosed not with AIDS but with pulmonary tuberculosis.

Calvin initially responded to a three-drug regimen, which he took for several weeks. He felt that one drug—it's not clear which one, though it was not isoniazid—made him itch, and so he stopped taking it. Cultures later revealed that his infecting strain was resistant to isoniazid. Thus, although public health officials believed that Calvin was taking two effective agents, he was actually taking only one. It is difficult to know, in retrospect, how much of the incorrect treatment Calvin received was physician-directed. It is clear that he reported his distressing itch to his private physician and was instructed to "take pyridoxine with isoniazid"—even though it had been demonstrated by then that his strain of TB was resistant to isoniazid. Calvin was also given conflicting information regarding the interaction of methadone with his antituberculous drugs: the public health nurse, who seemed concerned and better informed than his doctor, worried about such an interaction; his internist dismissed this possibility.

About six months into therapy, Calvin noted that his cough was worsening. A chest radiograph suggested relapse, although sputum studies, urged by a tuberculosis outreach worker, did not reveal the tubercle bacillus in his lungs. His internist then added another drug to Calvin's regimen. Although his laboratory results were reviewed, his documented resistance to isoniazid must have been missed again, because the drug was continued.

Calvin felt better, but his improvement was short-lived. By December 1992, reported the tuberculosis outreach worker, Calvin "felt as sick as he had ever been." He continued to take his medications, but he did not return to either the public health clinic or the VA clinic. In January, quite possibly with active pulmonary disease, Calvin "took off," by bus or by train, for New York City.

Calvin's internist, an affable but busy man, subsequently attributed his patient's poor response to "his HIV infection." When reminded that, in fact, multiple serologies had revealed Calvin to be HIV-negative, the physician recalled that his patient's infecting strain of M. tuberculosis was "mildly resistant." He further ventured that Calvin, "notoriously noncompliant," was just "not with the program."

In any case, Calvin's doctor never heard from him again. When New York public health authorities created a central information bank about tuberculosis patients, Calvin Loach's name was not among those listed.

MAKING SENSE OF MISERY:
CRITICAL PERSPECTIVES ON TUBERCULOSIS

Jean, Corina, and Calvin all had unfavorable outcomes. At what point in the trajectories of their lives were their fates sealed? Were their experiences typical of what it's like to have tuberculosis at the end of the twentieth century?

Dr. García, who met Corina near the end of her life, remarked that her experience revealed to him "the significance of external factors and their effects on the lives of poor people. These factors determined whether Corina lived or died." Critical perspectives on tuberculosis must ask how social forces become manifest in the morbidity of unequally positioned individuals in increasingly interconnected populations. Poverty, social inequality, economic policy, war, discrimination along lines of race and gender and class, medical incompetence—which forces were significant in structuring the risks faced by Jean, Corina, and Calvin as well as their poor outcomes?

Take the cases one by one. Jean's experience is typical of those who suffer from tuberculosis in Haiti. As Haiti produces few nonagricultural products, it's safe to say that Jean is a member of its only truly productive class: the rural peasantry. But membership in that class brought him certain "birthrights." For example, Jean is, de facto, a member of the poorest class in the hemisphere. From the day he was born, he was ensured the "right" not to attend school, to have no access to electricity or safe drinking water, and to have little access to medical care. Jean was also ensured no role whatsoever in the running of the country that he and those like him were supporting. He was born, as the Haitians say, with a *baboukèt*, a muzzle, on his mouth. In fact, Jean fared better than many Haitian peasants, since tuberculosis is the leading cause of death in his age group. But delays in therapy meant permanent damage to Jean's lungs, forever compromising his ability to feed his family—a precarious enough enterprise in contemporary Haiti, even for the hardy.

Corina similarly typifies the experience of Latin Americans living with multidrug-resistant tuberculosis. Although she may have been originally infected with a drug-resistant strain of *M. tuberculosis,* it is equally probable that her disease became resistant during the course of intermittent and poorly conceived therapy. Her son Jaime, however, was likely to have been infected with a drug-resistant strain from the beginning. How common are such experiences in Peru? The country has been praised for its greatly improved tuberculosis-control program, which has systematized the diagnosis and treatment of the disease, made first-line medications more widely available, and instituted directly observed therapy.[13] But

Corina did not fit into the prevailing algorithm, which does not take account of increasing drug resistance on the part of the bacillus; subsidized retreatment schemes, while available, are inadequate for patients like her.

Indeed, while attention is focused on the detection and control of susceptible tuberculosis disease, cases such as Corina's will inevitably take on greater epidemiologic significance. Corina was sick and infectious for at least six years, as Jaime's tragic death reveals. She worked during most of those years, taking crowded buses across Lima twice a day. At this writing, hundreds of cases of highly resistant tuberculosis have been documented in northern Lima; with the exceptions noted in Chapter 1, virtually none of these patients are receiving appropriate therapy. All of them may be presumed to be infectious.

What of Calvin's experience in the United States, a country vastly more wealthy than Peru (although Peru itself boasts a per capita income ten times higher than that registered in rural Haiti)? Calvin was probably registered as one of the thousands of "excess cases" in 1991. As an African American and an injection drug user, he fit the bill: the brunt of the recent epidemic has been borne by U.S. citizens living in poverty, many of them people of color, as a review by McBride makes clear.[14]

Nor was Calvin's clinical course atypical of the lot of the U.S. poor with tuberculosis. Although his fate is unknown, he clearly received inappropriate care and was "lost to follow-up." This was much less common in Massachusetts than in New York, where dismantling of the tuberculosis-control program had made it difficult to ensure successful completion of therapy. In 1989, for example, fewer than 50 percent of New York tuberculosis patients who began treatment could be declared cured.[15] In one study conducted in Harlem Hospital, almost 90 percent of patients did not complete therapy for their disease.[16] An overview from the New York City Department of Health paints a grim picture:

> By 1992, the situation in New York City looked bleak. The number of cases of tuberculosis had nearly tripled in 15 years. In central Harlem, the case rate of 222 per 100,000 people exceeded that of many Third World countries. Outbreaks of multidrug-resistant tuberculosis had been documented in more than half a dozen hospitals, with case fatality rates greater than 80 percent, and health care workers were becoming ill and dying of this disease.[17]

Did Calvin also have multidrug-resistant tuberculosis? Although resistance to more than one drug was never documented, Calvin was put at high risk of developing resistance and of infecting others when his physician continued to give him a medication to which the strain was resistant and later added a single drug to an already failing regimen—a well-known recipe for generating drug resistance. In reviewing the histories of patients with drug-resistant tuberculosis who had been referred to a leading hospital in Colorado, Mahmoudi and Iseman discovered an average of 3.9 physician-directed errors per patient.[18]

Medical errors are readily discerned in the other cases as well, and this mismanagement is linked to the patients' poverty. Jean saw a nurse and two physicians and spent two weeks (along with all his family's savings) in a hospital before receiving effective antituberculous therapy elsewhere. Furthermore, the long duration of his active disease, including his time on an open ward, helps to explain why transmission continues apace in settings like Haiti. Corina's initial sputum sample was lost, and her providers mistook drug resistance for noncompliance. When she was at last correctly diagnosed, she was prescribed an inadequate regimen, which she took when she could afford it—a good way to engender resistance to even second-line drugs.

In each case, the patients were blamed for their failure to respond to therapy. In each case, the patients' agency—their ability to comply with costly and difficult regimens—was exaggerated. Certainly patients may be noncompliant. But how relevant is such a notion in the case of Jean Dubuisson? Biomedical practitioners told him to eat well. He "refused." They told him to drink clean water, and yet he persisted in drinking from the only stream near his village. He was instructed to sleep in an open room and away from others, and here again he was "noncompliant," as he built no such addition onto his two-room hut. Most important, he was instructed to go to a hospital. Jean was "grossly negligent" and dragged his feet for months.

One can also exaggerate the effects of medical mismanagement, which does not by itself explain skewed rates of tuberculosis distribution. Physician-directed errors do not create poverty or social inequalities, and it is along these lines that rates of tuberculosis vary. Other questions raised by these cases are harder to answer but nonetheless worth considering. For example, did Peru's structural-adjustment plan increase Corina's risk of a tuberculosis death? Corina was driven from the Peruvian Central Sierra by the collapse of the agrarian order and other complex economic transformations. But once in Carabayllo, she and her family were subjected to a new set of vagaries; they were beset no longer by drought and storm but rather by equally uncontrollable, and even less predictable, shifts in economic policy. Decisions made in far-off World Bank headquarters, for example, led to significant changes in the employment structure of Lima and to massive fluctuations in the price of key commodities. Corina soon found herself the maid to a woman who was to become only slightly less poor than she—*fujishock* took its toll on schoolteachers, too. When Corina became ill with drug-resistant tuberculosis, she and her family were in essence helpless to combat it.

In Calvin's experience, what role did racism play? He more than once wondered about its contribution to his care. In the VA hospital, he felt punished because of his history of drug use, and he was irritated by the predominantly white staff's relative tolerance of alcoholism—the ranking substance-abuse problem of most of the other patients, who were also largely white. But the more important effects of racial discrimination may have been those that led to his becoming infected with tuberculosis in the first place. As a black Vietnam veteran living in the inner city and injecting drugs, Calvin was certainly in a high-risk group. Furthermore, conscription for this war was to some extent distributed by the same forces that drove his parents out of the Jim Crow South, as the army ranks were disproportionately filled with young African American men. And among the troops, those with the grimmest prospects back home seemed to be those most likely to use heroin or opium.

A LOOK BACK

In reflecting on tuberculosis mortality in the world today, a troubling question comes to the fore: does TB's association with poverty damn it to irrelevance in the eyes of the powerful, who, after all, control funding for everything from treatment to research? In August 1994, an official of the International Union Against Tuberculosis and Lung Disease seemed to say as much. "You never hear about TB in North America," he commented to a journalist, "because of who gets it these days: immigrants, natives, poor people and AIDS patients for the most part."[19] It would appear that diseases predominantly afflicting the poor are unlikely to garner funding for research and drug development—unless they begin to "emerge" into the consciousness and space of the nonpoor.

A look back over past professional commentary on the differential distribution of tuberculosis reveals that this neglect was not always the case. A huge literature documents the pernicious synergy between poverty and tuberculosis. During its first 150 or so years, the United States, like Europe, counted tuberculosis as its number one killer. Lemuel Shattuck's *Report of the Sanitary Commission of Massachusetts, 1850* named consumption as the leading cause of U.S. deaths, and this remained true even in the latter part of the century, when rates began to fall sharply.[20] But tuberculosis rates differed variably between the sexes and reliably along lines of race and class.

Perhaps not surprisingly, given TB's importance, differences in mortality and susceptibility among various social groups occasioned much comment. In fact, notes historian Georgina Feldberg, "concern about differential susceptibility *dominated* American discussions of tuberculosis from the mid-nineteenth century onward."[21] But interpretations of these differences, continues Feldberg, depended on the social perspectives of the commentators: "As each generation attempted to make sense of this preferential, or differential, susceptibility, the explanations they offered reflected and reinforced their uncertainties about a changing scientific and social order."[22]

For example, "Southerners commonly believed that blacks suffered from a distinctive form of consumption, known as 'negro consumption.'"[23] Susceptibility, in this view, was genetically determined. This construct not only demonstrated a vested interest in an agrarian, slaveholding social order but also reflected, to some extent, prevailing medical views. An 1844 editorial in the *Boston Medical and Surgical Journal* noted that the "reality of hereditary influence on the production of phthisis [as tuberculosis was then known] is so universally admitted, that it would seem a sort of scientific heresy to doubt it."[24] Feldberg summarizes these views:

The hereditarian/environmental debate persisted as Northern commentators regularly attributed excessive mortality to the "general insalubrity of the sections of the city inhabited by [blacks], the crowded conditions of their dwellings, insufficient nourishment, and the other influences of poverty," while Southerners more typically cited the "habitual improvidence" of the black races.[25]

Similar theories abounded in discussions of why such great numbers of Native Americans died of tuberculosis. Although solid evidence from Peru documents TB's pre-Columbian existence in the hemisphere, there is less evidence of tuberculosis among the native population in North America before the arrival of the Europeans, and there is little doubt that rates increased dramatically after contact. But TB's rise among the native peoples was so clearly linked to a rapid decline in their standard of living that hereditary arguments were widely seen as less compelling.[26]

The belief that tuberculosis was hereditary was dealt a near-lethal blow by Robert Koch's discovery of the tubercle bacillus in 1882. "One has been accustomed until now to regard tuberculosis as the outcome of social misery," Koch wrote, "and to hope by relief of distress to diminish the disease. But in the future struggle against this dreadful plague of the human race one will no longer have to contend with an indefinite something, but with an actual parasite."[27]

Paradoxically, perhaps, but fortuitously, the idea of tuberculosis as "the outcome of social misery" was not undermined by the discovery of its etiology. In the latter part of the century, persistent poverty and rising inequality were increasingly believed to contribute to differential mortality. One prominent physician "venture[d] to assert that the necessary privations of poverty on the one hand, and the absurd excesses of wealth on the other, tend more to the formation of tubercles in children than all other causes combined."[28]

By 1900, observe Dubos and Dubos, "it had become obvious that tuberculosis was most prevalent and most destructive in the poorest elements of the population, and that healthy living could mitigate its harmful effects. Reformers could attack the disease from two directions, by improving the individual life of man and by correcting social evils."[29] Both of these approaches, never neatly demarcated, were advocated by public health officials, most of whom were physicians.

Many in the nascent antituberculosis movement, which in the earlier part of the twentieth century was linked to the establishment of sanatoriums, believed that education was the key to curing the disease. One side effect of this belief was a habit of infantilizing the sufferers. Reformers wrote of "careless consumptives" who needed above all to be trained. As one classic statement of this view would have it, "People are now infected by consumption through ignorance on the part of those who give and receive infection. Each man whose habits have been corrected, even by a short residence in the sanatorium will neither do nor willingly permit to be done by others acts which before would have seemed perfectly natural."[30]

But other medical reformers continued to argue that "tuberculosis is closely associated with all the social problems of housing, food, wages, rest, clothing, and insurance and can in no way be separated from them."[31] Feldberg, whose excellent work has restored to the historical score the voices of physicians whose understanding of tuberculosis was firmly biosocial, points out that "well into the twentieth century, American physicians held fast to an etiology that included microbes but also found room for malnutrition, unemployment, crowding, the living conditions in slums, and other social ills."[32] As one example, she cites a 1921 publication by pathologist Allen Krause, director of the Johns Hopkins University tuberculosis laboratories: "The solution of the tuberculosis problem is partly dependent on the removal of other evils and inequalities which constitute, no doubt, a more fundamental problem than does tuberculosis itself."[33]

Hybrids of these positions also emerged. Barbara Rosenkrantz writes of Ellen N. LaMotte's *The Tuberculosis Nurse (Handbook for Practical Workers in the Tuberculosis Campaign)*, published in 1915:

> LaMotte assembled facts showing that tuberculosis was principally a disease of the poor, afflicting both those who were "financially handicapped and so unable to control their environment," and "those who are mentally and morally poor, and lack intelligence, will power, and self control." Her conclusion that "people of this sort . . . constitute almost the entire problem—otherwise the situation would be so simple that the word problem would not apply" conflicted uncomfortably with her intention of encouraging nurses to go forth and help the poor to defend themselves against tuberculosis.[34]

The increased susceptibility of the African American population continued to engender racial speculations. Huber's popular 1906 text derided discriminatory "phthisophobia" but argued that "the negro's small lung capacity, as compared with that of the white, and his deficient brain capacity render him less resistant to the disease when once acquired." Huber concluded by warning that "unless the hygienic and moral surroundings of the race are improved there is danger of its extinction."[35] In a 1925 paper called "The Vital Capacity of the Negro Race," two Alabama physicians published their findings (based on research conducted on prisoners and children) that "low vital capacity is a racial characteristic, and that vital capacity standards applied to white people cannot be directly applied to the negro race."[36]

When anatomic considerations could not be invoked, commentators speculated about the "bizarre beliefs" of the afflicted. In seeking to explain the persistence of tuberculosis among the urban poor, Edward Livingston Trudeau wrote of "the blind love of 'the average proletarian . . . for the chorus of citylife.'"[37] High rates of tuberculosis among immigrants were commonly blamed on their "lifestyles" and lack of cleanliness.[38] It was widely argued that "superstition" and "conjuring" were to some extent responsible for poor health outcomes among African Americans, views that were echoed even among black professionals. For example, a survey titled "Superstition and Health," conducted in 1926 by the National Urban League, cites a young black physician practicing in New York:

> Ignorance, cherished superstitions and false knowledge often govern Negroes in illnesses and hamper recoveries. Young Negroes show patriarchal obeisance to the aged—the aged are, in a large measure, fatalists. They are willing to leave all to whatever their fate may be, the fatalism that has cursed the Orient for centuries. This fatalism exasperates the physician, for it ties his hands and tends to nullify his efforts.[39]

Strong associations between tuberculosis and race and class did not weaken as the century progressed, but calling attention to such associations did not often lead to compassionate responses. Changing conceptions of tuberculosis transmission—a result in part of the frenetic campaign against spitting in public places—led many to regard with hostility and fear those who were popularly held to have high rates of tuberculosis, such as black people or foreigners.[40] In a 1923 address to a state medical society, one physician observed that "tuberculosis continues to be a serious problem with [Negroes], and because of their association with whites . . . as cooks, nurses, maids, [and] laundresses," black people represented a "menace to whites."[41] Such interpretations were common well into the 1960s. "In the South," McBride points out, "segregationists attempted to turn blacks' excessive tuberculosis mortality rates into justification for keeping white and black youths from attending integrated schools."[42]

Racial differentials, tightly tied to class divisions, became further entrenched as effective therapies were developed. Although tuberculosis continued to decline among all U.S. citizens, rates among black people remained relatively high, particularly among young black adults, for whom tuberculosis remained the leading cause of death even during World War II. Deaths were highly concentrated in the large industrial cities that had attracted black workers throughout the first decades of the century:

> From 1938 to 1939 black TB mortality rose in New York City from 949 deaths to 1,036. In numerous other major cities, blacks were more than one-half of those dead from TB in 1939. That year blacks suffered 50 percent of the TB deaths in Baltimore; 58 percent in New Orleans; 72 in Washington, D.C.; 78 in Birmingham; 78 in Atlanta; and 79 in Memphis. Nationally, blacks suffered 5,925 deaths or 32 percent of the TB deaths reported in the nation's 46 largest cities.[43]

In 1946, one prominent Harlem physician took city, state, and federal authorities to task for ignoring the tuberculosis problem among African Americans, which during the war years had claimed thousands of lives: "Here is a contagious disease killing people in the low income brackets at an outrageous rate, yet health authorities don't get excited. Several days ago, a plane flew experts from Boston to Texas because of 5 children ill with infantile paralysis—not a death but just becoming ill. They wanted to protect the other children. We in Harlem want protection too, not from just a paralyzed limb but from death itself."[44]

But afflicted communities had never been less likely to be construed as such. With the development of effective therapy, which began in 1943, energies turned increasingly toward treatment of the *individual* case. "At the national meetings of public health officials and TB experts," recounts McBride, "this optimistic and narrow concept of public health, which

focused on the patient and not groups at risk or conditions and social behaviors that created this risk, prevailed."[45] By the late 1950s, tuberculosis
was regarded as a disease well on its way to being eradicated, and little
interest remained in attacking the disease at its roots.

If individuals, and not the conditions endured by entire communities
or classes, are increasingly seen as the sole repositories of risk, has there
at least been a corresponding decrease in the differential risk so well described for the pre-antibiotic era? On the contrary, inequalities of risk
seem to be increasing. For example, tuberculosis rates have dropped substantially among Native Americans, but less rapidly than among other
groups. Michael and Michael, in reviewing the health status of contemporary Native Americans, note, as do others, their increased morbidity
and decreased life expectancy. And although tuberculosis plays a small
role in these grim figures, it takes on a new significance if disparities of
risk become the focus. In looking at age-adjusted mortality rates, for example, 1987 tuberculosis deaths among Native Americans exceeded
those among "all races" by 400 percent. Thus tuberculosis still tops the
list of disorders *disproportionately* killing Native Americans.[46]

The story is similar for other minorities in the United States, where "the
decrease [in tuberculosis] has been considerably greater among whites
than nonwhites. As a result, the ratio of the annual risk of tuberculosis
among nonwhites to the risk among whites has risen from 2.9 in 1953 to
5.3 in 1987."[47] Increasing inequalities of risk belie the claim of a "national
problem" of excess cases; instead they reveal a scenario in which long-
standing inequalities of risk are now being further accentuated.

As the next two chapters document, similarly desocialized readings of
tuberculosis continue to hold sway today. The reasons for treatment failures and for TB's persistence are often sought in the psychological traits
of individual "defaulters" or in the cultural attributes of groups held to
be "at risk." And yet in no instance has it been clearly demonstrated that
rates of tuberculosis vary by beliefs or by psychological makeup. In no
instance have educational interventions for those deemed "at risk" been
shown to inflect trends in tuberculosis incidence. The occurrence of tuberculosis has varied primarily with economic development; tuberculosis case-fatality rates have varied with ready access to effective therapy.
Pierre Chaulet put it well: as an "index of poverty, [tuberculosis] under-

lines inequalities of income and in the distribution of wealth. . . . In a world both off-track and 'deregulated,' TB persists and spreads, striking always the poor."[48]

THE ROLE OF PRAGMATIC SOLIDARITY

At the close of the twentieth century, we are challenged not only to explain the uneven distribution of tuberculosis but also to explain poor therapeutic outcomes in a time when effective treatments have existed for decades. Between 1943, when Selman Waksman and co-workers discovered streptomycin, and the late 1970s, over a dozen drugs with demonstrable effectiveness against tuberculosis were developed. New diagnostic methods, including immune-fluorescence staining and new culture methods, are equally impressive. In fact, in 1997 the FDA approved a test that can identify and amplify mycobacterial gene sequences in a matter of minutes. Now in the pipeline are tools that might identify resistant strains in less than twenty-four hours. We indeed have the scientific knowledge—but the hard truth is that the "we" in question does not include the vast majority of the three million people who died from tuberculosis in 1996. We must acknowledge that our guilt surpasses that of earlier generations, who lacked our resources: Michael Iseman, one of the world's leading authorities on tuberculosis, is right to use the word "shameful" in describing our failure to touch tuberculosis prevalence in much of the world.[49]

Looking toward the next millennium, it is difficult to be optimistic. The arrival of strains of *M. tuberculosis* that are resistant to all first-line and many second-line drugs is surely a harbinger of pan-resistant strains to come. And HIV looms: ever-increasing numbers of co-infected individuals, most of them poor, promise millions of cases of reactivation tuberculosis. These "excess cases" will in turn infect tens of millions. In failing to curb tuberculosis before the advent of these truly novel problems, it seems clear that a window of opportunity has slammed shut.

Although tuberculosis is inextricably tied to poverty and inequality, experience shows that modest interventions have effected dramatic changes in outcome. Pragmatic solidarity means increased funding for tuberculosis control and treatment. It means making therapy available in a systematic and committed way. For example, we now know that short-course, multidrug regimens can lead to excellent outcomes in even the most miserable settings. In rural Haiti, as Chapter 8 explains, we learned that cure rates could increase from under 50 percent to nearly 100 percent if comprehensive supports, including financial and nutritional aid, are put in place while patients are being treated.[50]

In San Francisco, one project addressed poor attendance at tuberculosis clinics by moving the clinics to the times and places desired by the patients and by replacing staff who placed the blame for poor outcomes on the patients.[51] In New York, where the chances of compliance among injection drug users with tuberculosis were wearily dismissed as hopeless, one clinic more than trebled rates of completion. Much of the success was due to directly observed therapy, but a comprehensive, convenient, and user-friendly approach clearly had an impact, too.[52] Especially critical—and important to underline when confronted with claims that treating susceptible disease will somehow make MDRTB go away—were efforts in New York to speed the rate at which resistant strains were identified and then treated with the antibiotics to which they had demonstrated susceptibility.[53]

Pragmatic solidarity means preventing the emergence of drug resistance whenever possible, but it also means treating people like Corina Valdivia. As this book goes to press, a massive pandemic of MDRTB in Russia and other countries of the former Soviet Union becomes even more massive—with minimal public comment and even less public action. Problems of this dimension call for public subsidies of costly second-line drugs as well as for the development of new drugs. "No new antituberculous compounds have been developed by the pharmaceutical industry since the 1970s," observed Cole and Telenti in 1995, although researchers have serendipitously found certain antibiotics that have activity against M. tuberculosis.[54] Reichman sounds a pessimistic note: "Most of the drug companies that publicly announced a quest for TB drugs at the time of the recent resurgence have been noticeably quiet. Few have even shown interest in developing such drugs."[55]

In identifying the microbiological cause of consumption, Koch had hoped to end the era in which tuberculosis could be addressed only "by relief of distress." But tuberculosis remains, at this writing, "the outcome of social misery." If it is true, as Feldberg argues, that "scientific professionalism . . . fundamentally eroded the therapeutic impulse to social reform,"[56] surely it would be an error to divorce efforts to confront tuberculosis from broader efforts to confront social misery. We still have something to learn from the analysis of those who did not have our tools at their disposal. In 1923, pathologist Allen Krause made this observation: "More or less poverty in a community will mean more or less tuberculosis, so will more or less crowding and improper housing, more or less unhygienic occupations and industry."[57] This statement remains as true today as it was seventy-five years ago.

At the same time, it is necessary to avoid "public health nihilism."[58] Even if we lack the formulas necessary to "cure" poverty and social inequalities, we do have at our disposal the cure for almost all cases of tuberculosis. Those who remain committed to addressing tuberculosis by championing increased access to effective drugs must resist restricting their field of analysis of the tuberculosis problem. We are told to choose, in Haiti and in much of Africa, between treating tuberculosis and treating malnutrition. We are told to choose, in Peru, between treating those with susceptible and resistant strains. We are told to choose, in Harlem, between more funding for tuberculosis and more funding for affordable housing. Calls for more ambitious interventions are trumped by a peculiarly bounded utilitarianism: such interventions, we're told, are not "cost-effective." The inadequacies, the multiple ironies, of such analyses are not lost on the poor. In Peru, for example, it is impossible to ignore that a much-praised tuberculosis program is supported in part by the World Bank, one of the institutions that mandated the structural-adjustment program that led to increased suffering—and perhaps increased tuberculosis risk—for the Peruvian poor.

It is possible, of course, to exaggerate the significance of any one policy change. To cite Dr. García again: "If there had not been *fujishock*, it would have been something else. In Peru, there's always something beating down the poor." Although Dubos and Dubos mistakenly identify tuberculosis with a time—the nineteenth century—rather than with the inhumane conditions faced by billions on this planet, on another score they are right: "It is only through gross errors in social organization, and mismanagement of individual life, that tuberculosis could reach the catastrophic levels that prevailed in Europe and North America during the nineteenth century, and that still prevail in Asia and much of Latin America today."[59] As decision-making power—about social organization *and* about individual life—comes to be increasingly concentrated in the hands of a very few, we must ask, Who gets to determine the boundaries of analysis? Who is to determine what is "cost-effective" and what is not? As a global economy is "restructured," is there no room for alternative strategies of development? Alternative visions of providing health care to the poor?

Addressing these questions may get at the heart of the meaning of tuberculosis at the close of the twentieth century. If tuberculosis could once be termed "the first penalty that capitalistic society had to pay for the ruthless exploitation of labor,"[60] what does it mean now? Is it perpetually the lot of the poor to pay this penance?

8 Optimism and Pessimism in Tuberculosis Control

LESSONS FROM RURAL HAITI

We know most things about it,

but TB still kills more people

than any other pathogen, far

more than alcoholism, AIDS,

malaria, tropical diseases and

Ebola combined, and nobody

seems to care. . . . Where is the

shame? Where is the outrage?

LEE REICHMAN, 1997

What the social world has made,

the social world, armed with

knowledge, can undo.

PIERRE BOURDIEU, 1993

A survey of the current literature reveals discordant views on the question of progress in the control of tuberculosis. On the one hand, optimistic observers point with understandable pride to advances in our understanding of mycobacterial pathogenesis and to the elaboration of shorter but more effective treatment regimens. Recent years have seen a growing consensus that even six-month-long, multidrug regimens will lead to high cure rates if therapy is directly observed by medical personnel or health workers. The World Health Organization's adoption of DOTS—directly observed therapy, short course—has been hailed as a victory by experts from around the world.[1] Indeed, the WHO claims that DOTS is "the most important public health breakthrough of the decade."[2] The cure for tuberculosis, in this view, has at last been discovered.

Pessimists, on the other hand, call attention to the widening gulf between the advances reported in the scholarly literature and the degree of effective control in those communities hardest hit by the disease. Some point to the increasing microbial resistance to our best drugs; some point to our lack of an effective vaccine. But deaths from tuberculosis, numbering in the millions, are the most compelling rebuke to optimism.

In fact, it is difficult to document any impact of the new treatment regimens on worldwide tuberculosis incidence: in the current decade, an estimated 300 million people will become infected with tubercle bacilli; 90 million will develop active tuberculosis; and, if access to care does not become a global priority, 30 million will die.[3] In projecting changes in the rank order of the fifteen leading causes of death, Murray and Lopez show that tuberculosis alone among infectious pathologies will hold its unenviable place for the next thirty years; with the exception of HIV disease, all other infectious diseases are projected to drop in rank over the coming three decades. According to a baseline projection, tuberculosis will be the fourth leading cause of death overall in developing countries by the year 2020. Tuberculosis and HIV, which both afflict young adults disproportionately, are the only infectious diseases expected to cause more life years to be lost in 2020 than they cause now.[4]

Because effective therapy for tuberculosis has existed for decades, it is necessary to explain—and, sometimes, to explain away—our failure to treat it. Such explanations are contested terrain, and the literature contains striking divergences of opinion. Although patient "noncompliance" generally heads the list of favored explanations,[5] the vast majority of tuberculosis deaths are registered in settings of great poverty with abysmal tuberculosis services. In such venues, noncompliance is often outweighed by massive numbers of drop-outs from treatment, the result in no small part of prohibitively high treatment costs. Visitors to programs in such settings also report substandard care, a failure to keep accurate records, a near-total lack of follow-up, and high mortality. One review noted that "the proportion of patients with active disease who complete therapy under standard conditions ranges from as little as 20–40 percent in developing countries."[6] And these are the patients who are brought to medical attention; in 1991, the WHO estimated that only about half of all tuberculosis cases are ever diagnosed as such.[7] In short, too few tuberculosis patients have access to care, and those who do often do not receive appropriate care.

This gulf between the ideal and the real engenders, in seminars and in print, much discussion about compliance—but also discussion about the need for culturally appropriate interventions, enhanced convenience for patients, and community-based care. Although a consensus has been reached regarding certain goals, there remains a basic disagreement as to how they might be met. Optimists underline the surmountable nature of cultural and logistic barriers. Pessimists signal the large-scale forces that immiserate entire communities, putting them at risk of tuberculosis infection and disease—and at risk of having no access to therapy. Others observe that interest in tuberculosis is at an all-time low, which is certainly striking if deaths are at an all-time high. Dixie Snider has remarked that "despite the magnitude of the world's tuberculosis problem, the disease no longer concerns people in the United States and other industrialized nations."[8]

Haiti, the nation in the Western hemisphere most affected by tuberculosis, offers a good deal of support for the more pessimistic assessment. But our experience there, described in this chapter, shows that many of the problems can be surmounted. This chapter also reports sociomedical research that gets to the heart of the compliance question. This research explored adherence to therapy among a group of patients with active tuberculosis in village Haiti, where local conceptions of tuberculosis are often strikingly at odds with conventional biomedical understandings. Comparisons between two groups who held similar beliefs about the disease but who received standard versus enhanced services call into question the immodest claims of causality staked by analysts and providers who seek to explain the persistence of tuberculosis in the era of antibiotics.

HOW TUBERCULOSIS RISKS ARE STRUCTURED OVER TIME

The experience of tuberculosis in rural Haiti is one strongly conditioned by historical contingencies and material constraints. Haiti is Latin

America's oldest nation, having declared itself independent from France after a slave revolt that began in 1791. Haiti had been France's most valuable possession; by 1789 the country was producing more wealth than all thirteen North American colonies combined. French wealth was made possible because Haiti's then-rich soil was tilled by half a million slaves. Most available documentation suggests that the slave forebears of contemporary Haitians were ill indeed: "The slaves brought from Africa to Haiti carried with them the remnants of their cultural systems, yellow fever, yaws and malaria. The Spanish gave them sugar cane, vicious slavery, a form of Catholicism, smallpox, measles, typhoid and tuberculosis. The French, in their turn, gave the Haitians a language, traces of French culture and continued vicious servitude."[9]

The introduction of tuberculosis, whenever it took place, would prove to be of enduring significance. By 1738, the disorder was widespread enough to alarm French doctors visiting the island.[10] Moreau de Saint-Méry noted in the late eighteenth century that the rainy season was particularly hard on the colony's *poitrinaires,* a term still commonly used in reference to tuberculosis in rural Haiti.[11] A later observer estimated that *les tubercules* were, after dysentery, the most common chronic illness.[12]

Despite the importance of Haiti to the French economy, France's investments in health care infrastructure had been negligible. On the eve of the revolution, only a few miserable military hospitals were in operation. Ill members of the white minority were treated at home. Members of the black majority, if they were treated at all, received care in plantation sickbays, of varying quality. Although one historian presents data suggesting that the slaves of one large plantation enjoyed robust enough health, most have noted differential mortality rates for newly arrived Africans and Creole slaves.[13] One plantation's records show that a third of the newly acquired slaves were dead within "a year or two."[14]

And what were the conditions a decade later, at the close of the war of independence? According to Bordes, all of the island's doctors and surgeons had fled. The majority of hospitals and other institutions had been destroyed; only the military hospitals in Port-au-Prince and Cap Haïtien (formerly Cap Français) remained. The towns were in shambles, without sewers or latrines. What little care could be delivered was offered by orderlies who had worked in hospitals or by midwives, herbalists, and bonesetters. Bordes writes of a "host of technically unprepared health workers in the presence of a population newly liberated from slavery, living for the most part in primitive huts, without water or latrines, and undermined and decimated by the infectious diseases against which they were so poorly protected. [This was the] oppressive legacy from our former masters, thirsty for profits, and little interested in the living conditions and health of the indigenous population."[15]

Today, this oppressive legacy is very much alive in rural Haiti. With a rural per capita income under $300 per year, Haiti has long teetered on the edge of famine, and its people are faced with a long list of health problems worsened by chronic undernutrition. "Primitive huts" describes existing housing well enough indeed. In 1980, the Département de Santé Publique et Population estimated that only 1.8 percent of rural Haitians had access to safe drinking water.[16] Latrines are rare. And if "decimated" is taken literally, then the toll taken by infectious disease has mounted: "Over 50 percent of deaths are among children under age five, with nearly 75 percent of deaths caused by or associated with malnutrition. Infectious diseases account for the majority of deaths. The major causes of childhood deaths are diarrhea, pneumonia and tetanus; tuberculosis is the leading cause of death among adults."[17]

These death rates are among the highest in the hemisphere. By conservative estimates, infant mortality exceeds 120 per 1000 live births.[18] A report released by UNICEF in 1987 asserted that "one Haitian child dies every five minutes of malnutrition and related diseases."[19] Diarrheal disease exacts a toll on children of all ages. It is the leading cause of death among poorly nourished preschoolers and the chief cause of missed school among those fortunate enough to attend.

Tuberculosis heads the list of diseases dreaded by adult Haitians. "Of all the health problems cited," observes Wiese, "one stands out from the others by virtue of its insidious onset, its tenacity, and its prevalence—pulmonary tuberculosis."[20] The prevalence of tuberculosis in Haiti is estimated to be the highest in the hemisphere. Little is known of the disease during the nineteenth century, but in 1941 Leyburn wrote that, in a series of seven hundred autopsies performed in the Port-au-Prince General Hospital, 26 percent of deaths were due to tuberculosis.[21] The United Nations reported that in 1944 in Haiti "tuberculosis was the most important cause of death among hospitalized patients." Linking the high incidence of the disorder to poor sanitation and poverty, the organization predicted that "for many years to come tuberculosis will, it is feared, continue to take a heavy toll of human lives in Haiti."[22]

This prediction has come true. In 1965, the Pan American Health Organization estimated prevalence at 3,862 per 100,000 inhabitants.[23] Available data indicate that tuberculosis remains the leading cause of death among individuals between the ages of 15 and 49. Studies from the Hôpital Albert Schweitzer suggest that, in this age group, tuberculosis causes two to three times as many deaths as the next most common diagnosis.[24]

In recent years, the situation seems to have worsened. The high prevalence of tuberculosis has been further augmented by the advent of HIV. In sanatoriums in urban Haiti during the mid-1980s, some 45 percent of all tuberculosis patients reportedly were co-infected with HIV. In a more recent survey of over 7,300 ostensibly healthy adults living in a densely populated slum, 70 percent of those screened were tuberculin-positive and over 15 percent were HIV-positive. More alarming, community-based screening detected a prevalence of 2,281 *active* pulmonary tuberculosis cases per 100,000 adults. Among the 1,629 HIV-seropositive patients, 5.8 percent of those screened were deemed to have active tuberculosis.[25]

These astoundingly high rates of tuberculosis raise questions about the noxious synergy between TB and HIV. One study conducted in rural regions found that 15 percent of patients diagnosed with tuberculosis disease were also infected with HIV.[26] In another rural setting, at the Hôpital Albert Schweitzer, 24 percent of all patients with tuberculosis were co-infected with HIV. Of tuberculosis cases diagnosed there in adults between the ages of 20 and 39, the hospital deemed 31 percent "attributable to HIV." The study's authors conclude that HIV seropositivity is a major risk factor for pulmonary tuberculosis among young adults in Haiti. Their data also suggest that at least one-fourth of the smear-positive pulmonary tuberculosis among young adult Haitians would be preventable if the spread of HIV were controlled.[27]

The emergence of resistance to first-line drugs is another concern. There are very few published studies of drug resistance in Haiti, in large part because it is difficult to culture *Mycobacterium tuberculosis* in settings with no reliable source of electricity. One of the only large series including culture data revealed that 22 percent of isolates were resistant to at least one first-line drug.[28]

Although drug resistance presents a new and potentially significant problem, most studies of treatment failure agree that the problem is predominantly one of designing and implementing programs that are appropriate to the needs of the population to be served.[29] In one large town in southern Haiti, fully 75 percent of all patients had abandoned treatment by six months after diagnosis, and over 93 percent had abandoned treatment before the end of one year.[30] Since short-course therapy did not exist at the time of this study, we must assume that the majority of patients in this series were left with partially treated disease.

The remainder of this chapter describes in some detail one community-based organization's efforts to implement a tuberculosis-control program that takes into account the crippling poverty that so often plays a central role in determining who does or does not benefit from interventions. In examining this program, I also want to oppose the "either-or" approach that has led some health advocates, tragically, to adopt a Luddite stance.[31] This position holds that it is acceptable to defer tuberculosis treatment while the "root causes" of the disease are addressed through development projects. But health policy is not a zero-sum game. One of the lessons from rural Haiti is that effective tuberculosis-specific interventions are both urgent and inexpensive and should not be regarded as somehow detracting from the broader development efforts that might well serve to reduce tuberculosis incidence.

THE PROJE VEYE SANTE EXPERIENCE

Since it was founded in 1984, Proje Veye Sante, the small community health program introduced in Chapter 5, has sought to serve the landless peasants and children of the Péligre basin of Haiti's Central Plateau. In recent years, the project has grown considerably as more villages seek to participate by sending community members to be trained as health workers. Although the project is centered around a large clinic staffed by myself and four other physicians (the Clinique Bon Sauveur), it is in the outlying villages that much of the work takes place: more than fifty village health workers form the backbone of Proje Veye Sante. All paid staff positions are filled by Haitians, most of them natives of the region.[32]

The catchment area of Proje Veye Sante includes the settlements scattered around the reservoir created by the hydroelectric dam, which flooded the valley in 1956, leaving most of the area's peasants landless and impoverished. Sector 1 of the catchment area rings the lake; at the time of this study it encompassed approximately twenty-five thousand individuals, almost all of whom were peasants living in small villages.[33] Sector 2, more loosely demarcated, consists of a large number of outlying villages and towns contiguous to Sector 1.

Although inhabitants of the villages in Sector 2 were offered the same clinical services available in Sector 1 (consultations with a physician, lab work, and all medications for about 80 cents), they were not served by community health workers, nor did they benefit from activities sponsored by Proje Veye Sante such as women's health initiatives, vaccination campaigns, water protection efforts, and adult literacy groups. These interventions, implemented by community health workers, had proven to be a powerful means of addressing malnutrition, diarrheal disease, measles, neonatal tetanus, malaria, and typhoid fever. Through the community activities, the health workers were able to identify the sick and refer them to the clinic, where, of note, all antituberculous medications were free of charge. (Isoniazid, ethambutol, pyrazinamide, and streptomycin were then on formulary at the clinic.)[34]

Although Proje Veye Sante was effective in identifying and referring patients with pulmonary tuberculosis to the clinic, it became clear during the late 1980s that detection of new cases did not necessarily lead to cure, in spite of our policy of waiving even the 80-cent fee for any patient diagnosed with tuberculosis. In December of 1988, following the deaths from tuberculosis of three HIV-negative patients, all in their forties, the staff of Proje Veye Sante met to reconsider how the care of these individuals had been managed. How had the staff failed to prevent these deaths?

Responses to this question varied. Some community health workers felt that tuberculosis patients who had poor outcomes were the most economically impoverished and thus the sickest. Others, including the physicians present, attributed poor compliance to widespread beliefs that tuberculosis was a disorder inflicted through sorcery, which led patients to abandon biomedical therapy. Still others hypothesized that patients lost interest in chemotherapy after ridding themselves of the symptoms that had caused them to seek medical advice.

Over the course of the next two months, we devised a plan to improve services to patients with tuberculosis—and to test these discrepant hypotheses. Briefly, the new program embraced the goals of finding cases, offering adequate chemotherapy, and providing close follow-up. Although contact screening and BCG vaccination for infants were included in the program, the staff of Proje Veye Sante was then most concerned with the care of smear-positive and coughing patients—believed by many to be the most important source of community exposure.

The new program was designed to be aggressive and community-based, relying heavily on community health workers for close follow-up. It was also designed to respond to patients' appeals for nutritional assistance. All residents of Sector 1 diagnosed with pulmonary or extrapulmonary tuberculosis would be eligible to participate in a treatment program featuring—during the first month following diagnosis—daily visits from their village health worker. These patients would receive financial aid of $30 per month for the first three months and would also be eligible for nutritional supplements.

Further, these patients were to receive a monthly reminder from their village health worker to attend clinic. "Travel expenses" (for example, renting a donkey) would be defrayed with a $5 honorarium upon attending clinic. If a Sector 1 patient did not attend, someone from the clinic—often a physician or an auxiliary nurse—would make a visit to the no-show's house. A series of forms, including a detailed initial interview schedule and home-visit reports, regularized these arrangements and replaced the relatively limited forms used for other clinic patients.

During the initial enrollment period, between February of 1989 and September of 1990, fifty Sector 1 patients joined the program.[35] Forty-eight of those identified had pulmonary tuberculosis. Seven individuals also had extrapulmonary tuberculosis (for example, tuberculosis of the spine), and two had cervical lymphadenitis ("scrofula") as their sole manifestation of tuberculosis. During the same period, the clinical staff diagnosed pulmonary tuberculosis in 213 patients from outside Sector 1.

Many of these patients were from Sector 2, although a few had traveled even greater distances to seek care at the clinic; at least 168 of these individuals returned to the clinic for further care. The first fifty of these patients to be diagnosed formed the comparison group by which the efficacy of the new interventions would be judged. They were a "control group" only in the sense that they did not benefit from the community-based services and the financial aid; all Sector 2 patients continued to receive free care. To test hypotheses regarding patients' beliefs and clinical outcomes, we interviewed all patients regarding their own explanatory models and their experience of tuberculosis.[36]

The mean age of our patients (forty-two years) and the sex ratio (both groups had significantly more women than men) did not vary significantly between the two groups.[37] But indirect economic indicators (for example, years of school attended, ownership of a radio, access to a latrine, a tin roof rather than a thatched roof) suggested that patients from Sector 2 may have been slightly less poor than those from Sector 1. This is not surprising, as several of the villages in Sector 1 are squatter settlements dating from the year the valley was flooded.

Results

The following discussion explains the findings of the Proje Veye Sante study in some detail. These findings are summarized in Table 8.

Mortality. One patient from the Sector 1 group died in the year following diagnosis, although she did not die from tuberculosis. Six patients from Sector 2 died, all, it seems, from tuberculosis; one of these was a young woman who was also seropositive for HIV.

Sputum Positivity. The clinical staff attempted to examine sputum for acid-fast bacilli (AFB)[38] whenever patients developed recrudescent symptoms as well as approximately six months after the start of anti-tuberculous therapy. None of the patients from Sector 1 were sputum-positive at six months. One young woman did become sputum-positive during a pregnancy in the subsequent year; we found that she was in-

Table 8.   Characteristics of Tuberculosis in Sector 1 vs. Sector 2 Patients

	Sector 1 (N = 50)	Sector 2 (N = 50)
All-cause mortality (18 months follow-up)	1 (2%)	6 (12%)
Sputum-positive for AFB after 6 months of treatment	0	9 (18%)
Persistent pulmonary symptoms after 1 year of treatment	3 (6%)	21 (42%)
Average weight gained/patient/year (lbs.)	9.8	1.9
Return to work after 1 year of treatment	46 (92%)	24 (48%)
Average number of clinic visits/patient/year	11.6	5.4
Average number of home visits/patient/year	32	2
HIV co-infection	2 (4%)	3 (6%)
Number denying the role of sorcery in their illness	6 (12%)	9 (18%)
One-year disease-free survival	50 (100%)	24 (48%)

fected with HIV and may have been reinfected with a second strain of tuberculosis. Of the Sector 2 cohort, nine patients had acid-fast bacilli demonstrable in their sputum about six months after the initiation of therapy.

Persistent Pulmonary Symptoms.   After a year of treatment, a thorough history and physical exam were used to screen for persistent pulmonary symptoms such as cough, shortness of breath (dyspnea), and hemoptysis. Only three patients of the Sector 1 group reported such symptoms, and two of them had developed asthma during the course of their convalescence. Twenty patients in Sector 2, however, continued to complain of cough or other symptoms consistent with persistent or partially treated tuberculosis. One additional patient in this group was an asthmatic without radiographic or other evidence of persistent tuberculosis.

Weight Gained.   Monitoring body weight revealed marked differences between the two sector groups in the amount of weight gained per patient per year. Correcting for fluctuations associated with pregnancy, Sector 1 patients gained an average of nearly ten pounds during the first year of their treatment. Patients from Sector 2 had an average weight gain of about two pounds per person per year.

Return to Work. The vast majority of patients from both groups were peasant farmers or market women whose families relied on their ability to perform physical labor. It is especially notable, then, that one year after diagnosis, forty-six of the Sector 1 patients stated that they were able to return to their work activities. In Sector 2, fewer than half (twenty-four patients) were able to do so.

Clinic Visits. As patients were given one month's supply of medication with each visit, the staff of Proje Veye Sante strongly encouraged monthly clinic visits, which served as an indirect measure of a patient's adherence to antituberculous therapy. In the Sector 1 group, the one-visit-per-month ideal was nearly achieved: these patients, who received a small sum for "travel expenses," averaged 11.6 visits per year. In the control group, the average number of clinic visits per year was 5.4.

Home Visits. Our treatment protocol at that time called for at least 30 grams of intramuscular streptomycin over the course of the first two months of therapy, and community health workers were asked to administer these injections to the patients living in their area. Most patients from Sector 2 had their streptomycin administered by local *pikiris*, or injectionists. (Some lived near licensed practical nurses and received this drug in other clinics.) This is perhaps the chief reason that the number of home visits by members of the Proje Veye Sante staff was far higher in the Sector 1 group than in the Sector 2 group: thirty-two visits in the former versus two visits in the latter.

HIV Seroprevalence. The rate of HIV seroprevalence was not substantially different between the two groups. Only two patients from Sector 1 showed serologic evidence of HIV infection; both had lived in urban Haiti for extended periods. One of these patients became smear-positive for acid-fast bacilli during a pregnancy that occurred over a year after she completed her initial course of therapy. She was treated with a new multidrug regimen and remained asymptomatic some sixty months after her initial tuberculosis diagnosis. In the Sector 2 group, similarly, three patients were seropositive for HIV and all had lived in greater Port-au-Prince.

Etiologic Conceptions About Tuberculosis.   Previous ethnographic research had revealed extremely complex and changing ways of understanding and speaking about tuberculosis among rural Haitians.[39] Open-ended interviews with patients in both groups permitted us to delineate the dominant explanatory models used by members of both groups. Because several physicians, nurses, and community health workers had hypothesized that a belief in sorcery as a cause of tuberculosis would lead to higher rates of noncompliance, we took some pains to address this issue with each patient. We learned that few from either group would deny the possibility of sorcery as an etiologic factor in their own illnesses, but we could discern no relationship between avowed adherence to such models and a patient's degree of compliance with a biomedical regimen.

Cure Rate.   In June 1991, forty-eight of the Sector 1 patients remained free of pulmonary symptoms. Two patients with persistent cough and/or dyspnea did not meet radiologic or clinical diagnostic criteria for tuberculosis (both had developed bronchospastic disease). Therefore, we judged that none had active pulmonary tuberculosis, giving the participants a cure rate of 100 percent. One of these patients, as noted earlier, was co-infected with HIV but remained asymptomatic sixty months after her initial diagnosis of tuberculosis. We could not locate all fifty of the patients from Sector 2, but of the forty patients we examined at more than one year after diagnosis, only twenty-four could be declared free of active disease based on clinical, laboratory, and radiographic evaluation. (Six patients from this group had died during the course of the study.) Even if the four patients lost to follow-up had in fact been cured, that would have left twenty-six others dead or with signs and symptoms of persistent tuberculosis—a cure rate of, at best, 48 percent.

Explaining Treatment Outcomes

In an important review of the significance of tuberculosis in developing countries, Murray, Styblo, and Rouillon estimate that 26 percent of avoidable adult deaths in these countries are due to tuberculosis, making it the greatest cause of avoidable death.[40] The experience of Proje Veye Sante speaks to the discrepant explanations of this colossal failure, since the majority of these deaths occur in settings not unlike Haiti. Although such small numbers do not permit any sweeping conclusions, the project described here suggests that *high cure rates are possible in settings of extreme poverty in which hospital-based care is unavailable even for the critically ill.*

Even after so small a study, we can also advance other pragmatic conclusions. First, projects designed to *treat* tuberculosis among the very poor must include financial and nutritional assistance, for many of these patients develop reactivation tuberculosis in the setting of malnutrition or concurrent disease. The Proje Veye Sante antituberculosis initiative indicates that, in Haiti at least, hunger and poverty are the prime culprits in treatment failure, just as they are so often responsible for the reactivation of endogenous infection. Countries held in underdevelopment would do well to invest resources in programs that address patients' nutritional needs while ensuring easy and reliable access to multidrug regimens.

In fact, these interventions may be more important than the choice of regimen: although we initially used traditional antituberculous therapy, rather than the short-course multidrug regimens shown to be effective in recent studies, our results are as encouraging as those of Styblo and colleagues, who report a 90 percent cure rate when a six-month course of INH and thiacetazone is preceded by two months of an *in-hospital*, strictly supervised three-drug regimen.[41] Given the high costs of hospitalization, a program that includes financial or nutritional aid may be less expensive—and far more feasible—than the tuberculosis-control programs now in place in many poor countries. Similarly, although directly observed therapy would seem to be almost always preferable to unobserved therapy, our experience suggests that high cure rates can be achieved even in sparsely settled, difficult terrain where patients are unable to make daily trips to clinics or health posts.

Second, projects designed to *prevent* tuberculosis among the very poor must keep in mind a central maxim of tuberculosis control: treatment is prevention. Although these projects may have different priorities than those of projects designed for low-prevalence, high-income settings, identification and complete treatment of patients with active pulmonary tuberculosis should be the top priority of tuberculosis control in settings like rural Haiti. Similar conclusions have been advanced in a review of data from throughout the developing world.[42] Experience among New York City's poor might also lead to such conclusions, since in one review of patients diagnosed with tuberculosis at Harlem Hospital, only 11 percent could be shown to have completed therapy.[43]

The eradication of tuberculosis would require that we halt transmission and also prevent the reactivation of quiescent TB infection. We have the tools to do both: treatment of all active cases and, in the majority of quiescent cases, "chemoprophylaxis" with isoniazid. Until there are major redistributions in the current partition of the world's wealth, however, chemoprophylaxis of contacts and of asymptomatic but infected (PPD-positive) patients has a limited role to play in poverty-stricken areas. Although a community may have a high level of tuberculosis *infection*—our own survey suggests that 70 percent of rural Haitian adults are PPD-positive—individuals with active pulmonary disease are those most likely to transmit the disease to others. They are also those most likely to die of tuberculosis. Ideally, however, resources available for tuberculosis control would be increased so that even chemoprophylaxis could be administered as directly observed therapy.

In a sense, the high cure rates we achieved also show that debates over whether to treat tuberculosis or to prevent it are essentially false debates, whose costs are borne, as usual, by the poor. Among those who correctly argue that poverty is the ultimate cause of tuberculosis, some make a serious error by advocating that development efforts should take precedence over tuberculosis treatment. As noted earlier, this Luddite trap remains a peril of modern tuberculosis control. After all, we know how to treat tuberculosis, but development efforts often go awry. The people of the Péligre area know this well, for the hydroelectric dam that immiserated them, and so increased their tuberculosis risk, was billed as a development project.

JUST WHO IS NONCOMPLIANT?

Let us return to the central question: if effective therapy has existed for decades, why does tuberculosis remain the world's leading infectious cause of death? There is no shortage of opinions on the subject. "The most serious problem hampering tuberculosis treatment and control," asserted three pulmonologists in a 1993 review, "is patient non-compliance with therapy." We find no mention, here, of any structural barriers to therapy. "Potential determinants of compliance," they continued, "include personal characteristics of patients, features of the disease and/or treatment, and patients' beliefs and attitudes."[44]

Other experts reach altogether different conclusions. In a searing overview of tuberculosis control, Lee Reichman concludes that "patient non-compliance is the least of our problems."[45] Those with long experience in combatting tuberculosis register similar opinions. "In developing countries," writes Chaulet from Algeria, "non-compliance with antituberculous chemotherapy is less often due to the patients' failure to comply with treatment than to other factors." The factors underlined by Chaulet are largely logistic and are closely linked to public health officials' inability to ensure the steady provision of services: "These factors are not abstract entities or forced and uncontrollable situations: they are people, men and women, who are not doing the jobs they have been assigned and for which they are paid."[46] In a similar vein, Horton writes of the "institutional inertia" impeding effective tuberculosis control, identifying not patients but rather national governments, science policy makers, the market, and national health infrastructures as the chief impediments.[47]

Obviously, the degree of confidence with which such opinions are proffered is no assurance of their accuracy. Because discrepant opinions about the same topic cannot all be correct, some are necessarily immodest claims of causality. At the heart of these debates is, once again, the "compliance" question. "The word compliant," observes Sumartojo in a sophisticated review of the topic, "has the unfortunate connotation that the patient is [ideally] docile and subservient to the provider."[48] But our experience in Haiti suggests that, even more unfortunately, the term exaggerates patient agency, suggesting that *all* patients possess the ability to comply—or to refuse to comply—with antituberculous therapies. Patient noncompliance as the chief explanation for poor treatment outcomes makes little sense, if the WHO is correct in suggesting that as many as half of all cases of active tuberculosis are never even diagnosed.[49] It also makes little sense when half of the national tuberculosis programs surveyed in 1992 reported "drug stock-outs" in their countries during the previous years.[50]

Experiences across boundaries of time and place have shown radical differences in the ability of different populations to comply with demanding therapies, whether they be admonitions to move away from "consumptive climes," as in the previous century, or exhortations to take a year's worth of several costly drugs. Most new studies describe program failure as alternatively patient-dependent, drug-dependent, or project-dependent. But underlying these distinctions are broader theories about the *nature* of these barriers.

Cultural, political, and economic factors, while inevitably important, cannot be of equal significance in all settings. Although cultural considerations—such as the nearly universal stigma attached to tuberculosis—may very well be extremely important in the industrialized, wealthy world, they matter less in Haiti. In Haiti, the factors that govern treatment success or failure—factors such as initial exposure to mycobacteria, reactivation of endogenous tuberculosis infection, complications, access to therapy, length of convalescence, development of drug resistance, degree of tissue destruction, and, finally, mortality—are determined chiefly by economic variables. In the Proje Veye Sante project, the relative insignificance of patients' understandings of etiology when compared to access to financial aid is one marker of the primacy of economic considerations in impoverished settings

A broad, biosocial view of tuberculosis brings into relief the political, cultural, and economic barriers to effective tuberculosis treatment (and chemoprophylaxis). Such a view reveals "compliance" to be an analytically flimsy concept in countries such as Haiti, where the poor are put systematically at risk for tuberculosis and then denied access to adequate care. All too often, the notion of patient noncompliance is used as a means of explaining away program failure. Patient-dependent failure should be a "diagnosis of exclusion"—invoked only after poor program design and lack of access are excluded.

9 Immodest Claims of Causality

SOCIAL SCIENTISTS
AND THE "NEW" TUBERCULOSIS

From the extreme inequality of

conditions and fortunes, from the

diversity of passions and talents,

from useless or pernicious arts,

and silly sciences would arise

hosts of preconceived ideas, all

contrary to reason, happiness,

and virtue.

JEAN-JACQUES ROUSSEAU, *1755*

The best lack all conviction, while the worst

Are full of passionate intensity.

WILLIAM BUTLER YEATS,
"The Second Coming," 1919

René Dubos, who began his career as a distinguished microbiologist but later turned toward the contemplation of the patterns of tuberculosis and other epidemic diseases, underlined the social nature of tuberculosis almost half a century ago: "Tuberculosis is a social disease, and presents problems that transcend the conventional medical approach. . . . Its understanding demands that the impact of social and economic factors on the individual be considered as much as the mechanisms by which tubercle bacilli cause damage to the human body."[1] Anthropologists and other social scientists have long argued that tuberculosis will not be eradicated without attention to these fundamentally social forces. But there is clearly dissent among social scientists concerning which social forces are involved in the persistence of tuberculosis and the emergence of multidrug-resistant forms of the disease, the differing impact of these forces, and the ways in which large-scale and impersonal forces come to be embodied as individual pathology and epidemic disease.

The major poles of thought among social scientists in fact resemble the two diametrically opposed positions that we can readily discern among physicians and the lay public. Simply put, on the one hand are those who believe that TB's persistence and increasing resistance are in large part the result of patient-related factors; on the other hand are those who primarily target structural barriers to the delivery of effective care. In Chapter 8, for example, these two opposing positions were clearly reflected in the discrepant hypotheses advanced to explain tuberculosis deaths in Haiti. Each argument has many variants—for example, both culture and personality may be subsumed under the "personalistic" pole—but these tendencies run through most debates about TB's "resurgence."

Chapters 2 and 7 outlined the lineaments of this resurgence—the millions of tuberculosis deaths each year throughout the world, the recent series of focal tuberculosis epidemics that have significantly altered local patterns of morbidity and mortality even in nations where tuberculosis deaths had steadily decreased throughout much of the century. (Witness the United States, where a decades-long downward trend in reported tuberculosis cases began to reverse dramatically after 1984.) Why has the promise of the 1950s—when tuberculosis, it was declared, would soon be a disease of the past—become only hollow words? Why does tuberculosis remain a leading killer of young adults when effective chemotherapy exists? Two factors are commonly cited to explain this setback: the advent of HIV and the emergence of tuberculosis strains that are resistant to multiple drugs (MDRTB). These two developments have had sufficient impact that several leaders in the field now speak of "the new tuberculosis."[2]

Earlier chapters have documented the rapidly growing spread of HIV infection. Through two major mechanisms, HIV and tuberculosis exhibit a synergy that is particularly noxious to their human hosts. First, in patients who carry quiescent tuberculosis infection—roughly a third of the world's population, by some estimates—subsequent infection with HIV often means that the immune system's ability to keep mycobacteria in check will wane. In this subgroup of doubly infected persons, dormant tuberculosis "reactivates" as cell-mediated immunity declines; in much of the world, reactivation tuberculosis heralds previously unsuspected HIV infection. Tuberculosis may in fact be the world's most common HIV-associated opportunistic infection: in late 1992, one leading source observed that, of the 11.8 million persons then estimated to be infected with HIV, 4.6 million of them were co-infected with *Mycobacterium tuberculosis*.[3]

The second mechanism of synergy follows naturally from these epidemiologic insights. Unlike many of the other opportunistic infections afflicting those with AIDS, and unlike HIV infection itself, the tubercle bacillus may be transmitted without sustained or intimate contact. When a patient with active tuberculosis coughs, viable bacilli are aerosolized and may remain in the air for hours. Perfectly immunocompetent persons may subsequently inhale these organisms and become infected. If HIV-infected persons are much more likely to develop active pulmonary tuberculosis than are controls who are HIV-negative but PPD-positive (a test result suggesting infection with *M. tuberculosis*), then it is obvious that the new disease will have an enormous impact on the old scourge.[4]

Into the midst of this already grim scenario comes MDRTB, which develops when naturally occurring mutants become favored during the course of intermittent or poorly conceived tuberculosis therapy. Individuals who develop MDRTB may expose others, who then suffer a primary infection with a resistant strain.[5] In cities throughout the world, the past decade brought reports of strains resistant to at least the first-line drugs isoniazid and rifampin. In the United States, significant outbreaks of MDRTB have been reported in homeless shelters, prisons, and medical facilities from Washington, D.C., to San Francisco. Though less well documented, outbreaks have been registered in large Latin American cities, as well as in the former Soviet Union.[6]

The city of New York was hit particularly hard by MDRTB, in large part thanks to HIV but also because the city allowed its tuberculosis infrastructure to crumble. In 1968, for example, some $40 million was spent to maintain New York City's one thousand designated tuberculosis beds, its twenty-one "chest clinics," and the staff of these facilities. Ten years later, the tuberculosis beds were gone, and annual funding for tuberculosis had been slashed by up to $17 million. Federal monies earmarked for tuberculosis surveillance and control in New York City also decreased. In 1979, tuberculosis incidence for the city began to climb for the first time in decades, and it continued to do so until 1992.[7]

By 1991, fully a third of the city's reported cases were resistant to at least one first-line drug; almost 20 percent were resistant to both isoniazid and rifampin.[8] New York City had become the epicenter of a significant outbreak of MDRTB. The cost-cutting backfired: "When all the costs of the 1989–94 MDRTB epidemic were totaled, it was clear that more than $1 billion was spent to rein in the mutant mycobacteria. Saving perhaps $200 million in budget cuts during the 1980s eventually cost America an enormous sum, not only in direct funds but also in lost productivity and, of course, human lives."[9]

The more highly resistant strains were notoriously difficult to treat, and the finest medical care in the world offered no assurance of cure. In the largest cohort study thus far reported, Iseman and co-workers detail their experience with 171 patients, all of whom were HIV-negative. Among these patients, the infecting tuberculosis isolates were all resistant to isoniazid and rifampin; most were resistant to three or more first-line agents. These patients were treated with an average of more than six drugs per person, had a mean hospital stay of more than six months, and received, in certain cases, adjunctive surgery. Treatment lasted, on average, more than four years. These heroic measures, which cost up to $250,000 per patient, yielded an overall response rate of only 56 percent.[10]

The story is even worse for those with both HIV disease and MDRTB. Among the HIV-infected who fall ill with drug-susceptible strains of tuberculosis, response to therapy is often excellent. When these patients do die, it is usually not from tuberculosis—unless they lack access to care. But the news has been bleak for HIV-positive patients who fall ill with multidrug-resistant strains. "Despite aggressive multidrug treatment," concludes one review, "72 to 89 percent of more than 200 patients were dead in 4 to 19 weeks, with 38 to 70 percent of the deaths caused by tuberculosis."[11]

Who is falling ill with these deadly strains of tuberculosis? In spite of the theoretical risk to the "general population," the majority of U.S. cases to date have, again, been registered among the inner-city poor, with significant outbreaks confined to prisons, homeless shelters, and public hospitals. This strikingly nonrandom occurrence of MDRTB speaks to some of the forces at work in the pandemic. The two factors central to the "new" tuberculosis—the advent of multidrug-resistant strains and HIV—are ostensibly biological in nature but are in fact best understood as *biosocial* phenomena. In one sense, to argue that drug-resistant tuberculosis is a socially produced biological phenomenon is simply to state the obvious, since resistance develops in response to chemotherapeutic agents recently created by humans. But, as I've argued earlier in this book, the rapid spread of HIV among certain populations has been shaped by social (political, economic, and cultural) processes—the structural violence that has also led, in large part, to the emergence of MDRTB.

To examine the relationship between structural violence and the emergence of drug-resistant tuberculosis, this chapter presents two case studies. One is from Haiti, which currently serves, I am sorry to say, as a natural laboratory for the ill effects of such violence on the health of a population. Although tuberculosis has usually been termed the leading cause of death in autopsy series of Haitian adults between 15 and 50 years of age,[12] MDRTB has not previously been reported in Haiti. Indeed, in the only large study in which drug susceptibilities were tested, we read that "no significant resistance to drugs other than isoniazid was seen even though streptomycin and thiacetazone have been widely used."[13] But, based on what we know, it is likely that MDRTB strains are already present and will emerge first among the poor, as the case of Robert David shows. The other case—that of an entire family—comes from urban Peru. The experience of Blanca Pérez and her family reveals how, in a setting marked more by inequity than by absolute deprivation, an epidemic of resistant tuberculosis may be fanned both by inequalities and by inappropriate policies.

ROBERT

In August of 1986, Robert David, then nineteen years old, noted the onset of a nonproductive cough, night sweats, and intermittent fevers and chills that were more marked in the evenings. Like most impoverished peasant families, the Davids lived in fear of tuberculosis, in part because of its high mortality rate and in part because of its tendency to leave survivors—or surviving kin—saddled with unpayable debts. And so Robert attempted, at first, to treat himself with readily available herbal remedies. But when his cough gave way to shortness of breath and marked weight loss, Robert's parents brought him to a referral hospital in the city of Hinche, the district seat of Haiti's Central Plateau. There he was diagnosed with pulmonary tuberculosis and placed on an unknown two-drug regimen that probably included isoniazid.

In order to receive care in this public facility, Robert had to commute from his home village. By truck, this trip took two hours; by donkey or on foot, it was an overnight trek. In spite of his heroic efforts to keep appointments, which included a full day of waiting inside the clinic, Robert's symptoms did not promptly respond to treatment.

In June of 1987, he sought care in a large market town closer to his home village. He was then treated for eighteen months, initially with a three-drug regimen (isoniazid, ethambutol, and streptomycin). During this second course of therapy, Robert recalled hearing from his doctor that he had organisms in his sputum (indicating possible resistance) on "several" occasions, but his regimen was never altered. Throughout this period, he had great difficulty acquiring his medications, even though family members made enormous financial sacrifices—including selling more than half of their land—in order to buy syringes and the prescribed medications.

Robert completed one and one-half years of irregular treatment in December of 1988, but he continued to experience the same symptoms. In January, he had an episode of massive hemoptysis but received essentially no biomedical care for this life-threatening complication. "We didn't have any money," he responded, when asked why he did not seek care, "and the bleeding had stopped by the time we could borrow some."

The other symptoms persisted. In May of 1990, Robert traveled to Port-au-Prince, where he was admitted to a sanatorium for six months of treatment with isoniazid, ethambutol, pyrazinamide, and rifampin. He was discharged to complete a total of eight months of this regimen, followed by two more months of isoniazid and ethambutol. Because of political difficulties—including but not limited to a bombing that destroyed a key pharmacy—Robert was unable to obtain many of his medications. He did, however, feel "much better" for more than a year.

Robert returned to central Haiti and remained there until June of 1992, when most of his symptoms (cough, weight loss, night sweats) recurred. In September, he was again admitted to a Port-au-Prince sanatorium, where he received only thiazina, the combination of isoniazid and thiacetazone. His symptoms did not lessen substantially, and, again, Robert was often unable to acquire medications because of political disruptions in the capital.

These same political upheavals drove Robert back to the Central Plateau and, eventually, to the Clinique Bon Sauveur. When we first saw him, in January of 1993, Robert explained that he had been unable to obtain his medications because he had no money. He reported to the clinic seeking relief of his chronic cough, night sweats, and weight loss. A thin young man with minimally labored breathing, Robert then weighed 110 pounds. Physical examination revealed temporal wasting, pale conjunctiva, and severe thrush. His neck was supple with no cervical lymphadenopathy. Examination of his lungs revealed abolition of breath sounds at the left apex. The remainder of his exam was unremarkable. Laboratory studies included examination of his sputum, which was laden with acid-fast bacilli, and a serologic test for HIV, which was negative. We could not perform mycobacterial cultures because we lacked regular electricity.

We found Robert to be highly motivated and desperate to recover from his refractory tuberculosis. He had made every attempt, he told us, to comply with his physicians' orders. MDRTB was raised as a possibility, although it had not been previously reported in Haiti. The only antituberculous drugs available in Haiti were isoniazid, thiacetazone, pyrazinamide, ethambutol, PAS, streptomycin, and rifampin, all of which we had in stock at the Clinique Bon Sauveur at the time. Based on the observation that Robert developed floridly positive sputum on thiazina, we elected to give him a cocktail of *all* the other drugs, although we were aware that PAS was the only drug he had not yet received.

In February of 1993, then, Robert began this difficult regimen. We stopped the streptomycin when he complained of buzzing in his ears; this symptom abated shortly thereafter. In both March and May, Robert had negative sputum exams, but he continued to lose weight, and his pulmonary symptoms diminished only slightly. He attributed his nausea and abdominal pain to the enormous number of pills he was taking each day. A repeat HIV test was again negative.

In August, Robert's sputum was again laden with the tubercule bacillus. We collected a sputum specimen for culture and sensitivity testing, which was performed in the United States. Tests found that the isolate was resistant to isoniazid, rifampin, ethambutol, streptomycin, and pyrazinamide but susceptible to kanamycin, cycloserine, capreomycin, ethionamide, and ciprofloxacin. None of the drugs in the latter group are readily available in Haiti, so we made arrangements to import them, and Robert eventually started a four-drug regimen consisting of cycloserine, kanamycin, ethionamide, and ciprofloxacin.

Robert showed marked clinical improvement—weight gain, decreased shortness of breath, and less coughing—within two months. His sputum became free of organisms two months after initiation of this therapy and remained so for six months. In August of 1994, however, Robert again began losing weight and coughing. He continued his treatment, in spite of side effects including epigastric pain and, at one point, an abscess at an intramuscular injection site. Repeat tests showed that his MDRTB had recurred and, furthermore, had become resistant to kanamycin. The organism continued to destroy his lungs in spite of his strict compliance with a demanding regimen. In December of 1995, Robert David died in his sister's home.[14]

BLANCA, ANDRÉS, AND THE *FAMILIA TEBECEANA*

As subtle as her initial symptoms may have been, Blanca Pérez had little doubt about what was coming when, in July of 1995, she began having fever, chills, and a productive cough. Blanca and her husband, Andrés, both then twenty-two years old, were living in her mother's house with Blanca's six siblings, two of whom were being treated for active tuberculosis. But they alone were not the reason that the Pérez family had been labeled a *familia tebeceana*—a tuberculosis family. Blanca was in fact the fifth in her family to be diagnosed with the disease. Of her nine siblings, two had already died of tuberculosis.

It all started in 1987, when Blanca's older sister Sonya was diagnosed with tuberculosis. Sonya received numerous treatments, which were unsuccessful despite what she described as "religious" compliance. Because tuberculosis treatment in Peru is supervised, it is highly likely that Sonya had primary drug resistance—that is, she had been infected initially with a drug-resistant strain, which is why her treatments failed. In any case, she remained smear-positive for years, living in a small house in the hills of Carabayllo with her mother, nine siblings, and a changing cast of spouses and partners and children.

It was not long, of course, before others in the household began to cough. Pablo, the family's only son, was diagnosed with tuberculosis in 1990. Pablo was a teenager at the time but was already the main breadwinner in the family. He worked as a street vendor, making a pre-dawn ride to Lima's central market to collect old limes from the trash and then returning to sell them in the Carabayllo market. On a crowded bus, the trip took almost two hours each way. Responsible for feeding his siblings, Pablo often missed his medications on days when he was unable to leave work. For years, he was in and out of treatment and was considered a classic "problem patient" by the health center.

As the disease destroyed more and more of his lungs, Pablo became increasingly short of breath. Eventually he was unable to work. In late November of 1994, Pablo was referred, after his repeated requests, to a pulmonologist. Although he eventually did see a specialist and was diagnosed presumptively with MDRTB, Pablo never had a chance to follow the pulmonologist's advice. He died the following day, still receiving first-line antituberculous drugs.

In 1991, Sonya's husband, Raúl, was also diagnosed with tuberculosis. Sonya continued to have positive smears throughout her directly observed therapy, but her illness was not recognized as MDRTB until 1993; Raúl's resistance was not confirmed until mid-1996. Sonya and Raúl made heroic efforts to buy the same second-line drugs that had been prescribed for Corina Bayona, whose story was recounted in Chapter 7. But, like Corina, they could do so only intermittently, since their work as street vendors could scarcely feed them and their daughter. Both remained smear-positive for years, and Sonya was terrified by life-threatening episodes of hemoptysis.

Luisa, another older sister, was also diagnosed with tuberculosis in 1991. She followed the same pattern of unsuccessful treatment and re-treatment as her siblings. After she saw Pablo die, Luisa gave up hope and refused any further treatment. She often said to Sonya: "Why do you go through all that to get those pills, when you know we're both going to die, just like Pablo did?" Luisa died one year after Pablo, in November of 1995.

Rosa was diagnosed with tuberculosis in the first months of 1995. While receiving her antituberculous treatment, she became pregnant but miscarried. Since completing her treatment, Rosa has been symptom-free. Blanca's mother was also treated for tuberculosis last year, and her symptoms have disappeared.

For all these reasons, then, Blanca suspected that she too was ill with tuberculosis when she began coughing in July of 1995. Initially, however, she did not seek either diagnosis or treatment. But one morning in August, about a month after her symptoms began, Blanca had an episode of massive hemoptysis. Blanca's sisters, by this time experts, rushed her to the local health post, where her sputum was found to be abundantly positive for the tubercle bacillus. In spite of her known MDRTB contacts, Blanca began receiving the *esquema único*, the standard six-month, four-drug tuberculosis treatment regimen sanctioned by the Peruvian national tuberculosis program.

In patients with fully susceptible tuberculosis, directly observed therapy with these four drugs leads to rapid response; patients generally feel better within a couple of weeks. Most are usually smear-negative—and likely noninfectious—within the first month of treatment. By mid-September, however, a full month into treatment, Blanca's symptoms had failed to improve. Her chest X-ray looked worse, and her sputum smear remained positive. In fact, during every month of treatment, Blanca had a repeat smear; every month it was positive.

During this entire period, the local health workers who gave Blanca her daily medications were concerned that she might be resistant to these drugs. They knew about her family history; they, in fact, were the ones who had coined the term *familia tebeceana* to describe the Pérez family and other families decimated by tuberculosis. Fearing MDRTB, the health workers collected a sputum specimen from Blanca in November and sent it for culture and susceptibility testing.

In early January of 1996, Blanca's drug sensitivity results finally revealed that her tuberculosis strain was, like that of her sister, resistant to isoniazid and rifampin, the two most powerful antituberculous drugs. Despite these laboratory results, and to the dismay of the health workers who visited her each day, the health authorities told Blanca that she must complete the *esquema único*, even though at that point it consisted of only two drugs—the exact two drugs to which she had confirmed resistance. Discouraged, indeed frightened, Blanca did as she was told. Her symptoms worsened.

In late January, when she had completed the daily six-month regimen, Blanca's sputum continued to show abundant tubercle bacilli. She was wracked by fevers and coughing and had experienced life-threatening hemoptysis; she weighed less than 80 pounds. In keeping with the rules of Peru's national tuberculosis-control program, Blanca was evaluated by a program pulmonologist, who placed her on an "alternative" three-drug regimen approved by the national program. In addition, this physician prescribed two third-line drugs, ciprofloxacin and ethionamide, explaining that if she could obtain these drugs, her treatment would be even stronger. Blanca recognized the names of these drugs, which had also been prescribed for Sonya and Raúl. Since these drugs were not part of the standard public health program's regimen, Blanca knew that she would have to buy them herself. But where on earth would she or Andrés—parents of two small children—obtain the $200 a month to buy the drugs? This sum was well in excess of her entire family's monthly income.

The extended family pulled together enough resources to purchase one week's worth of the drugs for Blanca. This only made her feel worse, she recalled, as she could see that it was not possible for her family to sustain this economic burden and survive. Blanca announced that she would find another way of getting the drugs. Desperate for effective treatment, and thinking of her small children, Blanca changed her name and moved to another catchment area in order to be accepted by another health center. Under the alias Blanca Rodríguez, she began a standard retreatment regimen in February of 1996—despite the laboratory documentation that she was resistant to the most powerful of the drugs she was receiving. Her symptoms improved, but she remained smear-positive throughout this second treatment as well.

After completing this regimen, Blanca's symptoms returned, then worsened. Without further treatment options, she spent the next two months bedridden, losing weight, and coughing blood—the classic picture of galloping consumption.

Just when things seemed as if they could not get worse, Blanca's husband fell ill. Andrés worked as a street vendor, selling books, but he had also assumed all the cooking and housekeeping chores as well. So the increased fatigue and muscle aches he felt were initially attributed to overwork. In August of 1996, however, he began coughing, and soon he was diagnosed with tuberculosis. Given his multiple MDRTB contacts, Andrés was reluctant to begin standard therapy with the drugs to which his wife, sisters-in-law, and brother-in-law had been resistant. But he too was pulled into the official algorithm; he too remained smear-positive for most of his treatment.

In October, Blanca's nineteen-year-old sister, Ana, was diagnosed with tuberculosis. She was in the first trimester of her first pregnancy. She was the sixth Pérez child to fall ill with tuberculosis.

The Pérez family did receive some good news, though: in October, Blanca, along with Sonya and Raúl, began receiving a treatment regimen with drugs to which their isolates had demonstrated susceptibility. These drugs were provided, along with nutritional support and daily visits from a community health worker, by Socios en Salud, the community-based organization described in Chapter 1, and the same organization that had tried to treat Corina Bayona. By mid-November, Blanca's sputum test was negative for the first time since her initial diagnosis. Raúl and Sonya were also soon smear-negative.

By the end of 1996, Andrés and his family were sure that he too had MDRTB, and he was angry that he was being forced to complete the standard regimen. The advent of therapy for MDRTB had engendered a certain amount of tension in the local "tuberculosis community," since many of the patients who had failed the official regimen understood, as did some of their providers, that they might have "knocked off" other potentially effective drugs in the process—Sonya, for example, had become resistant to five drugs, although she had initially been resistant to only two. Blanca was initially resistant to two drugs, but by the time she finished her empiric retreatment regimens, she was also resistant to five. Still other patients had died while waiting, as one patient put it, "to be liberated from *esquema único*." In addition, the drugs made Andrés nauseated: "Why should I take drugs that make me sick if they're ineffective?"

Laboratory studies done by Socios en Salud revealed that Andrés did in fact have resistant disease. In January of 1997, a few days shy of completing *esquema único*, Andrés refused to take his medications. He was forced to sign a statement acknowledging that he was "abandoning treatment." For this reason alone, Andrés will never figure in national data as a case of primary MDRTB. Instead, he will be mislabeled, as were all members of the Pérez family, as having acquired MDRTB though erratic compliance. They were "problem patients."

DNA fingerprinting of the strain infecting Andrés shows, of course, that he is sick with the same strain that almost killed his wife. He too is now improving on appropriate therapy, which he began in late January of 1997.

POVERTY, INEQUALITY, AND MDRTB: MYTHS AND MYSTIFICATIONS

How does the biomedical literature explain the emergence of resistance? In an influential review published in the *New England Journal of Medicine*, Michael Iseman writes: "In the circumstances of monotherapy, erratic drug ingestion, omission of one or more of the prescribed agents, suboptimal dosage, poor drug absorption, or an insufficient number of active agents in a regimen, a susceptible strain of *M. tuberculosis* may become resistant to multiple drugs within a matter of months."[15] In this one sentence, Iseman suggests a host of "risk factors" for MDRTB. Each is inescapably a part of the lives of millions like Robert David—poorly nourished adults who develop reactivation tuberculosis, which is treated (when it is treated) with a small number of erratically available drugs. In this sentence, too, are condensed the experiences of Blanca Pérez, who has seen her family decimated by ever more resistant tuberculosis even as blame is heaped on such *familias tebeceanas*.

Social circumstances account for biomedical outcomes; there is, clearly, a "political economy of MDRTB." That is, there are large-scale forces that make monotherapy and erratic drug ingestion much more likely in settings such as Haiti or Carabayllo or Harlem than in the affluent communities where MDRTB has not yet become a problem. With this in mind, how do the experiences of Robert David and the Pérez family address the central thesis of this chapter, that the emergence of MDRTB (and of the "new" tuberculosis in general) is inextricably linked to structural violence?

Like most patients with MDRTB, Robert had been previously treated for tuberculosis. He was treated inappropriately, with a two-drug regimen that he could ill afford. When he relapsed, he was not started on a regimen consisting of drugs that he had never received before. During the second course of treatment, he was technically "noncompliant"—but how useful is such a term in describing the experience of a young man whose family was willing to sell all its land to treat him? Even while in a sanatorium, he was unable to purchase his medications, a problem worsened by the incessant political violence of the period. Errors were also made in Robert's more recent medical management at the Clinique Bon Sauveur. Although we suspected MDRTB early in 1994, the lack of electricity meant that no cultures were obtained until after he had failed another empiric regimen. When he finally received tailored therapy, he may even then have received too few drugs.

Robert David's lamentable experience clearly shows the complicated relationship between individual agency and structural violence. In most settings where tuberculosis is prevalent, the degree to which patients are able to comply with treatment regimens is significantly limited by forces that are simply beyond their control. The biomedical literature displays a certain delicacy in discussing this problem. In the largest Haitian series in which drug susceptibilities were examined, we read only that "primary drug resistance in Haiti has many probable causes, including the availability of isoniazid without prescription, past inclusion of isoniazid in cough remedies and a high default rate."[16] Nowhere do we read about the insurmountable barriers to effective biomedical care faced by the overwhelming majority of Haitians. Nowhere do we read about the absence, at that time, of an efficient national tuberculosis program that could ensure detection and treatment of cases.

The tragic history of the Pérez family, like that of Corina Bayona and her family, is not merely a tale of medical mismanagement and ill-advised tuberculosis-control policy, although it is certainly all of that. The cases from Carabayllo demonstrate how high grades of social inequality serve to amplify strain resistance. In settings of shared wealth, transmission of M. *tuberculosis* is usually interrupted quickly; in settings of shared poverty, like Haiti, few have access to antituberculous drugs, and thus acquired resistance is less likely. The settings characterized by the most highly resistant organisms are those like urban Peru, where access to many drugs, including newer agents such as the fluoroquinolones, is possible but not ensured.

In such cities throughout Latin America and Asia and in South Africa, where great wealth is juxtaposed to poverty, most second-line antituberculous agents are available for purchase; access to them is neither controlled nor ensured by national tuberculosis programs, which control only first-line drugs—if drugs are controlled at all.[17] The poor of these middle-income countries often have intermittent access to second-line drugs, ranging from the fluoroquinolones to kanamycin, but they are not able to obtain *regular* access. Thus may patients who are initially resistant to isoniazid and rifampin eventually come to have the spectacularly resistant patterns seen in some of the patients in Carabayllo.

The history of the extended Pérez family, like that of other *familias tebeceanas,* also reveals how important primary infection with MDRTB can be. The experience of Andrés shows how primary infection can be misdiagnosed as acquired MDRTB—"acquired," that is, through supposed noncompliance.

As is the case with AIDS, myths and mystifications about tuberculosis have had an important impact on organized responses to this disease. Although MDRTB is a new phenomenon, we can already discern a series of curiously potent myths about the illness that are now taking shape. In our work in Haiti, Peru, Mexico, Russia, and the United States, we have uncovered a great deal of received wisdom about the disease, but the following six myths seem to predominate.

1. MDRTB Is Untreatable.

The high costs of medications, hospitalization, and surgery have led many international health experts to declare MDRTB treatment "cost-ineffective" or simply impossible in poor countries. In our own experience in urban Peru, we've already analyzed outcomes among the first fifty patients treated through our collaboration with the national TB program. These patients were, on average, resistant to five drugs and had long-standing disease and significant lung damage. All received directly observed, individualized therapy with drugs to which their isolates had demonstrated susceptibility. Although side effects were universal, most patients tolerated high doses and long durations of even the more toxic second-line drugs. All patients smear- and culture-converted; only one abandoned therapy; and over 85 percent remain smear- and culture-negative as they near the end of protracted courses of therapy. They are apparent cures.[18]

2. MDRTB Is Too Expensive to Treat in Poor Countries; It Diverts Attention and Resources from Treating Drug-susceptible Disease.

Current recommendations for treating MDRTB depend on the resistance pattern of a given isolate and on the presence of co-morbid disease, but in general they include therapy with a minimum of four or five drugs, preferably for up to twenty-four months or more. Most authorities recommend that initial therapy include a parenteral (injectable) drug, and directly observed therapy is strongly advised. Other recommendations, including strict isolation of infectious patients in negative-pressure airflow rooms and the use of ultraviolet light, are intended to decrease nosocomial and community transmission of MDRTB. New, individually fitted masks are suggested for health care providers who are exposed to patients with pulmonary tuberculosis.[19]

Even in settings with significant resources, such as Mexico, Brazil, and Peru, it is clear that not all of these recommendations can be followed. It may well be true that ultraviolet light and negative-pressure airflow rooms are far from being priorities for most countries in Latin America. But providing effective treatment to patients with MDRTB is decidedly not out of the question, even in Haiti, the poorest country in the region. Nor are simple and inexpensive measures that could immediately decrease nosocomial transmission of MDRTB.

It is time that we question the analyses underpinning these confident pronouncements that MDRTB is "too expensive" to treat. If tuberculosis control is to be governed by the gurus of cost-effectiveness, it is easy to show that the most serious costs are incurred when we fail to diagnose and treat MDRTB. Certainly this is the lesson to be learned from the New York City experience, but the example was never really local. In 1990, the

CDC reported the case of a patient with MDRTB who exposed nine family members and friends. Care for these ten persons, who lived in Texas, California, and Pennsylvania, exceeded $1,000,000.[20]

"Transnational" cases provide additional support for this argument. Our own tuberculosis work in Peru stems from a transnational case—a U.S. relief worker who died in Boston of MDRTB acquired in Carabayllo (a story that is recounted in Chapter 1). Failure to diagnose MDRTB cost not only his life but also, in the United States, hundreds of thousands of dollars in direct medical and contact-tracing costs. We believe that nosocomial spread was probable in this case, with skin-test conversion noted in hospital staff. Similar stories are well documented in the literature.[21] These transnational cases will only increase in the coming years, especially if the large epidemics of Russia and the former Soviet Union are not addressed promptly. "The globalization of currencies," as Pierre Chaulet points out, "carries with it the globalization of TB transmission."[22] Accordingly, our analyses *and* our responses must be equally transnational.

It would seem that a rigorous cost-effectiveness analysis should lead us to address MDRTB outbreaks promptly, wherever they happen to occur. But we should not abandon other arguments, including the fundamentally moral stance that the poor and those otherwise disenfranchised—including prisoners—have a right to high-quality tuberculosis treatment. It is worth noting that in the previous decade, as MDRTB became a ranking problem in Mexico, the country claimed the world record for the creation of new billionaires. Unless these developments are reconciled with claims that MDRTB is too expensive to treat, we should be wary of double or triple standards based on misleading indices, such as the GNP of the country in question. For most of us, mention of "triple therapy" does not suggest what clearly is a triple standard for MDRTB: treatment for some populations, neglect in others, and outright denial of outbreaks in still other settings.[23]

3. Treating Drug-susceptible Tuberculosis Is the Best Way to Address Epidemics of Drug-resistant Disease.

It has frequently been observed, in conferences if not in print, that by treating drug-susceptible disease, it is possible to stem outbreaks of MDRTB. This is false. It is true, however, that better treatment of drug-susceptible disease is likely to decrease the incidence of resistance *acquired* during therapy, as Weis and co-workers have shown in Texas and as Frieden and co-workers are now showing in New York City. But in both settings, aggressive attempts to *diagnose and treat cases of MDRTB have also been central to these efforts.*[24]

What will happen if tuberculosis programs greatly improve their ability to treat drug-susceptible tuberculosis but do not treat existing cases of MDRTB? This is precisely the situation that prevails in many of the countries now justly lauded for their tuberculosis-control programs, which are increasingly successful at treating patients with drug-susceptible disease. It is also the situation in certain prisons in Siberia. It stands to reason that in such settings there will be less and less transmission of drug-susceptible strains, since improved detection and treatment of patients with drug-susceptible tuberculosis means that these patients are smear-positive and coughing for shorter periods of time. Even where MDRTB cases are currently a very small proportion of all tuberculosis cases, however, the *relative importance* of primary infection with MDR strains should thus increase because these patients remain effectively untreated for years, often have cavitary disease,[25] and continue, in most cases, to frequent health establishments ranging from hospitals to local health centers.

Experience from Spain demonstrates what happens when we do not address MDRTB. Spain, said to have the highest new-case rate of AIDS in Europe, also has high rates of reported tuberculosis. In Madrid in 1994, the rate of reported tuberculosis cases was 33.5 per 100,000 inhabitants. Rullán and co-workers recently reported the country's first major nosocomial outbreak of MDRTB, which occurred in an infectious-disease facility in Madrid. Between September 1991 and May 1995, 47 cases of MDRTB were diagnosed in HIV-infected patients hospitalized in an HIV-dedicated ward, and one case was diagnosed in an HIV-infected hospital employee who worked on the ward. All but one of the patients died, with mean survival after diagnosis of MDRTB a mere seventy-eight days. "The epidemiologic curve," observe the authors of the study, "suggests a propagated transmission pattern of MDRTB among HIV ward patients, starting in 1991 and continuing until June 1995. By the first 6 months of 1995, 65% of *Mycobacterium tuberculosis* strains seen among HIV ward patients were multidrug-resistant."[26] Failure to diagnose and treat MDRTB aggressively meant that, in less than five years, MDRTB had become the dominant strain in the hospital.[27]

4. MDRTB Is Less Infectious Than Drug-susceptible Tuberculosis.

Although it is often suggested that drug-resistant tuberculosis strains may not be as transmissible or infectious as drug-susceptible strains, the available data do not support this claim.[28] On the contrary, pulmonary MDRTB appears to be as easily transmitted as are drug-susceptible strains, even though in the few studies we have the index cases are often co-infected with HIV. Although cavitary lesions are less common in patients with HIV, we now know that HIV-infected patients are efficient transmitters of tuberculosis, even without the massive microbial burdens associated with cavitary disease.[29]

Many studies report high levels—18 to 50 percent—of transmission to, and several cases of MDRTB among, health care providers.[30] When an outbreak of MDRTB in a referral hospital in urban Spain led to employee screening, a startling 80 percent of hospital employees were found to be already infected with *M. tuberculosis.* Of tuberculin-negative employees, the incidence of conversion (infection) during the thirty-month study period was fully 26 percent, and the relative risk of conversion had a dose-response relationship with the amount of time spent on the HIV-dedicated ward.[31]

But the Latin American and Russian experiences strongly suggest that HIV is by no means a required co-factor for outbreaks of MDRTB. In fact, long delays in diagnosis and treatment—or, more commonly, no treatment at all—mean more cavitary disease and more smear-positive and coughing patients. In order to explore the ease with which MDR strains are transmitted in the absence of HIV, Brazilian researchers prospectively followed HIV-negative close contacts of sixty-four patients who themselves had MDRTB. They found that, over four years, almost 8 percent of 218 previously healthy contacts developed tuberculosis—1.6 cases per 1000 person-months of contact. Of these, the majority of patients had drug-resistant disease—and 46 percent had strains with resistance patterns identical to those of their contacts.[32] In Peru, as noted, resistance patterns have suggested high rates of transmission to close contacts; this impression has been confirmed by DNA fingerprinting.

5. Patient Noncompliance Is the Chief Cause of MDRTB.

We often hear the argument that patient noncompliance is the major reason for TB's persistence and resurgence—a claim contested throughout this book. Similar strategies are used to "explain" MDRTB, as this quotation from a 1994 study reveals: "Non-compliance on the part of patients is the most serious remaining problem in the control of tuberculosis and the chief cause of relapse and drug resistance."[33] Other authorities, writing from poor countries, offer a quite different picture, however.

In Latin America, as in the United States, physician-directed errors are common, as is uncontrolled use of the most effective antituberculous agents. In our experience in various settings in Latin America and the former Soviet Union, it appears that individuals with active MDRTB who followed medical advice are at increased risk for poor outcomes—that is, for acquiring further drug resistance, or for death. Certainly, patient noncompliance has not been central to the major MDRTB outbreaks in North America and Europe, which to date have been nosocomial (or institutional) and the result of inappropriate infection-control procedures.

*6. Since Poverty Is the Problem, the Best Approach
to Tuberculosis in Poor Countries Is to Promote Development.*

Throughout the hemisphere, epidemics of MDRTB are inevitably patterned, disproportionately afflicting the poor. As Brudney and Dobkin write, "Regaining control of epidemic tuberculosis will be difficult and will require effective approaches to hardcore issues also common to the AIDS epidemic: poverty, homelessness, and substance abuse."[34] Such sound conclusions about the *dynamics* of the epidemic have led, in some circles, to the erroneous conclusion that tuberculosis is best addressed by support for "development projects." But even the best-intentioned efforts at reducing poverty will not cure the millions of cases of active tuberculosis in the world today and would thus be an altogether insufficient response to the problem.

Debate also focuses on what might constitute effective strategies for reducing poverty. Some of the large-scale development projects deplored in these pages and elsewhere—the Péligre hydroelectric dam, for example—were touted as such. Fortunately, other levels of intervention are indisputably effective for curing tuberculosis and are the responsibility of physicians and other health care workers. As Weis and co-workers argue, "There are no easy solutions to the problems of drug addiction, alcoholism, homelessness, psychiatric illness, or indifference on the part of the patients, but immediate solutions to the problems of drug resistance and relapse are needed."[35] These immediate solutions are not easy, but many of them are straightforward, for they involve an unswerving commitment to delivering effective treatment for all patients with active tuberculosis.

SOCIAL SCIENCE AND
IMMODEST CLAIMS OF CAUSALITY

Clearly, a great deal of confusion exists regarding MDRTB, although various, discrepant hypotheses about its causes and management tend to be advanced with great assurance. How have social scientists discussed the various forces that conspire to render certain groups vulnerable to tuberculosis while shielding others? What have we written about the recent trends outlined earlier in this chapter? How have we discussed the discrepant claims of causality apparent in the clinical and epidemiologic literatures?

Although we have a large sociomedical literature on tuberculosis, social scientists have yet to comment on the "new" tuberculosis. Let us examine, then, a handful of studies of tuberculosis published in the socio-medical or anthropologic press. Each was conducted in a poor country, and each makes certain claims of causality in attempting to explain why tuberculosis remains a major cause of death in the setting under study and why patients fail to comply with medically mandated regimens. Sometimes, the studies echo trends in the clinical literature by attributing program failure to patients' beliefs or behavior.

In important research conducted in southern Haiti and published in *Social Science and Medicine*, Weise devotes most of the discussion to the "health beliefs" of tuberculosis patients and their families. This is certainly a legitimate preoccupation for an anthropologist, especially one who has given us the most detailed study of the experience of tuberculosis in rural Haiti. She argues that the failure of a tuberculosis-control program in the region was largely the result of "the clinic's lack of knowledge about the local culture and consequent failure to operate within it."[36] Here, however, Weise assumes a linkage between culture and outcome that is simply not apparent. While Weise notes that the cost of ten weeks of treatment was equivalent to half a peasant family's annual income, the article offers no further discussion of this significant economic barrier to care—it is simply listed, below several other, apparently more important, "cultural" factors that led to the failure of the program. One could more easily argue that tuberculosis-control programs in Haiti have failed not because of cultural insensitivity but rather because of a lack of commitment to the destitute sick.

In the Proje Veye Sante initiative described in Chapter 8, we interviewed one hundred tuberculosis patients regarding their own understanding of their illness, which almost all agreed was tuberculosis. The majority of patients believed that sorcery might have caused their illness. Both the medical anthropologic literature and many of the Haitian health care providers queried predicted that these individuals would be the ones most likely to abandon antituberculous therapy. We found, however, that holding the belief that sorcery might have caused their sickness did not predict half-hearted compliance with chemotherapy. In Haiti's Central Plateau, what *did* predict adherence to therapy? Among patients who were offered free and convenient care, compliance and outcome were strongly related only to whether or not patients had access to supplemental food and income. We were led to conclude that cultural, political, and economic factors, although inevitably important, are not equally significant in all settings.

Similar disjunctions between anthropologists' expectations and treatment outcomes are found elsewhere in the literature. For example, Rubel and Garro reported high rates of compliance in California among migrant Mexican farmworkers with tuberculosis, who attributed their symptoms to disorders ranging from bronchitis to "folk illnesses" such as *susto:* "Interestingly, interviews with these patients show a continued denial of their diagnosis of tuberculosis despite faithful adherence to lengthy treatment regimens and extensive education by clinical staff members."[37]

To take an example from South Africa, where black people of all ethnic backgrounds have much higher rates of tuberculosis than do whites, a recent anthropologic study identified several reasons for the high default rate seen among Xhosa-speaking patients with tuberculosis. Chief among these were the patients' "deep-seated mystical beliefs," including the understanding that tuberculosis may be caused by witchcraft and is thus best treated with the help of a diviner who can explain who caused the sickness. The author listed several other reasons as well, from the side effects of the medications to the "carelessness" of certain patients, but nowhere was there any mention of the poverty of black South Africans or of apartheid and its effects on the delivery of services. Small wonder, then, that the investigator's conclusions focus so exclusively on patients' cognitive profiles:

> As an anthropologist it is therefore possible to plead that health care personnel who treat black patients with tuberculosis be aware that their patients' perceptions of the disease may differ from their own, that the patient may already have consulted a non-western practitioner, or that they are merely seeking time before they embark on a different strategy for seeking a solution for what troubles them.[38]

This is eminently sensible, but one could as readily argue instead that the proximate cause of increased rates of morbidity and mortality among black South Africans is not their "mystical beliefs" but rather lack of access to resources, as a study by a team of physicians concluded: "Poverty remains the primary cause of the prevalence of many diseases and widespread hunger and malnutrition among black South Africans. The role of apartheid in creating and maintaining this poverty has been well documented."[39]

Even here, a more extensive social analysis is necessary. Poverty and apartheid are not to be discounted, but high rates of tuberculosis in South Africa are closely linked to a "racial capitalism" far older than apartheid itself. The historian Randall Packard has shown that institutionalized apartheid alone is inadequate to explain the skewed incidence of the disease. Indeed, differential patterns of onset and outcome were emerging well before the enactment of apartheid laws, which are merely decades old:

> It is not enough to invoke apartheid, racial discrimination, and black poverty, for they themselves are symptoms of more fundamental politi-

cal and economic transformations that have been associated with the rise of industrial capitalism in South Africa. Ultimately the answer to why TB remains such a serious problem in South Africa lies in understanding the history of these transformations.[40]

Packard has since been proven correct, because tuberculosis is an even greater problem in South Africa than in many of the poorer countries on the continent. What's more, the inequalities formalized in the South African economy have fostered rising rates of MDRTB, just as forced removals to "homelands" may have ruralized the tuberculosis epidemic more than in other settings.

In Latin America, another region characterized by high grades of inequality, similar conditions obtain. But again these features of society escape comment even in the social science literature on tuberculosis. Another study, set in Honduras and published in *Medical Anthropology*, begins with a telling vignette:

> One day, in an important health center in Tegucigalpa, the capital city of Honduras, Central America, the general practitioner identified ten patients suffering from symptoms of tuberculosis. He asked them to go up to the laboratory, which was one floor above, to get the authorization for laboratory exams. Only five of them arrived at the laboratory; of those, only three brought the sputum sample the following day. Only one of them returned to pick up his result: it was negative. The results of the other two, who had given false addresses, were positive. They were suffering from tuberculosis. They were never located.[41]

A team of investigators set off to interview some five hundred Hondurans to uncover the reasons for this noncompliance. The study began with the formulation of six hypotheses that might explain noncompliance. None of these hypotheses linked treatment failure to a failure of the public health system or to Honduran society at large; none mentioned poverty or social inequality at all, although the individuals surveyed, in contrast, correctly associated tuberculosis with "extreme poverty, filth, and malnutrition."[42]

The researchers found the patients and the public to be full of strange "knowledge, attitudes, and behaviors" as well as suffering from a "great lack of education about the disease." When patients were interviewed, many "maintained a careful distance when speaking to the investigators, and seemed fearful and distrustful." (They had, speculates the author, "feelings of isolation . . . accompanied by guilt.") Above all, of course, the patients were noncompliant, "refus[ing] to accept [TB's] existence, and attempt[ing] to remedy the symptoms with self-prescribed medications." Some of the patients were downright refractory "and obstinately refused the visits of health personnel." "Even when the patient can no longer ignore the evidence of his symptoms," adds the author, "he is willing to die rather than undergo treatment."[43]

Nevertheless, consultants such as the author were prepared to remedy the situation. They designed a flip chart explaining "the measures that should be taken by the patient and his family" and had sputum cups "printed with attractive and clear illustrations." Sadly, though, "the Ministry [of Health] had not yet improved its tuberculosis program services, and the necessary sample cups were not available in time," nor were the flip charts. But a series of radio spots, posters, and a pamphlet served to "clear up the patient's immediate confusions about the disease."[44] The author seems confident that Honduras—which in his account sounds more like Sweden than one of the poorest countries in Latin America—is well on its way to solving its tuberculosis problem.

Even in a more thoughtfully conceived investigation, with more robust data, we can easily discern the same circular logic. Working in Wardha District in central India, Barnhoorn and Adriaanse compared fifty-two compliant TB patients with fifty noncompliant patients in an effort to determine what factors were responsible for failure to take medications. They found that "three socioeconomic variables, i.e., the monthly income per capita in a family, the type of house in which a family lived, and the monthly family income" were the strongest predictors of compliance with antituberculous chemotherapy. "It is noteworthy," the authors add, "that the highest ratings were followed by three additional socioeconomic variables, i.e., place of residence, fuel used, and education."[45]

Etiological beliefs about tuberculosis did not correlate strongly with adherence to therapy in this study. Although a number of "health beliefs" were felt to be strong predictors of compliance, these "beliefs" also sound much more like indirect socioeconomic indicators: "Compliers also tended to clean their body, ate good foods, visited a Primary Health Centre, whereas noncompliers tended to isolate themselves and prayed to God for a cure." Similarly, other items classified under "family attitudes" included having someone to prepare meals and "eating breakfast regularly."[46]

In essence, the researchers found that the only strong predictors of compliance were fundamentally economic, not cognitive or cultural. However, their conclusions would seem otherwise: "Concerns with the determinants of [noncompliance] might improve the care of tuberculosis patients by giving directions for *educational interventions*." And although Barnhoorn and Adriaanse insist that socioeconomic obstacles to treatment do exist and are fundamental, these obstacles become secondary in much of the discussion: "Before obstacles to a treatment regimen can be cleared away, patients have to develop health beliefs and social norms consistent with it." When the investigators call for the patients to be "liberated," it is not from the structural violence that creates and sustains a significant and growing tuberculosis epidemic among the world's poor. Instead, they propose that "future health education programmes aimed at the public at large should be focused on the liberation of the masses from false thoughts and burdens."[47]

In another paper published in *Social Science and Medicine*, a prominent anthropologist reported that, in one city in the Philippines, children's respiratory symptoms are often attributed to *piang*, a folk illness best treated by traditional healers: "Such a lay diagnosis *leads to* long delays before tubercular children are brought to a physician."[48] If this claim is true, then little short of changing the culture would lead to a change in compliance. But Valeza and McDougall, working in a nearby area, were able to double compliance with antituberculous medications by merely making drugs readily available and easy to take.[49]

In East Africa, another region characterized by extreme poverty, a weak medical infrastructure, and high rates of tuberculosis, "attribution of tuberculosis symptoms to witchcraft or other folk illnesses is associated with delays in seeking professional treatment as well as remarkably high rates of default once treatment has begun."[50] Similar claims are often made in Haiti, where we found no association, except in the minds of most physicians surveyed, between sorcery and tuberculosis *outcomes*—even though compliant patients often attributed their tuberculosis to sorcery.

These discrepancies bring us back to the sociology of knowledge. What is it, exactly, that medical anthropologists are expected to say and do? For many physicians and public health specialists, anthropologists are expected to "do the cultural piece." We're expected to elicit the local beliefs and customs that hamstring sensible efforts to treat or prevent illness; we're supposed to reveal what it is that makes the natives tick. This role is crystallized in the "knowledge, attitude, beliefs, and practices" surveys that crop up so often in AIDS research. These surveys are not designed to reveal the messy contingencies of everyday life or the large-scale forces that may at times render cognitive considerations irrelevant to outcomes; nor are funders looking for such information, which is often regarded as useless or worse. They're looking for "rapid ethnographic assessments" with distilled kernels of cultural wisdom. And very often, we have been willing to fill this restricted role, even if it means not talking about the forces and structures that ultimately determine tuberculosis outcomes.

It is inappropriate, of course, to generalize on the basis of such a small number of papers. But a more thorough review of the sociomedical literature on compliance with antituberculous therapy does little to gainsay the impressions made by the articles cited here. Such research tends to be conducted in settings—called "cultures" in these studies—characterized by high rates of tuberculosis and by extreme poverty, which a priori calls into question conclusions regarding the impact of the patients' culture on treatment failures. The common denominator among these patients is tuberculosis and poverty, not their culture. They also share, often enough, spectacularly bad tuberculosis services, such as those described by Friemodt-Möller, working in rural India:

> The treatment began when a sufficient number of patients had been collected to justify sending out a drug-issue team the long distances. To begin with, there was an interval of 2 months from the time the sputum was found positive until treatment began. Forty-seven patients died before the treatment could begin, 14 left the towns, 20 refused treatment from the beginning, 26 stopped after the first or second drug issue, two preferred to take their own drugs.[51]

Strenuous insistence on the causal role of culture or personality in explaining treatment failure runs the risk of conflating cultural (or psychological) difference with structural violence, leading to the immodest claims of causality evident in the studies described. In theory, it would be necessary to ensure full and ready access for all persons before ascribing blame for the failure to complete treatment to patient-related shortcomings. And in none of the places in which this research was conducted is full and ready access ensured. On the contrary, these settings are crying out for measures to improve the quality of care, not the quality of the patients.[52] *Throughout the world, those least likely to comply are those least able to comply.*

In each of the sociomedical studies I have critiqued, a well-intentioned effort to incorporate the patients' points of view has served, paradoxically, to shift the blame onto the sick-poor by exaggerating their agency. In so doing, researchers echo the received wisdom of many physicians and other providers. Their explanations tend to focus on local actors—most notably, on patients—and local factors. Curiously, many of these studies take it as a matter of faith that educational interventions will have significant effects on rates of tuberculosis in a particular population. No one, as far as I know, has ever shown this to be true. Historical reviews, such as that by McKeown, suggest that, in England and Wales at least, death rates from tuberculosis have varied quite independently of patients'—and healers'—understandings about the disease.[53]

Sociomedical research shows not merely the expected divorce between patients' and healers' etiologic conceptions of tuberculosis but also great dissensus regarding treatment failure.[54] Collando reported that when Mexican district health officials were asked, "To what do you attribute the problematic nature of tuberculosis control in your jurisdiction?" those surveyed "overwhelmingly laid the blame at the door of their patients' shortcomings: 'poverty,' 'lack of education,' 'poor motivation,' 'superstition,' and 'failure to comprehend the importance of compliance with treatment recommendations.'"[55]

A similar pattern was described in a San Francisco chest clinic, where in the 1960s up to 34 percent of the patients failed to keep their appointments. Again, the providers and the patients had very discrepant ideas about this failure. The physicians and nurses tended to focus on the patients' shortcomings—"the social and cultural characteristics of the user population"—while the patients listed structural barriers ranging from the inconvenience of the clinic's hours and location and a "rigidity in taking patients in order of registration regardless of extenuating circum-stances" to a failure to treat affected families as a unit, with adults and children seen instead on different days and by different physicians.[56] Ad-dressing these structural problems by moving the clinics to more conve-nient times and places, as well as "an improved attitude on the part of the professional staff," led to a drop in missed appointments from 34 percent to 6 percent after five years.[57] The social and cultural characteristics of the user population were not altered.

Anthropologists and other social scientists have long complained that their perspectives are not incorporated into tuberculosis-control efforts. While it is true that physicians and their biomedical colleagues have often disregarded the social forces at work in the changing epidemiology of tu-berculosis, a review of the biomedical literature suggests an increasing willingness to incorporate social factors in their explanations of why tu-berculosis control has failed. Indeed, specialists from the CDC and from academic departments are all likely, these days, to speak of social and eco-nomic determinants. Medical anthropologists have often been less willing to take account of basic biomedical insights, including the following: among their poor informants, untreated tuberculosis disease may have a case-fatality rate of over 80 percent; in drug-susceptible tuberculosis, at least, over 95 percent of patients can be cured with appropriate therapy. Nevertheless, drug-susceptible tuberculosis will kill tens of millions in the coming years, and it will kill them slowly, allowing many of them to serve as culture media for the induction of resistant strains. This, and not a fail-ure to incorporate the concept of culture in efforts to prevent or treat the disease, is the obscenity of late-twentieth-century tuberculosis.

These assertions are rooted in the hopeful belief that social science might well hold some of the keys to halting the spread of these new pan-demics. But if we are to be other than academic Cassandras, we would do well to acknowledge the largely structural causes of persistent tubercu-losis and ask why we have not had much influence in past attempts to prevent or treat the disease. In other words, the research tasks before us are more likely to be accomplished if we can avoid the traps of the past. As I examine my own field—similar exercises would be welcome in each of the sociomedical sciences—five such pitfalls, summarized in the fol-lowing sections, come quickly to mind.

Conflating Structural Violence with Cultural Difference

Each of the sociomedical sciences—medical anthropology, medical sociology, health economics, and so on—tends to stake out its specific turf. Representatives of these fields then tend to claim that their disciplinary focus is of paramount importance in explaining the phenomenon under scrutiny—regardless of what that phenomenon happens to be. In medical anthropology, often enough, "culture" is held up as the determinant variable. Because culture is merely one of several potentially determinant factors, anthropologists and other researchers who cite cognitivist "cultural" explanations for the ill health of the poor have been the object of legitimate critiques:

> Medical anthropologists and sociologists have tended to elevate the cultural component into an omnibus explanation. The emphasis is on cultural determination. Even when social relations receive more than reflexive recognition, medical social scientists restrict the social relations to small "primary" group settings, such as the family, and factions at the micro unit. . . . Little or no attempt is made to encompass the totality of the larger society's structure.[58]

One side effect of such cognitivist approaches to culture is the conflation of structural violence and cultural difference. Related trends are apparent in medical psychology, where personality attributes—the turf of that discipline—are held to explain risk for such disorders as AIDS, alcoholism, and addiction to drugs.

Minimizing the Role of Poverty and Inequality

Many anthropologists, regarding their turf to be the "cultural piece," also tend to underplay the economic barriers to effective care. Poverty has long been the chief risk factor for both acquiring and dying from tuberculosis; this was true long before MDR strains appeared. It was true when the likes of Lord Byron and Keats died from tuberculosis, for even then "the white plague" found the great majority of its victims among the poor. Dramatic shifts in local epidemiology aside, a global analysis does not suggest major decreases in the importance of tuberculosis as a cause of death. In fact, it is only with a significant proviso that tuberculosis may be said to be an emerging disease.[59]

Almost unexamined has been the relationship between the social reproduction of inequalities and the persistence of tuberculosis. To my knowledge, there have been no studies of the mechanisms by which steep grades of inequality might exacerbate resistance to antituberculous drugs. Our failure to discern a political economy of risk both for the development of MDRTB and also for suboptimal treatment may be related to a desire to link our (perfectly legitimate) investigations of the shaping of personal experience by culture to (inaccurate) claims of causality.

Exaggeration of Patient Agency

The praiseworthy effort to incorporate the patients' point of view can serve, at times, to obscure the very real constraints on agency experienced by most, but not all, patients with tuberculosis. Clinicians make their own immodest claims. One influential editorial in *Chest* declared patient noncompliance to be "the most serious remaining problem in the control of tuberculosis in the United States."[60] Assumptions regarding human agency underlie most discussions of treatment failure and noncompliance. In tuberculosis clinics throughout the world, patient-related factors top providers' lists of explanations for treatment failure. These lists, as Sumartojo politely and acutely notes, reflect providers' "observations and experience, but exclude environmental, structural, and operational factors that are beyond the patient's control."[61]

Calls to change "lifestyle and behavior" are often directed to precisely those persons whose agency is most constrained. The same exaggerations took place in earlier eras, as the historian Barbara Rosenkrantz observes in examining the elaborate treatment protocols at the turn of the century: "The disease-oriented hygienic regimen dictated by bacteriologic research came to grief when a patient's poverty made it unlikely that such advice would be followed."[62]

Exaggeration of patient agency is particularly marked in the biomedical literature, in part because of medicine's celebrated focus on individual patients, which inevitably desocializes. Strong behaviorist trends mar much of the psychological literature on tuberculosis. Similar critiques of modern epidemiology have also been advanced.[63] But it is social science that has underlined the importance of contextualization, and so our failure to complement clinicians' views with more robustly contextualized ones is all the more significant.

Who better than social scientists to find sad irony in the fact that a rhetoric of patient "agency" is applied only *after* populations have been subjected to a series of external attacks, of which contagious disease is only one? The poor have no option but to be at risk for tuberculosis; thus tuberculosis is merely one factor in an environment of structural violence. For most populations, as we have seen, the chances of acquiring infection, developing disease, and lacking access to care are structured by a series of systematic forces. In South Africa, say, these forces include poverty and racism; in other settings, gender inequality conspires with poverty to lead to higher incidence of tuberculosis in poor women.[64] Throughout the United States, increased indices of economic inequity seem to favor epidemics in blighted inner cities, already ravaged by related epidemics of AIDS, intravenous drug use, homelessness, and racism. Overt political violence and war—themselves usually a reflection of long-sustained structural violence—have well-known associations with increased rates of tuberculosis.

Romanticism About "Folk Healing"

A strong vein of commentary in medical anthropology depicts folk healing as somehow superior—perhaps by virtue of its deeper roots in local cultures?—to biomedical therapies. Although some within the field have called these claims into question, the issue has since assumed importance far beyond the boundaries of anthropology.[65] But nonbiomedical treatments for active pulmonary or extrapulmonary tuberculosis have thus far proven to be spectacularly ineffective. They do not change case-fatality rates.

If folk healing were so effective, the world's wealthy would be monopolizing it. When the privileged do use folk healing and other nonbiomedical modalities, it is as adjunctive therapy, often for chronic illnesses refractory to biomedical intervention. (As an aside, I have personally treated dozens of Haitian folk healers for tuberculosis, malaria, and typhoid.) We live in an increasingly interconnected world. Robert David's use of herbal remedies to treat tuberculosis is emblematic not of his cultural integrity but of the unfair distribution of the world's resources.

Persistence of Insularity

We medical anthropologists, like other subspecialists, are usually familiar with the arcane debates of our own field. Yet we are too often unwill-
ing to learn the basics of infectious disease or epidemiology, even when
they are related to our chosen arenas of intervention. This sectarian approach to research can be costly when we are examining pandemics with
demonstrable relation to both biological and social forces—which is to
say all pandemics, as far as I can tell.

Why, for example, have anthropologists been generally ignored in the
AIDS pandemic? Perhaps because we too often and too loudly made immodest claims of causality: in the first years of the pandemic, the refrain
at many of our professional meetings was that anthropology had "special knowledge" about the "cultural practices" then held to be related to
the high incidence of AIDS in certain areas where we worked.[66] Regarding Haiti, for example, there was much talk about the role of voodoo.
Long after "exotic" cultural practices proved irrelevant to the spread of
HIV, these red herrings continued to figure prominently in our professional meetings. Meanwhile, important multidisciplinary research fal-
tered or was based on slipshod social theory.

FUTURE RESEARCH ON MDRTB

The emergence of MDRTB is a terrible vindication for those who predicted earlier in this century that a social disease could not be eradicated
without social action. But that clairvoyance is no occasion for celebration.
MDRTB is a biologically and socially complex development. To check it,
we must treat and prevent it, which requires an understanding of the
forces promoting and retarding its advance. How, more precisely, might
anthropology (and the other social sciences) contribute to efforts to control the new scourge of MDRTB?

Several research tasks come to mind. First, who is better qualified than social scientists to discern the mechanisms by which social forces (ranging
from racism to political violence) promote or retard the transmission or recrudescence of tuberculosis? Since several fairly obvious mechanisms have
already been brought forward, it is incumbent on us to offer a hierarchy of

factors and to understand how, in different settings, these might be differentially weighted. New research technologies, such as DNA fingerprinting techniques, promise new insight into the dynamics of transmission but will also lead to new social dilemmas that will demand innovative responses.[67]

Second, ethnographic research will be important in identifying and, again, *ranking* the barriers that prevent those afflicted with MDRTB from having access to the best care available. The best available care, regardless of the etiologic beliefs of the patient, seems to consist of multiple-drug regimens, accompanied by adequate nutrition, for at least eighteen months, and probably longer. Adopting a patient-centered approach, though important, is insufficient: "The challenge to researchers is to acknowledge that adherence is influenced by a complex array of factors, many of which are beyond the patient's control, and to begin identifying and describing these factors."[68]

Third, social scientists must become more engaged in multidisciplinary research and trials. We have much to offer those who seek to design programs that increase access to optimal therapies. In settings in Latin America and Russia, where effective therapy is urgently needed, we must critically examine confident claims that treating MDRTB is not cost-effective. Outcomes research on community-based MDRTB treatment efforts must be linked to innovative research on the dynamics of the transmission of this disease. Such explorations will link ethnography to both conventional and molecular epidemiology.

Fourth, research that exposes—and deplores—the mechanisms by which entrenched medical inequities are buttressed may help to redress these inequities. In so doing, we would no doubt also be exposing the real co-factors in this emerging epidemic of "social disease."

These suggestions are more crassly utilitarian than those usually heard in calls for social science research, but it is clear that we should act quickly to make common cause with those on the side of the sick-poor, regardless of profession—whether we are community health workers, or folk healers, or physicians, or bench scientists. Certainly, some of these will be stop-gap measures, but such measures matter a great deal to those sick with tuberculosis. "It is useful to remember," remarks Rosenkrantz, "that a 'social disease' typically affects the socially marginal, who can ill afford to wait for the fundamental insights and social transformations that challenge the well-established associations of disadvantage and disease."[69]

10 The Persistent Plagues

BIOLOGICAL EXPRESSIONS OF SOCIAL INEQUALITIES

Are you unaware that vast numbers of your fellow
men suffer or perish from need of the things that you
have to excess, and that you required the explicit and
unanimous consent of the whole human race for you
to appropriate from the common subsistence
anything besides that required for your own?

JEAN-JACQUES ROUSSEAU, 1755

We don't have to be expert in foreign affairs to have
an opinion as to how much security the
industrialized nations of the world bought with the
$300 million they spent over ten years to eradicate
smallpox, as compared to what was achieved with
the $28 billion spent in 1983 alone for arms exports
to Third World countries. Perhaps a few million
dollars given to improve the health of the children
of Central America would bring more security to
the area than the billions we have spent to arm the
parents—and often the children.

HOWARD HIATT, 1987

TWO WORLDS, TWO HOPES?

Suppose that you're a physician caring for patients infected with HIV. Perhaps your patients are typical of the more than thirty million people living with HIV in the world today.[1] That is, your patients are young— with a mean age of less than thirty years—and have the hopes and dreams of most young people. Half of them are women, most of them raising children. And the clear majority of your patients live in poverty.

This certainly describes my own patients. Some of them live in a U.S. city; the rest live in rural Haiti. On the one hand, these two groups of patients have little in common. They don't share language or culture. They acquired HIV in different ways. The health care systems in their countries are radically different, as are the relative availabilities of medications and diagnostic capabilities. On the other hand, what they do have in common—poverty and HIV—is becoming increasingly determinant as the clock ticks on.

Nowhere was this more clear than at the Eleventh World Conference on AIDS, held in Vancouver, Canada, in July 1996. The meeting's theme was "One World, One Hope," and the mood, as many noted, was unlike that at any of the preceding gatherings. "In contrast to the almost un-remitting gloom of the previous 10 AIDS conferences," reported the *Boston Globe*, "there is suddenly a giddy optimism that science has at last gained the upper hand against HIV."[2] The medical press concurred. "Mood Upbeat at International AIDS Conference," read a headline in *Infectious Disease News*, and similarly encouraging reports surfaced in the refereed journals.[3] On its 2 December 1996 cover, *Newsweek* went even further, asking simply, "The End of AIDS?"

The wellspring of this optimism was the announcement of "revolution-ary" new antiviral agents. Acting with unprecedented speed, the U.S. Food and Drug Administration approved three protease inhibitors in 1996; sev-eral more agents were already in the pipeline.[4] The wonders of combina-tion therapy—specifically, a three-drug cocktail that includes reverse tran-scriptase and protease inhibitors—were widely extolled in Vancouver and seem to have captured the imagination of providers, pharmaceutical companies, and, especially, patients. David Sanford, an editor at the *Wall Street Journal*, opens an affecting account of his own resuscitation by combination therapy by observing that "the year 1996 is when everything changed, and very quickly, for people with AIDS."[5] *Newsweek* wrote of "the Lazarus effect" seen among some living with HIV: "More drugs keep coming, more options, more time, more hope. It is a circle of life: all you have to do is stay alive until the next drug comes out, and the next, and the next."[6]

The concurrent development and approval of viral-load testing, which offered the first convenient index of viral activity, seemed only to buttress the extraordinary claims made about the new medications. In patients with high viral loads, instituting combination therapy usually led to a marked decline in detectable HIV.[7] Enthusiasm peaked when respected researchers spoke of patients in whom the virus was simply no longer detectable. Researchers announced an intense quest for "sanctuary sites" where the virus might be hiding, further fueling hopes of radical cures or "ablative treatments."[8] These hopes were echoed and amplified in the popular press and in clinics and AIDS service agencies throughout the United States and Europe.

That was the good news. The bad news, which undermined illusions of "One World, One Hope," concerned money. Annual costs of combination therapy can exceed $20,000, when laboratory tests and provider fees are added to the bill. This figure might not mean much in and of itself, but it takes on enormous significance in the absence of strategies to make these therapies available on the basis of need. This is precisely the situation faced by most of my patients in both Haiti and the United States. It is the situation faced by most people now living with HIV.

Let's say you permitted yourself, while in Vancouver, a brief moment of exhilaration and hope. This was powerful news. After all, what practitioner of modern medicine is at heart a Luddite? The advances of the past few decades have usually been laboratory-based, stemming from cumulative basic research rather than serendipitous discoveries. A decade of hard work has yielded the protease inhibitors and other antiviral agents. New tests of viral load are the logical sequels to a previous generation of tests. The significance of these findings, and of the research on which they are based, is enormous.

But one can be impressed by the power of modern medicine and yet dejected by our failure to deliver it equitably.[9] For me, one of the quickest ways to burst the "One World, One Hope" bubble was to return to Haiti, where HIV, unhampered, has continued to spread. And this is as true in certain U.S. settings as it is in Haiti. AIDS is already the leading cause of death of young adults in many U.S. cities, as it is in most cities in the developing world. Moving along the fault lines of society, HIV continues to entrench itself among the world's poor and marginalized, making enormous gains in parts of Asia, Africa, and Latin America. Some fairly sober scholars estimate that by the year 2000 as many as forty to one hundred million people will be infected with HIV.[10]

What accounts for our failure to prevent the spread of HIV? What forces promote its transmission? As I've argued throughout this book, social inequalities are central to the distribution of HIV infection. In the United States, as elsewhere, the disease is settling into poor or otherwise marginalized communities; previously bounded "risk groups" have in some settings melted into insignificance. The incidence of AIDS among women is increasing more rapidly than the incidence of AIDS among men: between 1985 and 1994, AIDS cases among women increased threefold.[11] Of cases of AIDS among women, 77 percent are registered among black and Hispanic women, most of them poor. Structural violence—gender inequality, racism, and poverty—is at the very heart of these trends.

There are not only striking differences in the distribution of HIV but also a great inequality of outcomes among those living with AIDS. In the United States, survival after a diagnosis of AIDS varies enormously, with women and people of color having shorter life expectancies than white men.[12] In the United States in 1994, death rates from HIV disease among black men were almost four times as high as for white men; for black women, death rates from AIDS were nine times as high as for white women.[13] What accounts for this variation? Some have suggested biologically based differences in susceptibility, noting that differences in viral type as well as differences in the biological makeup of men and women may contribute to poor outcomes.[14] Other conventional wisdom has it that cultural and psychological factors are important to differential survival.

When I and a group of colleagues recently spent a year reviewing these outcome data, we found no shortage of similar hypotheses; what was in short supply was research confirming them. Indeed, the best empirical research suggests just the opposite: regardless of cultural and psychological factors, patients with poor outcomes—those living in poverty, by and large, with minorities and women overrepresented— had them because of barriers in access to effective care.[15] Strong support for this hypothesis comes from the work of Chaisson, Keruly, and Moore, who reported that when these barriers were removed in one inner-city AIDS cohort, survival differences between blacks and whites as well as those between men and women disappeared. Their conclusion: "access to medical care is a more important predictor of survival than are sex, race, and income level."[16] In other words, ensuring equal access to effective medical interventions can efface the biological expression of social inequalities. This is a remarkable claim and, if true, heartening news for physicians and other providers.

Heartening news, yes, but also a challenge: surely the effacement of outcome inequalities achieved by Chaisson and colleagues serves as a rebuke to all of us who now countenance deepening inequalities of access. If "One World, One Hope" were an apposite slogan, the advent of effective new therapies should signal new opportunities to diminish the outcome gap so richly documented in the literature on HIV and AIDS. Alas, one does not need to work in Haiti to grasp the magnitude of the problem. One thinks less about combination therapy's price tag and more about the example offered by tuberculosis. Fifty years after the introduction of almost 100 percent effective combination therapy, tuberculosis remains the world's leading infectious cause of preventable deaths.[17] If the World Health Organization is correct, tuberculosis killed some three million people in 1996—more than died from complications of HIV infection, and more than have died of tuberculosis in any one year since 1900.[18] If we've done such a poor job delivering effective and inexpensive cures to people in the prime of their lives, what are our chances with medications that are less effective and hundreds of times as costly?

AIDS already seems to be following the trail traced by tuberculosis. In the case of AIDS, too, the inequitable distribution of effective therapies is likely to deepen the divide between the haves and the have-nots, as Paul Wise observes: "Regardless of their preventive or therapeutic character, new interventions—particularly those with great efficacy—can widen disparities in outcome if differentials in access to these new interventions are allowed to persist."[19] This is the dark side of medical progress: the better the therapy, the more injustice meted out to those not treated. About one hundred thousand U.S. citizens are receiving protease inhibitors at this writing; perhaps a million are infected. In Europe, the situation is worse.[20]

In the developing world, where the majority of potential beneficiaries live, virtually no one is receiving, or is even slated to receive, the new drugs. Protease inhibitors, we're told, are not "appropriate technology" for the residents of poor countries. In this view, antiviral therapy is "pie in the sky" for those with the ill fortune to be both African and living with HIV. From outside of the sprawling international health bureaucracies, at least, it seems as if the health-care-for-all movement has run out of steam. In Geneva and Paris and Bethesda, few have made anything of the fact that Africa is the continent that could most benefit from these drugs. Again, where are the Virchows of global public health?

"GOTTA CLEAN UP YOUR ACT"

From inside health bureaucracies, the view is of course different. Here, one hears plenty of reasons why universal access to combination therapy is deemed "unrealistic," "impractical." And one does not have to travel to Africa to hear these reasons. Because failure to treat is regarded by many as medical injustice, the "justifications" for inequalities of access can become rather baroque. This is especially true when inequities are obvious to the naked eye. Often, in settings of poverty and persistent disease, failure to treat is transformed into "treatment failure." In this manner, the burden of responsibility for poor outcomes may more easily be laid at the feet of the untreated rather than on the shoulders of those who manufacture, sell, or prescribe therapies.

Take the city of New York, perhaps the wealthiest city in the world and at the same time home to a population that is among the most devastated by AIDS. It is a city marked by economic inequity, which seems to undercut AIDS care even as it promotes HIV transmission. Under the banner headline "Precious Pills," the *Wall Street Journal* ran a front-page story in 1996 about protease inhibitors and the city's poor. A subheading read: "Gotta Clean Up Your Act." The editors were quoting an AIDS outreach worker, who asserted, "A lot of people are saying they've heard something about this new kind of medicine that's different, more powerful, that's not like AZT. But I tell them, 'If you want the medicine, you first gotta clean up your act.'"[21]

The thoughtful report included conversations with some of the people who, in theory at least, might most benefit from combination therapy. Many were having enormous trouble acquiring the new drugs. The essay echoed rumors of noncompliance among the poor, recounting the story of one woman who sold her precious pills in order to buy narcotics. Such behavior, the article pointed out, was risky not only for the patient: "researchers fear that suspending treatment for even a few days, due to the loss of insurance coverage, simple forgetfulness or an episode of narcotics use or crime, may generate dangerous new drug-resistant strains."[22] Thus are reservations about the compliance of the poor recast as public health concerns, with the suggestion that medications "wasted" on the poor may only strengthen the disease's hand.

We already have anecdotal evidence that physicians in New York City are acting on their assessments of the likelihood that patients will adhere to therapy. "It is definitely happening," commented the director of planning of one AIDS service agency in lower Manhattan. "There is frustration on the part of social workers, case managers and such because they know some doctors won't prescribe to people who are drug users." The justification for withholding treatment is to protect the public: "The doctors maintain that poor compliance with the drug-taking regimen could not only spell disaster for an individual patient, but also create a potential public-health risk through the spread of a virus resistant to so many drugs."[23]

The specter of multidrug-resistant strains is often raised in the popular press and is widely cited as a reason to limit the use of combination therapy to those who can be relied upon. On the one hand, such observations seem eminently sensible. On the other, what do I tell Gloria, who at age thirty-nine is already blind in one eye (a complication of a viral opportunistic infection of the retina)? Never an addict herself, Gloria was in love with one once; he was the father of her two children, both uninfected. She wants, she says, to see at least one of them graduate from high school. She's without insurance and was not allowed to enroll in one protease-inhibitor study because she had previously failed to adhere to an AZT trial. (The drug gave her headaches, she reported, and made her anemic.) Discussions of her past "noncompliance" invariably played a role every time she was considered for combination therapy.

A great deal is at stake, clearly, in this intense focus on patient noncompliance. Those who argue that entire classes of HIV-infected people lacked the personal discipline to abstain from health-threatening activities—the fact of infection is here turned into a character flaw—now point to the unsuitability of these people for combination therapy. After all, if people can't get their acts together, they certainly won't be up to taking combination therapy, which demands rigorous scheduling. *Newsweek* recently cited Dr. Doug Dietrich as an AIDS specialist who helped write AIDS reimbursement guidelines for Blue Cross/Blue Shield. "If you give protease inhibitors to people who are not compliant," he claimed, "they're really wasted. It's tantamount to flushing them down the toilet."[24]

So goes the conventional wisdom. The casting-pearls-before-swine take on distribution of therapies is a staple of commentary whenever care is rationed. We read of people who "live in the present" and are thus incapable of taking prophylaxis designed to prevent adverse events. We read of "erratic noncompliers" who breed resistant strains, making the situation worse for everyone else. Worried about patients who can't get their acts together, Dr. Dietrich spoke of "screening for compliance." But careful research has revealed that physicians are incapable of identifying noncompliers.[25]

Furthermore, past noncompliance does not necessarily predict poor adherence to a new regimen. David Sanford, the *Wall Street Journal* editor, would certainly be described as a "model patient." Yet listen to his story. As he tells it, he was prescribed AZT and dapsone—"a drug for lepers"—after his CD4 count dipped below 200. Asked by the pharmacist if he wanted counseling, Mr. Sanford declined. "I also didn't want to take the medicines," he continued. "Definitely not a drug for lepers. And not AZT, which had potentially bad side effects, including liver damage. I took the pills for five days and quit." And yet Mr. Sanford was scrupulously adherent to his subsequent combination therapy, which he credits with bringing him back from the grave. Not only was Mr. Sanford noncompliant, he also displayed tendencies to "live in the present," and he tended, by his own description, to be impulsive: "I had blown my mother's estate, about $180,000, on living for the moment, eating in the best restaurants and taking three or four foreign vacations a year."[26] Somehow none of this was held against him—and rightly so, since Mr. Sanford subsequently complied with a new and better antiviral regimen.

Can we, in good conscience, blame the failure to make new technologies available on our patients? Is the locus of blame to be found in the hearts and minds of the sick? Can we claim that personal motivations or cultural beliefs will determine the efficacy of medical interventions when we can readily document that economic and logistic barriers to access continue to play a major role in the delivery of health care? In a medical system riven by inequities, willful noncompliance should always be a diagnosis of exclusion, made only after other extrapersonal barriers to access have been removed.

Working in Haiti makes this even clearer. What, exactly, do I tell my Haitian patients, many of whom, like Gloria, are as likely to lack "day planners" as they are day care? In Haiti, I suppose I'll have to pray that my patients don't ask me about protease inhibitors. I doubt they'll buy the it's-not-appropriate-technology argument that is already conventional wisdom in most international health circles. In Haiti, the concept of "appropriate technology" is already regarded as a means of justifying the unfair partition of the world's wealth. What if they ask whether I have access to such medicines? Surely the candid answer would be *yes*. I can get on an airplane and, in less than the time it took them to walk to our clinic, have my hands on indinavir, saquinavir, or any other drug I want. Some months from now, if past experience is any guide, I won't even have to leave Haiti to find these drugs—at a price. Wealthy Haitians have access to more or less the same medications as wealthy people anywhere else.

This question runs through my mind as I read and hear about patient noncompliance being *the* factor that limits the utility of combination therapy. There are many things I'd like to tell my patients, but somehow I cannot bring myself to recommend that they "clean up their acts." If I could acknowledge that their lives have been damaged by poverty, by racism, and, often enough, by gender inequality, if only I could say this in an appropriate way, I would. If I could tell them that they deserve the best medical care I can deliver, I'd tell them that, too.

Gloria eventually received her combination therapy. And she's doing much better—*almost as if she had a treatable infectious disease.* Others living in the wealthiest city in the world have not been so fortunate. A recent survey of seven hundred New Yorkers with AIDS revealed "sharp racial differences in the use of drug cocktails. While 35 percent of white patients surveyed were not taking any antiretrovirals, 54 percent of African American respondents were on no antiretroviral medications."[27]

CLEANING UP OUR ACT

Today the stakes for those living with both HIV and poverty are increasingly clear. The *Wall Street Journal* summed it up: "At a time of intense focus on the high cost of health care, the new treatments are certain to raise anew the question of how far the nation is willing to go to care for many of its sickest, especially those who live on society's fringes."[28]

If you're a physician working with people who inhabit these "fringes," it's possible to recast the question: how far are we willing to go in doling out health care only to those who can pay for it? Increasingly, the inequalities that we're called upon to countenance are inimical to good medicine. Even stop-gap measures, such as the federal program designed to make AIDS therapies available to the poor, are under heavy fire by politicians who have probably concluded, perhaps correctly, that they and theirs are never likely to need such drugs. More than half of all states, in administering these programs, do not include protease inhibitors among "reimbursable" therapies. Other states use lotteries to dispense the new antivirals. In Missouri, for example, where 2639 patients need the drugs, 75 lucky individuals will be chosen to receive them.[29] Nor are those who have already responded to the new therapies exempt. In May 1997, many AIDS patients in Mississippi received a notice from the Health Department: their antiviral cocktails would be cut off in thirty days. The state government was apparently uninterested in matching funds available through the federal drug program.[30]

Upon reflection, perhaps we physicians are the ones who need to clean up our act. In saying this, I do not wish to exaggerate the power of doctors and other providers; increasingly, it is the pharmaceutical and health care industries, and also federal governments, who call the shots on questions of access to effective medical care. But the power of medicine stems not merely from the wonders of science. It stems, too, from the power of moral suasion. We can call for certain measures not because they are cost-effective—the current and unchallenged mantra—but because they are the best we can do for our patients, especially our poor patients. For our success in confronting AIDS will not be measured, ultimately, by how well we do in treating the nonpoor. Ten years ago, Allan Brandt offered the following prediction, which now reads more like a final warning than a prophecy:

> In the years ahead we will, no doubt, learn a great deal more about AIDS and how to control it. We will also learn a great deal about the nature of our society from the manner in which we address the disease. AIDS will be a standard by which we may measure not only our medical and scientific skill but also our capacity for justice and compassion.[31]

"TAILORING A TIME-BOMB"

As the century draws to a close, we are faced with a troubling conundrum: our ability to detect and treat infectious disease grows, but less quickly, it seems, than do certain pandemics. Let us reconsider tuberculosis. The numbers, often reviewed, are nothing if not staggering: in this decade, several hundred million new infections and possibly as many as thirty million deaths.[32] Reichman has deplored the lack of "outrage" over our failure to confront tuberculosis; if tuberculosis treatment were taken seriously, he argues, discussions about it "would have to be moved to the local football stadium to accommodate all interested parties."[33]

One ominous possibility is that highly resistant tuberculosis will become an important cause of death. More than a decade ago, Michael Iseman signaled the "inadvertent genetic engineering" wrought by ineffective tuberculosis-control programs and warned of a time-bomb waiting to explode. In failing to prevent or contain resistance to first-line drugs, "we are unwittingly transforming an eminently treatable infection into a life-threatening disease that is exorbitantly expensive to treat."[34] Iseman's editorial called for increased attention to turning the tide in international tuberculosis, noting that a "proactive multi-national program" might defuse the time-bomb.

The stimulus for Iseman's commentary was the report of two large surveys of tuberculosis outcomes in Peru. In 1984, Hopewell and colleagues estimated the overall rate of success in treating 2510 patients diagnosed in 1980 at only 47 percent, largely because 41 percent of the patients failed to complete more than ten months of treatment. But even among those who completed more than ten months of fully supervised therapy, more than 21 percent had treatment failure, relapsed, or died. The authors concluded that these unfavorable outcomes among the treated were the result of "many years of poor chemotherapy resulting in a high prevalence of patients with drug-resistant organisms."[35]

Peru still has high rates of tuberculosis, but a great deal has happened in the years since Hopewell and colleagues presented their overview of the Peruvian experience. Following WHO guidelines, the government of Peru reorganized its national tuberculosis program in 1991. In the past several years, the program can point to significantly increased rates of therapy completion, in part because of the adoption of directly observed therapy with a short-course, four-drug regimen (DOTS). All patients with new diagnoses of tuberculosis are treated with the *esquema único*, the same regimen. Recent unpublished data also suggest a decrease in acquired resistance—a laudable trend often registered where directly observed therapy is used.

Peru has been singled out for special praise from the international tuberculosis community. But what happened to the "treatment failures" described by Hopewell and colleagues in 1984? Since they were not effectively treated and the natural history of untreated tuberculosis is well known, we can safely advance certain hypotheses. Most of the patients with resistant disease were young adults; most had cavitary disease, with high microbial burdens—in Hopewell's series, approximately 50 percent of the patients who abandoned treatment were defined as having positive sputum at the time of abandonment.[36] Most were thus highly infectious, often for years. When these patients had tuberculosis-related complaints—respiratory distress, hemoptysis, constitutional symptoms, paroxysms of coughing—they presented to area clinics and hospitals, where respiratory precautions were not followed. Eventually, many—perhaps most—died, but not before infecting many others.

Our own work in urban Peru confirms these hypotheses. In parts of Lima, an MDRTB epidemic of troubling proportions threatens recent gains in tuberculosis control. Contact tracing and ethnographic research reveal that this epidemic is by no means contained in this region of the city. Many patients with active MDRTB work as long as they can, usually to pay for the second-line drugs they know they need but can only intermittently afford. They also continue to frequent clinics and hospitals for their tuberculosis-related symptoms. Nosocomial spread continues apace; 10 percent of our patients are former health care workers. Further, these patients are highly mobile within the city of Lima and within the country, since many have close ties to the rural regions from which they came. The northern Lima epidemic has been felt beyond Peruvian borders as well: at least two cases of tuberculosis resistant to all first-line drugs, both apparently acquired in Lima's northern cone, have recently been reported in Boston and suburban New York. The time-bomb, it would seem, has already exploded.

COST-EFFECTIVENESS
AND THE EXCUSES OF OUR TIMES

What does the World Health Organization, a key architect of the Peruvian national program, say about these extraordinary and troubling developments? In materials published in anticipation of World TB Day 1997, WHO's Global Tuberculosis Programme announced that in Peru "TB is being defeated by a model DOTS program." As for MDRTB, the same publication argues that "DOTS makes it virtually impossible to cause a patient to develop the incurable forms of TB that are becoming more common. Other treatment strategies are actually causing multidrug-resistant TB and may be doing more harm than good."[37] The answer to MDRTB, in this view, is more short-course DOT with first-line drugs, with fairly overt opposition to efforts to manage drug-resistant MDR strains: "The WHO Tuberculosis Programme has recommended that treatment of chronic cases with [second-line] drugs remain a low priority for national tuberculosis programmes in developing countries due to their high costs and the limited prospects for cure of these cases."[38]

For clinicians, the fatal flaw of these arguments is apparent: those now sick with MDRTB cannot be so lightly dismissed. Milagros, for example, is a thirty-year-old woman who formerly worked in a tuberculosis clinic in a public health hospital in Lima. She used to love to care for children, she told me, especially those with tuberculosis, since they were often shunned. When I first met her, Milagros was gravely ill with MDRTB. She was emaciated, wasted by daily fevers and drenching sweats. Part of her right lung, destroyed by the disease, had been removed; the other lung was severely affected. She'd been told that nothing further could be done; in keeping with WHO recommendations, it had been determined that the treatment of MDRTB was not cost-effective in poor countries.

Needless to say, Milagros did not much appreciate this logic. Neither did her three sisters, also suffering with MDRTB. (Another sister had already died of this disease.) As a tuberculosis worker, Milagros knew that there were, in fact, antibiotics to which her infecting isolate was susceptible. When she received them, she soon began to respond—*almost as if she had a treatable infectious disease.* Milagros seemed particularly pleased that her treatment and improvement occurred against a tide of official opinion. She announced her intention to prove this opinion misguided. Efforts on her behalf may ultimately fail, but they will not have failed to call into question the cynical calculus by which some lives are considered valuable and others expendable.

QUESTIONING THE ANSWERS

If MDRTB is already a problem in the middle-income countries of Latin America, to say nothing of the former Soviet Union, why do current recommendations from the international health bureaucracies discourage tackling this problem? Opposition to the aggressive treatment of MDRTB in developing countries is justified as public health *realpolitik*—that is, the world is the way it is, with vast disparities in the amount of resources available for tuberculosis control. For developing countries, noneradicating control that focuses on DOTS is held to be the best way of addressing tuberculosis.

At least four sets of reasons—one clinical, one epidemiologic, one analytic, and one moral—lead me to conclude that ignoring MDRTB is an unacceptable strategy. The clinical reasons are straightforward and not unlike those advanced in discussing antiviral therapy. People like Milagros and others introduced in these pages exist, and they matter. They're sick with resistant tuberculosis, for which short-course therapy is wholly ineffective.

But arguments against treating MDRTB are also epidemiologically flawed. Untreated MDRTB creates a series of subepidemics in a susceptible population. One type of subepidemic is a "fast" MDRTB outbreak, in which progressive primary infection comes to invade households, factories, classrooms, and, especially, clinics, hospitals, and prisons. In the face of a growing global HIV pandemic, we can expect an increased fraction of MDRTB to be fast, since those concurrently infected are far more likely to progress to active disease. Even larger, however, will be the "slow" epidemic, since the majority of those infected with MDR strains do not develop progressive primary infection. Instead, those with latent MDRTB ensure that future epidemics, both fast and slow, will be resistant to our best drugs. We can also expect that malnutrition, high rates of HIV and other concurrent disease, crowding, and social disruption of various sorts will fan both types of outbreaks.

When susceptible disease is effectively treated while MDRTB is ignored, the relative contribution of resistant strains to the overall caseload can only increase each year. The day may come when DOTS generates more resistance than cures. Such "perverse" outcomes may occur in settings where levels of resistance—whether primary or acquired, since the dynamics of transmission are the same in either case—are sufficiently high. In such cases, DOTS will be insufficient to cure active tuberculosis, but it *will* serve to amplify resistance to first-line drugs.

Theoretical models of noneradicating control have already predicted such occurrences. "To prevent perverse outcomes," assert Blower, Small, and Hopewell, "the treatment failure rate should be <35 to 40% in developed countries and <10% in developing countries. Thus, higher standards (lower treatment failure rates) should be required of control programs in developing countries than of control programs in developed countries." Higher treatment failure could be tolerated, they argue, only "if the relative efficacy of treatment of drug-resistant tuberculosis could be increased in developing countries."[39] Thus, failure to treat MDRTB may well be the Achilles heel of national tuberculosis programs now labeled "success stories."

For those who counter that only incidence, not proportions, matter, other features of the Peruvian epidemic raise the specter of rising case rates. The encroachment of HIV and the massive urbanization registered there will surely hamper future efforts to decrease incidence, since both processes are likely to adversely alter the dynamics of tuberculosis transmission. As urbanization progresses, ties to rural roots are rarely severed. Instead, complex social webs not only link the city and the countryside but also link one country to another. It is for these reasons, and because of the often indolent nature of the disease, that tuberculosis epidemics are only briefly local. An estimated one-third of U.S. tuberculosis cases occur among those born in another country, and this proportion is growing.[40] With a third of the world's population infected with viable *M. tuberculosis*, there will be no closing the gates—certainly not in the global era. The ways in which tuberculosis is transmitted mean that a "local" MDRTB outbreak constitutes a global concern.

The insistence that it is too expensive to treat MDRTB in poor countries is also a failure of social analysis, in at least two ways. First, "large-scale," political-economic arguments against MDRTB treatment are fraught with error. Although we have obvious confirmation of our failure to effectively confront tuberculosis, little evidence exists to support the hypothesis that we lack sufficient means to cure all tuberculosis cases, everywhere and regardless of susceptibility patterns. In fact, the degree of accumulated world wealth is altogether unprecedented. This accumulation has occurred, however, in tandem with growing inequality and the draining of resources away from regions where tuberculosis is most endemic. Simply following the money trail reveals both the degree of available capital and also the degree to which resource flows are transnational. For example, in 1996, Peru made debt payments, largely to U.S. banks and the international financial institutions, of $1.25 billion—over 14 percent of total government expenditures. Projections for 1997 estimated that debt payments would total $1.85 billion, representing 18.7 percent of all government outlays.[41] And is it merely polemical to observe that, even as MDRTB was deemed too costly to treat in Peru, the government spent $350 million for a dozen fighter jets, calling the deal "a terrific bargain"?[42]

Second, the head-in-the-sand approach represents a failure of ethnographic analysis. Social scientists who study the therapeutic itineraries of tuberculosis patients know that a slow death from the disease is not quietly accepted by the young adults who are its chief victims. With ever-increasing access to information, patients and their loved ones know that MDRTB can be treated with second-line drugs, just as AIDS patients in many poor countries now know about the existence of effective antiviral therapies. In middle-income countries like Peru, which are in reality inegalitarian settings where wealth and poverty are in close juxtaposition, second-line antituberculous drugs are in fact already available—for sale at exorbitant prices. As we have seen, private pulmonologists prescribe these drugs to families who are willing to go to great lengths to save their sick. But because these families are poor, they cannot purchase these medications in a regular manner. In this way, intermittently acquired second-line drugs "knock off" even more potentially effective agents.

Finally, arguments against treating MDRTB in settings of poverty are morally unsound. Through analytic chicanery—the claim that the world is composed of discretely bounded nation-states, some rich, some poor—we're asked to swallow what is, ultimately, a story of growing inequality and our willingness to caution it. But careful systemic analysis of pandemic disease leads us to see links, not disjunctures. When these failures of analysis are pointed out, the real reason that MDRTB is treatable in the United States and "untreatable" in Peru or Haiti comes into view. Opposition to the aggressive treatment of MDRTB in developing countries may be justified as "sensible" or "pragmatic," but as a policy it is tantamount to the differential valuation of human life, for those who advocate such a policy, regardless of their nationality, would never accept such a death sentence themselves. It is because MDRTB's victims tend to be poor, and thus less valuable, that such policies appear reasonable. Where are the Virchows of international tuberculosis control?

In Virchow's day, with germ theory ascendant, the war against infectious diseases became a rallying cry for progressive forces working to improve the conditions endured by the poor.[43] In fact, throughout the history of medicine, physicians and other healers have honored a "social contract" that includes care for the destitute sick. The degree to which this duty is deemed central to the goals of medicine and public health has varied with time and place. Often enough, plagues of communicable disease have served as a warning to a society that dismisses the illness of those living in poverty. Writing of typhoid fever in early Victorian England, Dr. William Budd put it this way:

> This disease not seldom attacks the rich, but it thrives among the poor. But by reason of our common humanity we are all, whether rich or poor, more nearly related here than we are apt to think. The members of the great human family are, in fact, bound together by a thousand secret ties, of whose existence the world in general little dreams. And he that was never yet connected with his poorer neighbour, by deeds of charity or love, may one day find, when it is too late, that he is connected with him by a bond which may bring them both, at once, to a common grave.[44]

From the perspective of the world's poor—necessarily the perspective one takes in Haiti—it may be that we have never made the care of the destitute sick central enough. But even in a country as wealthy as our own, commitment to the health problems of the poor, never robust, is flagging. In the United States, at least, investor-owned health plans have rapidly transformed the way we confront illness. "Medicine became big business," observes one report. "Patients turned into profit centers; their many ailments, product lines." For-profit hospital chains now offer doctors "equity partnerships."[45] Writing in the *New England Journal of Medicine*, one of the cheerleaders for these new trends argues that "there is no longer a role for non-profit health plans in the new health care environment."[46]

If there is no role for any but the profiteers, what sort of "health care environment" have we created? Granted, there is nothing wrong with doing well by doing good. But in letting our guard down, we now find ourselves in a peculiarly modern situation: as the promise of science and technology at last yields the tools that could prevent early deaths, we have broken the social contract that could ensure that these tools are used wisely. And so the "thousand secret ties" that bind us to the destitute sick will become largely the pathogens that plague them. By the crude calculus of modern public health, will self-protection become the sole justification for effective measures to contain the plagues of the poor?

LAST WORDS

Jean-Jacques Rousseau knew that he could never provide enough detail to "unmask all the various faces behind which inequality has appeared up to the present." But some faces, though often hidden, are too grotesque to cloak for long. "It is manifestly contrary to the law of nature," he wrote in 1755, "that a handful of men should gorge themselves with superfluities while the starving multitude goes in want of necessities."[47] His observations are no less true today; they may be, in fact, even more apposite to our peculiarly modern inequality. Clearly we live in a time of unprecedented wealth and technological advancement. But a growing and globalizing market economy has not, as promised, lifted all boats. Instead, increasing world wealth has been linked to a sharp rise in inequalities of various sorts.[48]

What have such trends meant for the health of those who've lost out in this "new world order"? Like Rousseau, I have attempted to "trace the march of inequality"—in this case, its march through the ranks, through the bodies, of the poor. Even as I seek to avoid closing with too philosophical a flourish, it is impossible not to underline the costs of the widening gap between the haves and the have-nots. A growing body of data—Wilkinson reviews ten separate sets of data from eight different groups of researchers—reveals that income distribution is related to national mortality rates in countries in North America, Europe, and Asia. This association, Wilkinson observes, "cannot be regarded as the result of one or two chance findings."[49]

From the point of view of my patients, the cost of modern inequality is even greater than that calculated by Wilkinson and others who define "societies" as nation-states. When he writes that "it is clear that the main problems of poverty (at least within the developed world) are problems of relative poverty," Wilkinson misses the worst of it.[50] As I have tried to show, the intense suffering of many of the people described in these pages cannot be understood as divorced from the suffering and surfeit documented within the borders of countries like the United States and Britain. The sick of rural Haiti, urban Peru, and sub-Saharan Africa may be invisible to those tallying the victims of modern inequality, but they are, in many senses, casualties of the very same processes that have led to crime and decreased social cohesion "at home."

Modern inequalities are both local and global. One of the central arguments of *Infections and Inequalities* is that a lack of systemic and critical analysis permits these global ties to be obscured. And yet new kinds of proximity make inequality, and the plagues that accompany it, very modern affairs. As the book's subtitle suggests, these sicknesses and inequalities are themselves best thought of as together constituting our modern plagues. That they are not widely viewed as indissociably linked is in part a result of the limitations of epidemiology and international health—disciplines that increasingly take shelter behind "validated" methodologies while ignoring the larger forces and processes that determine why some people are sick while others are shielded from risk. McMichael, cited elsewhere in these pages, puts it succinctly: "Modern epidemiology is oriented to explaining and quantifying the bobbing of corks on the surface waters, while largely disregarding the stronger undercurrents that determine where, on average, the cluster of corks ends up along the shoreline of risk."[51] Some disciplines have trouble distinguishing rigor from rigor mortis.

In a sense, these shortcomings redeem anthropology, critiqued at the outset of this book, as they redeem other contextualizing disciplines. "Anthropology and social history," argues Kleinman in writing of international health, "offer a needed complement because they critique the deep-grained assumptions that need to be recast. Only through the concrete understanding of particular worlds of suffering and the way they are shaped by political economy and cultural change can we possibly come to terms with the complex human experiences that undermine health."[52]

It is patently unacceptable that we fail to see sociologically, for the events and processes and pathologies chronicled here, biological though they may be, are all of fundamentally social origin. They are biosocial. The many immodest claims of causality interrogated throughout this book are born largely of a failure to see sociologically. Taking on such claims is central to the work of demystification that might justify the existence of scholars in a world riven by inequality. As Bourdieu concludes in *La Misère du Monde:*

> To subject to scrutiny the mechanisms which render life painful, even untenable, is not to neutralize them; to bring to light contradictions is not to resolve them. But, as skeptical as one might be about the efficacy

of the sociological message, we cannot dismiss the effect it can have by allowing sufferers to discover the possible social causes of their suffering and, thus, to be relieved of blame.[53]

Girded by conviction and by critical reassessments of what inequality means for health, there is much to be done, particularly on behalf of the destitute sick. That is, we see sociologically, but we may act medically. The new millennium is a particularly good time to do so. Ironically, perhaps, it is technology that will redeem medicine and the healing arts. But technology, as we have seen, needs social medicine and other disciplines that might resist the seemingly ineluctable pull of inequality.

Three decades after the Surgeon General claimed that "it's time to close the book on infectious diseases," these pathogens, most of them treatable, remain the world's leading killers. Is this the best we can do? If we fail to improve on our past performances and to resist the current trends, we risk sapping modern medicine of its vast power. If we lived in a utopia, simply practicing good medicine or conducting quality research would be enough. But, no matter how you slice it, we live in a dystopia. Increasingly, inequalities of access and outcome characterize our world. These inequalities could be the focus of our collective action as engaged members of the healing and teaching professions, broadly conceived. We have before us an awesome responsibility—to prevent social inequalities from being embodied as adverse health outcomes. We have the technology.

The poor, we're told, will always be with us. If this is so, then infectious diseases will be, too—the plagues that the rich, in vain, attempt to keep at bay.

Notes

INTRODUCTION

1. For a review of my conclusions, see Farmer 1992, chap. 18.
2. World Health Organization 1996.
3. Bloom 1992, p. 538.
4. These estimates are from the World Health Organization, which further reports that acute lower respiratory infections, diarrhea (including cholera, typhoid, and dysentery), tuberculosis, malaria, hepatitis B, HIV/AIDS, measles, neonatal tetanus, pertussis, and intestinal helminthiases top the list of infectious killers; see "Infectious Diseases" 1996.
5. Friedman, Williams, Singh, and Frieden 1996.
6. Sen 1992, p. ix.
7. Fineberg and Wilson 1996, p. 859.
8. There are, of course, many exceptions to this general rule. There are also signs that an anthropology of suffering and a greater attention to the sicknesses of the poor are of increasing importance in anthropology and medicine, respectively; see, for example, Kleinman, Das, and Lock 1997. That growing numbers of U.S. physicians are impatient with a health care system that fails to address the

needs of the poor is suggested by statements such as that recently made by the Ad Hoc Committee to defend Health Care (1997).

9.   Scheper-Hughes 1992, p. 21.

10.   Wagner 1975, p. 2.

11.   Starn 1992, p. 168.

12.   Ibid., p. 163.

13.   See Fabian's 1983 essay on "how anthropology makes its object." On ethnographic writing and its canon, see Geertz 1988, which offers a fairly complete, if somewhat dismissive, listing of other studies of the subject.

14.   Asad 1975, p. 17.

15.   Marcus and Fischer 1986, p. 134.

16.   For a review of this literature, see Farmer, Connors, and Simmons 1996, chap. 5.

17.   I have used the term "exaggeration of personal agency" throughout this book to indicate the failure, widespread in the social sciences and in popular commentary, to incorporate an understanding of how individual agency is constrained by poverty and inequality. In anthropology, such exaggeration was linked to the use of the notion of a "culture of poverty" (see Lewis 1969 and Valentine 1968). For a helpful overview of the ideological legacy of the "culture of poverty" debate, see Morris's trenchant 1996 essay.

18.   It is important to note that risk for coronary artery disease, at least in the United States, is borne disproportionately by men in lower income brackets, not by prosperous businessmen with so-called Type-A personalities. For a review of the association between heart disease, race, and social class, see Ayanian, Udvarhelyi, Gatsonis, Pashos, and Epstein 1993; Escobedo, Giles, and Anda 1997; Giles, Anda, Caspar, Escobedo, and Taylor 1995; and Ferguson, Tierney, Westmoreland, Mamlin, Segar, Eckert, Zhao, Martin, and Weinberger 1997. See also two editorials on this topic by John Ayanian (1993, 1994). Some of the mechanisms underlying these associations are explored in Kawachi, Kennedy, Lochner, and Prothrow-Stith 1997.

19.   Again, note that in the United States local inequalities—along lines of race, for example—are clearly associated with poor access to interventional cardiology. See, for example, the studies by Ayanian, Udvarhelyi, Gatsonis, Pashos, and Epstein (1993) and Giles, Anda, Caspar, Escobedo, and Taylor (1995).

20.   Eisenberg 1984, p. 526.

21.   Farmer 1992, p. 8.

22.   I will draw upon this vast and heterogeneous literature throughout this book. For overviews, see Antonovsky 1967; Bunker, Gomby, and Kehrer 1989; Dutton and Levine 1989; Evans, Barer, and Marmor 1994; Haan, Kaplan, and Camacho 1987; Hahn, Eaker, Barker, Teutsch, Sosniak, and Krieger 1995; Kitagawa and Hauser 1973; Kosa, Antonovsky, and Zola 1969; Krieger, Rowley, Herman, Avery, and Phillips 1993; Pappas, Queen, Hadden, and Fisher 1993; Syme and Berkman 1976; Thiede and Traub 1997; Wilkinson 1992. A special issue of Dædalus (Fall 1994, vol. 123, no. 4) also reviews the subject of "health and wealth."

23.   Lerner 1969, p. 111. See also Adler, Boyce, Chesney, et al. 1994, p. 15.

24.   Dutton and Levine 1989, p. 31.

25.   Ryan 1971, p. 163.

26.   The often linear relationship between poverty and sickness changes as basic nutritional and sanitary needs are met. Wilkinson (1996) offers a critical overview of the association between income distribution—a key marker of social inequality—and health outcomes in wealthy and middle-income nations. In many of these settings, he argues, "health is almost unrelated to measures of economic growth and yet closely related to income distribution" (p. 221). For more on the association between high grades of inequality and increased morbidity and mortality, see Kawachi, Kennedy, Lochner, and Prothrow-Stith 1997; and Kennedy, Kawachi, and Prothrow-Stith 1996. In *Infections and Inequalities,* I have attempted to explore this topic from a transnational perspective, shedding light on some often obscured links between Latin America and the industrialized countries.

27.   Nardell and Brickner 1996, p. 1259.

28.   Wise 1993, p. 9.

29.   Compare Paul Wise on infant mortality: "In a setting of profound poverty, the intention of clinical interventions is not to alleviate poverty but reduce its power to alter health outcomes; thus, clinical interventions' attack on the tragedy of infant mortality will be successful only when social influences are no longer expressed in differential outcomes" (ibid., p. 12).

30.   See, for example, Farmer, Robin, Ramilus, and Kim 1991.

31.   Chaisson, Keruly, and Moore 1995.

32.   Sen 1992, p. 69.

33.   Wilkinson 1996, p. ix.

34.   Kadlec 1997, pp. 59–60.

35.   In keeping with convention, all of the names of patients and informants have been changed, as have certain identifying details and place names.

CHAPTER 1

1.   Weise 1971, p. 6.

2.   Diederich and Burt 1986, p. 366.

3.   Feinsilver 1993, p. 103.

4.   See Feilden, Allman, Montague, and Rohde 1981. For a review of health conditions in rural Haiti, see also Farmer 1992, chap. 5, and Farmer 1996a.

5.   The lack of interest in tuberculosis has been the subject of much commentary. Laurie Garrett also captures nicely some of the professional attitudes toward other topics of interest to me: "If many young scientists in the mid-1960s considered bacteriology passé—a field commonly referred to as 'a science in which all the big questions have been answered'—the study of parasitology was thought to be positively prehistoric" (Garrett 1995a, p. 37). The young scientists of the mid-1960s

were, of course, my professors in the early 1980s. I should add, however, that any faculty as large as that of Harvard Medical School has committed and enthusiastic exceptions to this rule, and I am grateful to Arnie Weinberg, Jamie Maguire, Ed Nardell, Bob Moellering, and the late Ed Kass for their steering.

6.   I have explored the differences between charity, development, and social justice efforts in Farmer 1995b.

7.   Calling such positions "Luddite critiques" is, in a sense, generous, since many who espouse them are discussing the health conditions of people living in poverty. That is, they deem advanced technologies too expensive (not "cost-effective") specifically for the poor. These positions are, as noted, frequently encountered in what is now termed "international health"; they are endemic among the development set. Too seldom do these professionals oppose the lavish deployment of expensive technologies in their own—our own—communities.

8.   See Chapter 5 for more information about the village. The history of the dam project and its effects on the people of Do Kay are documented in Farmer 1992.

9.   For an attempt at drawing a Wallersteinian analysis of Haiti's place in the global economy, see Farmer 1988b. Like many anthropologists, I was attempting to show that locales such as Haiti are not merely "swept up" into global capitalism, but rather formulate local (and quite unforeseen) responses to large political-economic systems. See Mintz 1977 and Roseberry 1988 for elaborations of this position. Dupuy (1997) offers a more comprehensive analysis of Haiti's place in the modern world economy.

10.   The work of some of the pioneers à la Wallerstein has since been complemented by a number of social theorists who study diverse "cultural phenomena." (One recent sampling is contained in King 1997.) Although it is difficult to classify these writers, "all share, to a greater or lesser extent, at least two perspectives: the rejection of the nationally constituted society as the appropriate object of [scholarly] discourse, or unit of social and cultural analysis, and in different ways and to varying degrees, a commitment to conceptualizing 'the world as a whole'" (King 1997, p. viii).

11.   Garrett 1995a, p. 618.

12.   Again, this disenchantment was not original; for a discussion of recent theoretical trends in anthropology, see Marcus and Fischer 1986, as well as Escobar 1992, Ortner 1984, and Roseberry 1988.

13.   Scheper-Hughes 1993, p. 967.

14.   In adopting such an approach, I was following trends widespread in my generation of anthropologists. We were responding to a lack of such analyses: Marcus and Fischer had argued, in a widely read essay, that "an interpretive anthropology fully accountable to its historical and political-economy implications . . . remains to be written" (1986, p. 86).

15.   We have jointly explored some of these questions (for example, in Farmer, Robin, Ramilus, and Kim 1991; Farmer and Kim 1991; Farmer and Kim 1996) but

know that others will necessarily remain unanswered. For instance, our own privileged status means that, although we have at times derided the "development set," we critics fit into our own lofty stratum. On this subject, Nancy Rose Hunt (1997) has written compellingly about "AIDS derivatives"—people whose livelihood depends somehow on the suffering of others.

16. For an overview of this work, see "Ten Years of Commitment" 1997. This article (and the *PIH Bulletin*) may be obtained from Partners in Health, 113 River Street, Cambridge, MA 02139.

17. De Cock, Soro, Coulibaly, and Lucas 1992.

18. Pape, Liautaud, Thomas, Mathurin, St Amand, Boncy, Pean, Pamphile, Laroche, and Johnson 1983. For example, we have seen HIV-TB co-infection presenting as tamponade (tuberculous pericarditis), paraplegia (tuberculous osteomyelitis of the spine), and even renal failure (a result of tuberculous nephritis rather than HIV nephropathy). For a detailed account of the presenting illnesses of two hundred patients with HIV disease, see Farmer 1997c.

19. Thanks are owed especially to the sustaining support of Tom White, who has made it possible for us to preferentially serve the destitute sick, and to the Episcopal Diocese of Upper South Carolina, who financed the new in-patient facility.

20. For a review of such patterns in poor urban communities generally, see Geiger 1992 and McCord and Freeman 1990.

21. See Martinez 1980 for an evaluation of the context of internal migration in Peru.

22. Starn 1992, p. 159.

23. Cited in "Peru: Politics and Violence; Sendero's Strategy from Close Up; Study Recommends Looking Beyond 'Terrorist' Label" 1989, p. 5. On the origins of Peruvian peasant revolt, see McClintock 1984 and Palmer 1986. For more on Sendero Luminoso, see Bourque and Warren 1989 and Degregori 1986.

24. These estimates vary. The figure cited comes from Paul Nunn, chief of the Tuberculosis Research and Surveillance Unit of the World Health Organization Global Tuberculosis Programme (see, for example, World Health Organization 1997b). See also Blower, Small, and Hopewell 1996.

25. Zimmerman 1997, p. 45.

26. Centers for Disease Control and Prevention 1992.

27. In a study of trends in U.S. tuberculosis from 1993 to 1996, 33 percent of patients with culture-positive tuberculosis and susceptibility results were foreign-born (Moore, Onorato, McCray, and Castro 1997).

28. See Farmer, Bayona, Becerra, et al. 1997. This work would not have been possible without the pragmatic solidarity of both Tom White and the Massachusetts State Laboratory Institute's Mycobacteriology Laboratory.

29. See Alexander 1997.

30. Farmer, Bayona, Shin, Alvarez, Becerra, Nardell, Nunez, Sanchez, Timperi, and Kim 1998.

31.   Whether the concept of nation-state functions as an analytic framework or an ideology is open to debate. Wallerstein observes that, in the current historical system, "one key geocultural value has been that every state should be a nation. This is what we mean by 'citizenship,' and it forms in turn the basis of the widely accepted myth of the primacy and sovereignty (with each state)" (1994, p. 9).

32.   See Angell 1997b; Angell justified her analogy by comparing, point by point, the AIDS trials to the infamous Tuskegee syphilis study. Angell was taken to task for this comparison by prominent figures in the scientific community (see, for example, Varmus and Satcher 1997), and two influential AIDS specialists resigned from the editorial board of the *New England Journal of Medicine* (see Saltus 1997). The debate continued on the front page of the *New York Times* with an exploration of the ironies of U.S.-funded AIDS research in the Ivory Coast (see French 1997). See also Lurie and Wolfe's original critique (1997) and Angell's editorial in the *New England Journal of Medicine* (1997a).

33.   A sharply worded editorial in *Lancet* questioned the "ethics industry": "Did ethicists know nothing about these trials (which seems unlikely, given their persistent rooting for ethically dubious medical practices), or was the fate of impoverished Africans thought not worthy of ethical consideration?" ("Editorial: The Ethics Industry" 1997).

34.   Anthropologists, in a zealous quest to promote cultural relativism, have at times contributed to this confusion. For example, Hammel (cited in Handwerker 1997, p. 799) asks, "By what principle short of imperialism do we insist on the application of civil or human rights in societies that have not come to these ideas through their own histories?" In so doing, he contributes to the two-worlds myth mentioned earlier. In most cases, the societies in question, and thus the ethically objectionable practices in question, are tightly linked to the (often powerful) society of the observing anthropologist. In an increasingly connected world, radical cultural relativism persists in the face of overwhelming evidence that we inhabit a single world. In adopting a world-systems approach to medical ethics, it is important not to erase the culturally specific experiences of any local moral world. As Kleinman notes, "Radical cultural relativism is a serious misinterpretation of what ethnography, cultural analysis, and cross-cultural comparison have contributed: the idea that before we apply an ethical category we hold to be universal, we had better understand the context of practice and ideas that constitute a local moral world" (1995a, p. 1672).

35.   Saba and Ammann 1997.

36.   Wallerstein 1995, p. 269.

CHAPTER 2

1.   Morse 1995, p. 9.

2.   Lederberg, Shope, and Oaks 1992, pp. 34–112. Oldstone (1998) takes a similar broad view of the emergence of viral hemorrhagic fevers.

3.   Morse 1995.

4.   Eckardt 1994, p. 409.

5.   Levine 1964.

6.   Ibid.

7.   Garrett 1995a, p. 47.

8.   Levine 1964, p. 3.

9.   For a helpful look at malaria as a reemerging disease, see Olliaro, Cattani, and Wirth 1996. For a critical review of recent malaria-control failures, see Garrett 1995a, chap. 2.

10.   Note that mine is a fairly innocent rereading of the term "tropical medicine," which has well-known roots in the colonial enterprise. Sheldon Watts offers a more trenchant and informed reevaluation of tropical medicine. He writes: "From its very onset tropical medicine was thus an 'instrument of empire' intended to enable the white 'races' to live in, or at the very least to exploit, all areas of the globe" (1998, p. xiii). See also Cueto 1992 and Solórzano 1992.

11.   See Frenk and Chacon 1991. See also Kleinman's excellent critique of "objectivity" in international health (Kleinman 1995b, pp. 68–93).

12.   See Gwatkin and Heuveline 1997.

13.   McCord and Freeman 1990.

14.   Satcher 1995, p. 3.

15.   MacKenzie, Hoxie, Proctor, et al. 1994.

16.   Lurie, Hintzen, and Lowe 1995.

17.   World Health Organization 1992a; McCarthy, McPhearson, and Guarino 1992.

18.   Goma Epidemiology Group 1995.

19.   McMichael 1995, pp. 633–34.

20.   Bifani, Plikaytis, Kapur, Stockbauer, Pan, Lutfey, Moghazeh, Eisner, Daniel, Kaplan, Crawford, Musser, Kreiswirth 1996.

21.   B. Kreiswirth, personal communication to the author.

22.   Johnson, Webb, Lange, and Murphy 1977.

23.   Lederberg, Shope, and Oaks 1992, p. 223.

24.   Preston 1994, p. 68.

25.   Ibid., p. 71.

26.   The 1978 report by the World Health Organization also underlined (if less eloquently than Richard Preston) the failure to follow contact precautions. "In some cases," observes Preston, "the medical system may intensify the outbreak, like a lens that focuses sunlight on a heap of tinder" (1994, p. 68).

27.   Garrett 1995b.

28.   Lederberg, Shope, and Oaks 1992, p. 213.

29.   Ryan 1993, p. 384.

30.   DiBacco 1998.

31.   Iseman 1985, p. 735.

32.   Bloom and Murray 1992.

33.   Murray 1991, p. 150.

34.   Snider, Salinas, and Kelly 1989, p. 647.

35.   Ibid.

36.   Friedman, Williams, Singh, and Frieden 1996.

37.   Ott 1996, p. 158.

38.   Ibid., p. 157.

39.   McKenna, McCray, and Onorato 1995, p. 1073. Historian Katherine Ott notes sharply, "It is not being foreign-born that puts a person at risk but the likelihood of repeated exposure to risk, compounded by poverty and ill health" (1996, p. 163).

40.   See Farmer 1992.

41.   Farmer 1990b.

42.   Mann, Tarantola, and Netter 1992, p. 1.

43.   Lederberg, Shope, and Oaks 1992, p. 39.

44.   United Nations Development Program 1992, p. 13.

45.   Sampson and Neaton 1994, p. 1100. They missed one study, however, as did my co-authors and I in our 1996 review (Farmer, Connors, and Simmons 1996). In a short communication published in 1990, Krueger, Wood, Diehr, and Maxwell reported from Seattle "an independent effect of self-reported income on HIV-antibody status." They get to the point in their conclusion: "Since poverty spans the lines of age, ethnicity and sexual orientations, programs targeted specifically to the impoverished may be difficult to devise and implement" (p. 813).

46.   Chaisson, Keruly, and Moore 1995; Farmer, Connors, and Simmons 1996; Fife and Mode 1992; Wallace, Fullilove, Fullilove, et al. 1994.

47.   Waldholz 1996. Some of the newer agents are even more costly.

48.   Zinsser 1934, p. 87.

49.   For case studies of the ways in which anthropologic methods and concepts can inform epidemiology, see Janes, Stall, and Gifford 1986; see also Inhorn and Brown 1997. In addition, I critically reexamine the epidemiology of HIV in the Caribbean in Chapters 4 and 5 of this book.

50.   Centers for Disease Control and Prevention 1993a.

51.   Field 1995; Patz, Epstein, Burke, and Balbus 1996.

52.   McMichael 1995, p. 634. See also Krieger and Zierler 1996.

53.   Garrett 1995b, p. 147. Garrett's comprehensive and engaging The Coming Plague (1995a) does an excellent job of highlighting many of the social factors central to disease emergence. See also the essay by Poinsignon, Marjanovic, and Farge (1996).

54.   In addition to the Institute of Medicine publications, see also the statements by the Centers for Disease Control and Prevention (1994a) and by the National Academy of Science (Roizman 1995).

55.   See Wilkinson's 1996 review of the mechanisms by which inequality and the resulting lack of social cohesion adversely affect health in "developed" societies. The topic has also been explored by Aïach, Carr-Hill, Curtis, and Illsley (1987) and by Fassin (1996a).

56.   Krieger, Rowley, Herman, Avery, and Phillips 1993, p. 99. On this topic, see also Navarro 1990 and Marmot 1994.

57.   Satcher 1995, p. 2.

58.   Wilson 1995, p. 39.

59.   Haggett 1994.

60.   Horton 1995, p. 790.

61.   Warner 1991, p. 242.

62.   Small and Moss 1993.

63.   Levins 1995, p. 50.

64.   Lederberg, Shope, and Oaks 1992, p. 33.

65.   Latour 1988, p. 243.

66.   World Health Organization 1992b.

67.   Berkelman and Hughes 1993, p. 427.

68.   Eisenberg and Kleinman 1981, p. 11.

CHAPTER 3

1.   Farmer, Connors, and Simmons 1996.

2.   Centers for Disease Control and Prevention 1981.

3.   See Oppenheimer 1988 for a review of how data gathering was structured in the early years of the epidemic.

4.   Langone 1985, p. 52. As Paula Treichler points out concerning this essay, "Though more vivid and apodictic (i.e., presented as unarguable), Langone's conclusion parallels the conclusion of many scientists" (1988, p. 250, n. 72).

5.   For a review of data documenting these trends, see Slutsker, Brunet, Karon, et al. 1992, pp. 610–14. It should be noted, however, that changing AIDS incidence was patterned among gay men: decreases were registered among those who were white and middle class, whereas for gays of color, as well as for those who were poorer, no such declines occurred. See Lemp, Hirozawa, Givertz, et al. 1994; Osmond, Page, Wiley, et al. 1994.

6.   Cited in Treichler 1988, p. 193. The image was epidemiologically inaccurate as far as HIV was concerned—white, yuppie couples were not those falling ill with heterosexually acquired HIV infection—but was probably accurate in its depiction of which "us" concerned the editors of the magazine.

7.   Treichler 1988.

8.   Fumento 1993, p. 32. The first edition of Fumento's book was published in 1990. The 1993 paperback edition is prefaced with unrepentant claims that heterosexual AIDS remains a myth.

9.   Slutsker, Brunet, Karon, et al. 1992, pp. 612, 613.

10.   See Selik, Chu, and Buehler 1993. In 1991, the CDC reported that in fifteen U.S. cities AIDS had become the leading cause of death among women of the ages 25 to 44.

11.   Treichler 1988, p. 193.

12.   An editorial in the *American Journal of Public Health* (Stein 1994) would seem to support these claims, as it notes that only at the 1994 HIV/AIDS conference in Yokohama were women's voices at last heard.

13.   See Centers for Disease Control and Prevention 1995; Gwinn, Pappaioanou, George, et al. 1991; Wasser, Gwinn, and Fleming 1993. For a comprehensive review, see Farmer, Connors, and Simmons 1996, chap. 2.

14.   These figures are taken from reports by the U.S. Centers for Disease Control and Prevention and from the overview by Mann, Tarantola, and Netter (1992). Also see Centers for Disease Control and Prevention 1997, p. 37, which details a male:female HIV infection ratio of about 3:1; as expected, this report merely confirms—tardily, in my view—the points raised in this text and in Farmer, Connors, and Simmons 1996.

15.   Global AIDS Policy Coalition 1995.

16.   United Nations Development Program 1992, p. 2.

17.   World Health Organization 1995b.

18.   For more ethnographic detail about Darlene's story and the effect of AIDS in this community, see Pivnick 1993 as well as Pivnick, Jacobson, Eric, et al. 1991. The sociography of AIDS in New York is compellingly detailed in the work of Mindy and Robert Fullilove (see, for example, Fullilove 1995; Fullilove, Fullilove, Haynes, et al. 1990; Fullilove, Lown, and Fullilove 1992), Michael Clatts (1994; 1995), Alisse Waterston (1993), Samuel Friedman (1993), Donald DesJarlais (DesJarlais and Friedman 1988; DesJarlais, Friedman, and Ward 1993; DesJarlais, Padian, and Winklestein 1994), and Rodrick Wallace (1988; 1990; Wallace, Fullilove, Fullilove, et al. 1994; Wallace, Huang, Gould, and Wallace 1997; Wallace and Wallace 1995), among others.

19.   For more on sexual unions in rural Haiti, see Chapter 5 of this volume as well as Allman 1980 and Vieux 1989.

20.   See the fine ethnographic study by Sarthak Das (1995), who collected the material presented here. For overviews of the AIDS situation in India, see Farmer, Connors, and Simmons 1996, chap. 2; Naik, Sarkar, Singh, et al. 1991; Mathai, Prasad, Jacob, et al. 1990.

21.   See Hunter 1995, p. 37.

22.   Mitchell, Tucker, Loftmann, and Williams 1992; cited in Schneider and Stoller 1995, p. 4.

23.   Centers for Disease Control and Prevention 1995. For a review of these data, see Lewis 1995, p. 57.

24.   Preliminary data from this study, known as the Human Immunodeficiency Virus Epidemiology (HER) study, suggest that 60 percent of the patients were African American, 17.5 percent Latina, and 21.5 percent white (Paula Shuman, personal communication to the author). See also Smith, Warren, Vlahov, Schuman, Stein, Greenberg, and Holmberg 1997.

25.   Wallace 1988.

26.   See Fullilove 1995, p. 46, and Fullilove, Fullilove, Haynes, et al. 1990. The Fulliloves draw heavily on the work of Wallace (e.g., 1988 and 1990). See also the 1990 study by McCord and Freeman, cited in Chapter 2, which reports that for some groups age-specific mortality rates are higher in Harlem than in Bangladesh. For an excellent and responsible ethnographic account of injection drug users in New York, see the work of Anitra Pivnick, cited earlier (1993; Pivnick, Jacobson, Eric, et al. 1991), and that of Alisse Waterston (1993). For an overview of AIDS in U.S. African American communities and public health responses, see McBride 1991 as well as Wilson and Pounds 1993.

27.   For an overview of the study, see Farmer 1995a.

28.   See the review by Das (1995).

29.   See the account by Shyamala Nataraj (1990) and the helpful review by Priscilla Alexander (1995).

30.   Denison 1995, p. 205.

31.   Ward 1993, p. 61.

32.   Schoepf 1993, p. 57.

33.   Ellerbrock, Lieb, Harrington, et al. 1992, p. 1707; emphasis added.

34.   The women in the HER study have even lower per capita incomes (Paula Shuman, personal communication to the author).

35.   On the rural-urban distribution of AIDS, see Wasser, Gwinn, and Fleming 1993. The HER study also suggests that geography as a determinant of AIDS risk is far less significant than many other criteria. Although results from this study have not yet been published, the "risk profiles" and AIDS outcomes of the women enrolled in it are similar to those of the women studied in Florida, although all the women in the HER study are from urban settings scattered across the United States (Paula Shuman, personal communication to the author).

36.   See, for example, Miller 1993.

37.   Zierler 1997, p. 209. Zierler later humanely adds: "These strangling forces of disenfranchisement are likely to include partners of women as well, given class and racial/ethnic distribution of women most at risk for HIV and violence. People who are violent against women may have experienced assaults against their own humanity, through racial discrimination, economic impoverishment and the social alienation that accompanies it" (p. 217).

38.   Treichler 1988, p. 194.

39.   Ibid., p. 207; emphasis added.

40.   For more about this group and about their AIDS prevention efforts, see Farmer, Connors, and Simmons 1996, chap. 8, "Zanmi Lasante" entry; see also Farmer 1997b. The document quoted in the text is my translation.

41.   Many other assessments concur: "It is worth noting that despite the portrayal of prostitute-as-vector, as of January 1989, in the United States, '. . . there [had] been no documented cases of men becoming infected through contact with a specific prostitute'" (Carovano 1991, p. 136).

42.   Ward 1993, p. 60.

43.   Wyatt 1995.

44.   Grover 1988, p. 30.

45.   The effects of these (witting and unwitting) obfuscations on explorations of suffering are examined in Farmer 1996b. For an overview on the inattention to class in U.S. health data, see Krieger and Fee 1994 as well as Navarro 1990.

46.   Schoepf 1993, p. 59. For a critical rereading of the literature on drug addicts in the United States, see Waterston 1993 and Bourgois 1995.

47.   See Krieger, Rowley, Herman, Avery, and Phillips 1993, p. 99.

48.   Nyamathi, Bennett, Leake, et al. 1993, p. 68.

49.   Ibid., p. 70.

50.   Holmes and Aral 1991, p. 337. It should be noted, however, that these interventions do not really square with these authors' excellent analysis of the nature of the problem. See, for example, the volume in which the Holmes and Aral essay appears (Wasserheit, Aral, and Holmes 1991).

51.   Denison 1995, p. 205. This phenomenon is by no means unique to AIDS. Waterston powerfully argues that street addicts, too, "have, de facto, joined hands with the larger public in *believing* the ideology of deviance and the myth of the defiant dope fiend. As such, their roles in social reproduction are obscured, actual resistance is subverted, and other alternatives are suppressed" (1993, p. 245).

52.   A 1994 study conducted in the state of Nebraska revealed that a single woman with two children needed an annual income greater than $21,887 to make ends meet—about $9,000 more than the 1994 federal poverty level. "These numbers are a conservative estimate of a decent but no-frills standard of living," noted the report's author. "There's no room here for savings to buy a home, pay for college or build up a nest egg for retirement—all items which have typically defined a middle-class standard of living" ("Federal Poverty Level" 1994, p. 9).

53.   Polakow 1995b, p. 592. See also Polakow 1995a. For more on this subject, refer to Lykes, Banuazizi, Liem, and Morris 1996, an excellent collection. Other important studies of this subject include those by Kluegel and Smith (1986) and Morris and Williamson (1982).

54.   In a moving and lucid essay, William Ryan (1971) explores the theme of blaming the victim and its significance in twentieth-century American thought. On blaming the victim in the context of the AIDS pandemic, see Farmer 1992, pt. 4. See also the studies by Brandt (1988), Kraut (1994), and Zyporyn (1988).

55.   See Plummer 1998. For more on the reduction of HIV transmission through effective treatment of sexually transmitted diseases, see Laga, Alary, Nzila, et al. 1994; Laga, Manoka, Kivuvu, et al. 1993; and Grosskurth, Mosha, Todd, et al. 1995.

56.   For an overview of these studies, which come from both Europe and North America, see the recent work of Don DesJarlais and co-workers (DesJarlais and Friedman 1988; DesJarlais, Friedman, and Ward 1993; DesJarlais, Padian, and Winklestein 1994).

57.   For examples of AIDS-related repression against sex workers, and for insights concerning the importance of organization among prostitutes, see the papers by Priscilla Alexander (1988, 1995) and Gloria Lockett (1995). It is important to underline the enormous differences in the constraints faced by sex workers in different settings. As Alexander (1995, pp. 107–13) shows, prostitutes have had an easier time organizing in Europe, North America, and Australia; the lot of women in the sex industry in poor countries has been far bleaker. Within poor countries, there is also immense variation in the nature of sex work.

58.   Alexander 1995, p. 105; Alexander provides an excellent overview of the effects of providing poor care to sex workers.

59.   Several studies have investigated the underrecognition of HIV infection among poor women living in the United States. Schoenbaum and Webber (1993), for example, reported that in one Bronx emergency room serving the poor, only 11 percent of women were assessed for HIV risks. Other studies continue to reveal significant variation in the knowledge of AIDS management in the United States, with the expected attendant results. See Farmer, Connors, and Simmons 1996, chaps. 4 and 7, for an overview.

60.   Centers for Disease Control and Prevention 1995.

61.   These are preliminary data from the HER study and were obtained unpublished from the CDC. Some of the data were published in Smith, Warren, Vlahov, Schuman, Stein, Greenberg, and Holmberg 1997.

62.   An important study by Chaisson, Keruly, and Moore suggests that if first-rate HIV care is provided to a cohort of poor persons, then "access to medical care is a more important predictor of survival than are sex, race, and income level" (1995, p. 755). This is a remarkable claim and, if true, heartening news for physicians and other providers. It is particularly important coming from one of the groups that in 1991 reported significant race-based differences in outcomes (Easterbrook, Keruly, Creagh-Kirk, et al. 1991).

63.   See Nina Glick-Schiller's 1993 study of this phenomenon.

64.   In July 1997, the CDC reported that 30,700 U.S. citizens died from AIDS during the period from January to September of 1996, which was 19 percent fewer than the 37,900 who had died during the same period in 1995. "We have entered a new era in the HIV epidemic," announced the CDC. As might be expected, however, these gains were not experienced evenly: AIDS mortality dropped 22 percent among gay men but only 7 percent among women; it dropped 28 percent among whites but only 10 percent among blacks and 16 percent among Hispanics. See "Significant Drop Seen in AIDS Cases" 1997; see also Fleming 1996. For more on the implications of these statistics for women, see Stolberg 1997.

65.   Although there are, as yet, no studies of the rates of HIV transmission in serologically discordant couples in which the infected partner is receiving highly active antiretroviral therapy, most AIDS clinicians believe that an undetectable viral load in plasma signals suppression in other tissues and fluids. It is of note,

however, that even among patients receiving these regimens, suppression of plasma viremia has not prevented recovery of replication-competent virus from CD4-positive T-lymphocytes. See, for example, Finzi, Hermankova, Pierson, et al. 1997; and Wong, Hezareh, Günthard, et al. 1997.

66.   Das 1995, p. 8.

67.   Hollibaugh 1995, p. 225. Hollibaugh's essay does not cite data to suggest that lesbians of color account for a large number of the U.S. women living with HIV, but her comments are helpful in their clarity and candor. Other writers do underscore divisions between white and black feminists. "When it came down to it," notes Veronica Chambers, an African American feminist, "I could not trust most white women to have my back" (1995, p. 25).

68.   Lee 1995b, p. 205. Nancy Krieger and Sally Zierler point out that "although women, as a group, may share experiences of being biologically female, these experiences occur in diverse gendered societies, located within a global economy, and simultaneously split, internally, by social class, race/ethnicity, and other social divisions" (1995, p. 251).

69.   Schoepf 1993, p. 70.

70.   Collins 1990, p. 10.

CHAPTER 4

1.   Viera 1985, p. 95. These speculations were republished in a subsequent revised edition of the book, rather unrepentantly, I thought.

2.   Kleinman and Kleinman 1997, p. 103.

3.   This phrase is the felicitous subtitle of an essay by Allan Brandt (1997).

4.   AIDS and Accusation (Farmer 1992) was published in a French edition in 1996 as Sida en Haïti: La Victime Accusée (Paris: Karthala).

5.   For an excellent, harrowing account of the experience of Haitians who were suffering from tuberculosis while in detention at the Krome Avenue facility, see Nachman 1993.

6.   Cited in Abbott 1988, pp. 254–55.

7.   Dr. Bruce Chabner of the National Cancer Institute, cited in the Miami News, 2 December 1982, p. 8A.

8.   The physicians also made the following, apparently offhand, comment: "If the syndrome originates in rural people, and it seems likely that it does, it occurs among those who have had little or no direct or indirect contact with Port-au-Prince or other urban areas" (Moses and Moses 1983, p. 565; emphasis added). As Chapter 5 describes, no data ever existed to suggest that AIDS spread from rural to urban Haiti.

9.   Métraux [1959] 1972, p. 15.

10.   Glick-Schiller and Fouron 1990, p. 337.

11.   The exoticization of Haiti, especially as regards U.S. foreign policy, is the subject of Farmer 1994. The elaboration of North American folk models of Haiti and Haitians is the subject of an excellent and comprehensive review by Lawless (1992).

12.   The first description is cited in Allman 1989, p. 81; the second is from Lief 1990, p. 34.

13.   In *The Uses of Haiti* (Farmer 1994), I explore the symbolic uses of Haiti over the course of the past five centuries.

14.   The World Bank defines "generalized epidemic" in the context of HIV as a situation in which "5 percent or more of women attending maternity clinics are infected" (World Bank 1997). According to the latest available statistics, Haiti's rate of infection was 8.4 percent (1993), Guyana's was 6.9 percent (1992), and Brazil's was 5.1 percent (1996); no other country in the Americas topped 3.6 percent (World Health Organization 1998).

15.   Liautaud, Laroche, Duvivier, and Péan-Guichard 1983.

16.   Oncologists initially suspected that Kaposi's was somehow related to previous infection with cytomegalovirus. For a review of data on this topic, see Groopman 1983. For a study revealing a lack of association of cytomegalovirus with endemic Kaposi's, see Ambinder, Newman, Hawyard, Biggar, et al. 1987. More recently, evidence has been reported for a causative role for human herpesvirus 8 in Kaposi's (André, Schatz, Bogner, et al. 1997).

17.   See Pape, Liautaud, Thomas, Mathurin, St Amand, Boncy, Péan, Pamphile, Laroche, and Johnson 1983.

18.   In rural Haiti, our own work eventually revealed a similar preponderance; see Farmer 1997c.

19.   Pape, Liautaud, Thomas, Mathurin, St Amand, Boncy, Péan, Pamphile, Laroche, and Johnson 1983, p. 949.

20.   Ibid., p. 948.

21.   Stephen Murray (personal communication to the author; see also Murray and Payne 1988 as well as Payne 1987) poses sharp questions regarding the statistics used in various publications by Haitian researcher-physicians, including Pape and his GHESKIO co-workers. For example, Murray notes that it is not possible to go from an N of 34, of whom 13 are bisexual, to an N of 38, of whom 19 are said to be bisexual (compare Pape, Liautaud, Thomas, Mathurin, St Amand, Boncy, Pean, Pamphile, Laroche, and Johnson 1984 with the 1986 study by the same authors). Dr. Murray's queries, which concern the relevance of bisexuality to the epidemic, deserve careful consideration and a reply in the scholarly literature. It should be noted, however, that the GHESKIO group worked with a gradually enlarging pool of ill informants, some of whom later and reluctantly revealed a history of bisexuality. In many countries, early reports on the AIDS epidemic were equally tentative and subject to revision (see Altman 1986, Oppenheimer 1988, Panem 1988, and Shilts 1987).

22.   In another review, Pape and Johnson state that "in 1983, the majority of male patients with AIDS were bisexuals who had at least one sexual encounter with visiting North Americans or Haitians residing in North America" (1988, p. 32).

23.   The Collaborative Study Group of AIDS in Haitian-Americans (1987) was similarly unable to find a single Haitian with AIDS who had a history of residence or travel in Africa

24.   Guérin, Malebranche, Elie, et al. 1984; Johnson and Pape 1989.

25.   Johnson and Pape 1989. Although the two populations are by no means comparable vis-à-vis established risk factors for HIV infection, it is instructive to compare these findings to contemporary studies from North America. In one retrospective study of 6875 "male homosexuals and bisexuals," 4.5 percent were already seropositive in 1978 (Jaffe, Darrow, and Echenberg 1985).

26.   Johnson and Pape 1989, p. 67.

27.   For example, in a letter of response to the 1983 article by Pape and co-workers in the *New England Journal of Medicine,* two researchers from Yale University suggested that "Pape *et al.* do not convincingly exclude malnutrition as a cause of immune deficiency and opportunistic infection in the patients described" (Mellors and Barry 1984, p. 1119). An earlier letter to the same journal suggested that "malnutrition is likely to be present in Haitians recently immigrated to Europe, Canada, or the United States," which might explain AIDS in Haitian infants (Goudsmit 1983, p. 554). The theory was echoed by Beach and Laura (1983) in the *Annals of Internal Medicine.* The advent of antibody tests put an end to suggestions that malnutrition or some other disorder was masquerading as AIDS: among the GHESKIO patients, fully 96 percent of those diagnosed with AIDS on clinical grounds were found to be seropositive for HIV.

28.   This is the thesis of Leibowitch's (1985) review, and it is reiterated in Shilt's (1987) best-selling account of the pandemic.

29.   Greenfield 1986, p. 2200.

30.   Moore and LeBaron 1986, pp. 81, 84.

31.   Chaze 1983.

32.   Gilman 1988, p. 102.

33.   Pape and co-workers also tested sera collected for other diagnostic tests and found that, of 1037 adults phlebotomized during the first six months of 1986 by three commercial laboratories in Port-au-Prince, 8 percent had antibodies to HIV (Pape and Johnson 1988). The health status of these persons was not known, but since none of the three laboratories performed HIV serology at the time of the phlebotomy, the samples had not been collected to diagnose HIV infection.

34.   World Health Organization 1998.

35.   A group of researchers based in Cité Soleil reported that 8.4 percent of 1240 healthy women receiving prenatal care in 1986 were seropositive for HIV (Halsey, Boulos, Brutus, et al. 1987; Halsey et al. 1990). In 1987, 9.9 percent of 2009 "sexually active women" in Cité Soleil were HIV-positive; in 1989, 10.5 percent of 1074

such women were found to have been exposed to HIV (Brutus 1989b). In Go-naïves, 9 percent of 1795 patients reporting to a clinic that served a predominantly low-income clientele tested seropositive in 1988 (Brutus 1989a).

36.   Pape and Johnson 1993, p. S344.

37.   Jean et al. 1997, p. 605.

38.   Pape and Johnson 1989, p. 70.

39.   Pape, Liautaud, Thomas, Mathurin, St Amand, Boncy, Péan, Pamphile, Laroche, and Johnson 1986, p. 7.

40.   Ibid.

41.   Early in the epidemic, it was noted that another mode of transmission of HIV was through the use of contaminated needles. In Haiti, intramuscular injec-tions may be given either by medical personnel or, in areas without access to medical facilities, by those known as *pikiris* ("injectionists"). Disposable needles and syringes, which are relatively rare in Haiti, are frequently reused without sterilization. Pape and colleagues (ibid.) found that during the five-year period before the onset of AIDS symptoms, 83 percent of male and 88 percent of female AIDS patients had received parenteral medications. Although the figure is by it-self suggestive, more than 67 percent of controls (seronegative siblings and friends) also reported injections, suggesting that other factors were involved in HIV transmission.

42.   Ibid., p. 6.

43.   An analogous mode of transmission has been described for HTLV-1—also a retrovirus   for which female to male transmission is thought to occur rarely, if at all. See Kajiyama, Kashwagi, Ikematsu, et al. 1986 and Murphy, Figeroa, Gibbs, et al. 1989.

44.   See Peterman, Stoneburner, Allen, et al. 1988. In a colloquium held at Har-vard University, Dr. Andrew Moss, director of the Department of AIDS Epidemi-ology at San Francisco General Hospital, observed that women are ten times as likely to become infected as men upon sexual exposure to HIV: "It worries me that the number of sexual partners is a risk factor for transmission [even among those who use intravenous drugs], and it worries me that the rate is twice as high in women as in men because this indicates that heterosexual transmission, not needle sharing, is responsible for new infections" (Harvard AIDS Institute 1990, p. 5). These data are reviewed in Farmer, Connors, and Simmons 1996.

45.   Mellon, Liautaud, Pape, and Johnson 1995. See also Deschamps, Pape, Hafner, and Johnson 1996.

46.   McBarnett 1988, p. 71.

47.   The persistent conception of women as "AIDS transmitters"—a result, in large part, as Anastos and Marte note, of "deeply ingrained societal sexism as well as racism and classism"—has skewed readings of U.S. epidemiology as well: women with HIV disease "are regarded by the public and studied by the medical profession as vectors of transmission to their children and male sexual partners

rather than people with AIDS who are themselves frequently victims of transmission from the men in their lives" (Anastos and Marte 1989, p. 10). The tendency of North Americans to "blame the victims" is further examined in Farmer 1992, chap. 21. For comprehensive studies of misreadings of HIV epidemiology among women, see Farmer, Connors, and Simmons 1996.

48.   The percentage of AIDS patients with Kaposi's decreased from 15 percent of cases occurring before and during 1984 to 5 percent in 1986–88, a shift later noted among North Americans with AIDS; see Franceschi, Dal Maso, Lo Re, Serraino, and La Vecchia 1997.

49.   Pape and Johnson 1988, p. 36.

50.   In Haiti, the decreasing *relative* significance of same-sex contacts in the spread of HIV is the cause, it seems, for a decreasing incidence of Kaposi's sarcoma. Among North Americans with AIDS, Kaposi's sarcoma is seen almost exclusively among gay men (rather than among injection drug users, for instance).

51.   Studies of U.S. press coverage of AIDS suggest some of the reasons for the public perception of Caribbean AIDS as largely a Haitian problem. When CBS News ran a story about HIV transmission in Australia on 25 July 1985, "it was the network's first mention of AIDS outside the United States, Africa, or Haiti" (Kinsella 1989, p. 144).

52.   Pape and Johnson 1988, p. 32. Ironically, given the extreme poverty of Haiti, Haitians with AIDS stand a better chance of receiving an adequate workup than do the citizens of several other Caribbean nations. Although Haiti has the weakest health infrastructure in the region, it has had the largest number of cases, and the greatest amount of international scrutiny as "the source of AIDS," and it has sustained the most substantial economic blows relative to GNP. Perhaps as a partial result of these negative forces, Haitian physicians and researchers have been centrally involved in the professional response to the epidemic. Haitians publish more HIV-related studies than do researchers in other Caribbean countries, and the GHESKIO-run national laboratories are among the most experienced in diagnosing AIDS and other forms of HIV disease.

53.   Lange and Jaffe 1987, p. 1410.

54.   Perez 1992.

55.   Garris, Rodríguez, De Moya, et al. 1991.

56.   Osborn 1989, p. 126; emphasis added.

57.   As my critique of conventional epidemiology suggests, it is perilous to classify people with AIDS into "risk groups." Efforts to do so, however, have supported the hypothesis that very similar trends occurred in the Dominican Republic. In a study by Perez (1992), for example, AIDS incidence among "heterosexuals" increased from 31 percent to 59 percent between 1987 and 1991, while "homosexual" cases decreased from 43 percent to only 6 percent. His conclusion: "The AIDS epidemic in the Dominican Republic seems to have completed its transition from WHO Pattern I to Pattern II."

58.   Pape and Johnson 1988, p. 36.

59.   Bartholemew, Saxinger, Clark, et al. 1987.

60.   Ibid., p. 2606.
61.   Merino, Sanchez, Muñoz, Prada, García, and Polk 1990, pp. 333–34. Such has also been the case in Denmark, where sexual contact with a North American gay man, rather than "promiscuity" per se, was an important risk factor in the first cases of AIDS (Gerstoft, Nielsen, Dickmeiss, Ronne, Platz, and Mathiesen 1985).
62.   Koenig, Pittaluga, Bogart, et al. 1987, p. 634.
63.   Ibid. When questioned by Payne (1987) regarding the ethnographic validity of their observations regarding homosexuality in the Dominican Republic, Koenig and co-workers replied that their "information on the Dominican Republic [came] from on-site visits to hotels that cater to the gay tourist trade. These places are frequented often by visitors from the United States and Caribbean countries" (Koenig, Brache, and Levy 1987, p. 47). In a retrospective assessment that seems to support Koenig's argument, García writes: "In the 1970s, [Puerta Plata] was favored by gay tourists and is considered to be one of the initial ports of entry for HIV in the Dominican Republic. During the 1970s, tourists were predominantly gay, over-sixty males who engaged in sex with local teenaged male prostitutes" (1991, p. 2).
64.   García 1991, p. 2.
65.   Ibid.
66.   Jean et al. 1997, p. 600.
67.   Hospedales 1989; Pape and Johnson 1993, p. S342.
68.   Carpenter 1930, p. 326.
69.   Haitians, notes Métraux, are "irritated—understandably—by the label 'Voodoo-land' which travel agencies have stuck on their home" ([1959] 1972, p. 359).
70.   Francisque 1986, p. 139.
71.   The protagonist of Graham Greene's *The Comedians* (1966) is a Port-au-Prince hotelier who in 1961 remembers fondly the days when tourists flocked to his bar and made love in the pool. "The drummer's fled to New York, and all the bikini girls stay in Miami now," he explains to two prospective clients. "You'll probably be the only guests I have" (p. 11).
72.   Cited in Trouillot 1990, p. 200.
73.   Barros 1984, p. 750.
74.   Cited in Altman 1983, p. 1.
75.   Abbott 1988, p. 255.
76.   Métellus 1987, p. 90.
77.   Greco 1983, p. 516.
78.   d'Adesky 1991, p. 31.
79.   Cited in Moore and LeBaron 1986, p. 82.
80.   Murray and Payne 1988, pp. 25–26. Payne had previously observed that "several gay travel guides, such as the *Bob Damron Guidebook* for 1982, contain as many as ten entries for the Bahamas, but only four for the Dominican Republic and one for Haiti" (1987, p. 47). Significantly, as Lange and Jaffe (1987) note, the AIDS attack rate in the Bahamas was then even higher than that in Haiti.

81.   Guérin, Malebranche, Elie, et al. 1984, p. 256.

82.   Ibid. Interestingly, Murray and Payne cite an American journalist's interview with Guérin and not the research published in the *Annals of the New York Academy of Sciences:* "At the Haitian end of the hypothesized transmission vector, Dr. Jean-Michel Guérin of GHESKIO told [journalist Anne-Christine] d'Adesky that 'all his patients—without exception—had denied having sex with tourists'" (1988, pp. 25–26). It is important to note that the *Annals* article, which brought together the research of ten physicians, clearly specifies which patients acknowledged sexual relations with gay tourists from North America. It is thus evident that Guérin meant that these patients *initially* denied such contacts. As described earlier, this initial denial was registered among other Haitians who were ultimately shown to have had histories of homosexual contact. It is not clear why such a misreading persisted, but d'Adesky has abandoned this tack, as her later essay underlines the sex-for-money exchanges that took place between tourists and poor Haitian men; see d'Adesky 1991, p. 31.

83.   Langley 1989, p. 175.

84.   Patterson 1987, p. 258.

85.   See the summaries of trade statistics and their directions in International Monetary Fund 1984. Similar exercises have helped reveal other socioeconomic webs that are important to the shape of the AIDS pandemic. For example, geographer Peter Gould links the density of air traffic in and out of Abidjan, Côte d'Ivoire, to the transnational spread of HIV in and across Europe and Africa (Gould 1993, p. 82).

86.   Liautaud, Pape, and Pamphile 1988, p. 690. Even by 1997, the HIV infection rate had increased only marginally in Cuba to 0.013 percent, with about 1,400 reported in a country of 11 million (World Health Organization 1998). Due largely to political upheaval during the late 80s and early 90s—events that have themselves favored increased transmission of HIV—there have been no recent serosurveys in Haiti. In 1997 the WHO estimated nationwide seroprevalence at 5 percent of the adult population, which would make Haiti one of the hemisphere's only countries with a "generalized epidemic" (World Health Organization 1998; see also Deschamps, Pape, Hafner, and Johnson 1996). Note that this figure of five percent aggregates rural and urban seroprevalence statistics; since rural areas are less affected, in relative terms, it may be taken as a certainty that the incidence of HIV in Haitian cities has risen significantly over the last decade. The forward march of HIV into rural Haiti will be explored in the next chapter.

87.   Wolf 1982, p. 4.

CHAPTER 5

1.   In their consideration of unequal exchange and the urban informal sector, Portes and Walton (1982, p. 74) designate Haiti as the most rural of all Latin Amer-

ican nations: in 1950, the nation was described as 88 percent rural; in 1960, 85 percent; in 1970, 81 percent.

2. Pape and Johnson 1988.

3. See Farmer 1992.

4. See Allman 1980 and Vieux 1989 for extended discussions of *plasaj*.

5. See Pape and Johnson 1988.

6. Desvarieux and Pape 1991, p. 275.

7. GESCAP (whose name is translated as "Study Group on AIDS in the Peasant Class") was founded with the generous support of the World AIDS Foundation.

8. Given that the staff of the clinic and of Proje Veye Sante are accountable to the communities served rather than to funding organizations or to research institutions, and given the poverty and non-HIV-related sickness in the region, it is not surprising that research as such is not seen as a high priority. In order to meet our obligations to the community, all serologic studies became part of a *dossier préventif*. This instrument included a series of laboratory examinations (such as hematocrit and RPR), a chest radiograph, and a physical examination. Any abnormal findings were to be pursued aggressively; free dental care was also offered as part of the program. This proposal was presented to members of the community in four different public meetings, engendering considerable enthusiasm for the undertaking.

9. One additional young woman, the regular sexual partner of a truck driver, was also found to be seropositive. She died suddenly during the course of the study, however, less than a week after a negative physical examination. Although the cause of death is unclear—she had explosive, watery diarrhea and presented in shock—she is not considered in this cohort.

10. Farmer 1992, p. 262.

11. Feilden, Allman, Montague, and Rohde 1981, p. 6.

12. Ibid., p. 4.

13. Locher 1984, p. 329.

14. Neptune-Anglade 1986, p. 150.

15. "Note that, in the cities, the [economically] active 10–14-year-old girls are essentially all domestics. . . . These 'restaveks' find themselves at the very bottom of the social hierarchy" (ibid., p. 209). My translation.

16. See Farmer 1988b for a review of data concerning the Haitian economy. In a personal communication on 18 September 1998, a desk officer at the US State Department's Haiti desk offered an annual per capita income estimate of $175 (not adjusted for Purchasing Power Parity); she cited internal IMF memos from April 1998 as her source.

17. Girault 1984, p. 177.

18. Ibid., p. 178. For a critical perspective on more recent "food security" issues, see Woodson 1997.

19. Trouillot 1986, p. 201. My translation.

20. Population Crisis Committee 1992.

21. Moral 1961, p. 173. My translation.

22. Allman 1980.

23. But see Laguerre 1982

24. This is a cursory discussion of a very complex—and changing—subject. For a more complete discussion of sexual unions in Haiti, see Lowenthal 1984, Murray 1976, Neptune-Anglade 1986, Sylvain-Comhaire 1974, and Vieux 1989.

25. United Nations Development Program 1992, p. 6.

26. See Mintz 1964, Neptune-Anglade 1986, and Nicholls 1985.

27. See Murray 1986.

28. Neptune-Anglade 1986, p. 155. My translation.

29. Maria de Bruyn offers a helpful review of these issues as they affect women in developing countries. She writes: "Even if they dare suggest avoiding risky sexual acts or using condoms, they often encounter male refusal, are accused of adultery or promiscuity (the desire to use condoms being interpreted as evidence of extramarital affairs), are suspected of already being infected with HIV or are said to accuse their partners of infidelity" (1992, p. 256). The mechanisms by which gender inequality conspires with poverty to enhance women's risk for HIV are the subject of Farmer, Connors, and Simmons 1996.

30. Desvarieux and Pape 1991, p. 277.

31. Farmer 1992.

32. Collaborative Study Group of AIDS in Haitian-Americans 1987, p. 638.

33. On American "folk models" of Haitians, see Lawless 1992 and, as related to AIDS, Farmer 1992.

34. The word *"sida"* is derived from the French acronym SIDA, for *syndrome immunodéficience acquise.* The French acronym is commonly rendered as S.I.D.A., SIDA, or Sida; *sida* is the Creole orthography. I have adopted the latter here in order to reflect the substantial difference between the terms as used in different national and cultural settings.

35. See Farmer 1996a for a more complete discussion of "Haiti's lost years."

36. Farmer 1996a examines the effects of the 1991 coup d'état on rates of HIV diagnosis in the Kay region.

37. de Bruyn 1992, p. 253.

38. See, for example, Laga, Manoka, Kivuvu, et al. 1993.

39. Poor, young women may be especially at risk of genital trauma: "Non-consensual, hurried or frequent intercourse may inhibit mucous production and the relaxation of vaginal musculature, both of which would increase the likelihood of genital trauma. A lack of control over the circumstances in which the intercourse occurs may increase the frequency of intercourse and lower the age at which sexual activity begins. A lack of access to acceptable health services may leave infections and lesions untreated. Malnutrition not only inhibits the production of mucus but also slows the healing process and depresses the immune system" (United Nations Development Program 1992, pp. 3–4).

40.   For example, see Liautaud et al. 1992; Deschamps, Pape, Williams-Russo, Madhavan, Ho, and Johnson, 1993; and Behets, Desormeaux, Joseph, et al. 1995.
41.   We do know that in one study of one hundred women presenting to our women's health clinic in 1991 fully 25 percent had trichomoniasis. GESCAP thanks Dr. Anna Contomitros for conducting this study, which included Pap smears. See also Fitzgerald 1996.
42.   Data from GHESKIO (e.g., Deschamps et al. 1992) suggest, however, that those ill with HIV disease continue to have sex.
43.   DiPerri, Cade, Castelli, et al. 1993.
44.   Lief 1990, p. 36.
45.   For a review of recent anthropological writings on AIDS, see Farmer 1997b.
46.   Benoist and Desclaux 1995, p. 363. My translation.

MIRACLES AND MISERY:
AN ETHNOGRAPHIC INTERLUDE

1.   Farmer 1992, pp. 43–45. I wrote myself out of this text not so much in naïveté as in reaction to the self-indulgent divulgences of reflexive anthropology, which has often confused the readers' interest in the subject at hand—presumably, the famous Other—with patience for the Self-referential writer.
2.   Geertz 1988, pp. 4–5.
3.   Kleinman 1995b, p. 76. He continues: "Context and interpersonal dialogue are understood to shape the knowledge so that it is always particular to a local world."

CHAPTER 6

1.   Several of the concepts in this chapter—cultural model, prototypical model, semantic network, social construction, and so on—have been used in different ways in medical anthropology. This chapter is informed by the critique of an "empiricist theory of language," offered by interpretive paradigms (for example, Good and Good 1982) and also by work in cognitive anthropology, which has begun shifting its attention from the formal properties of illness models to their relation to natural discourse and thus to context and performance characteristics of illness representations (see, for example, Price 1987). A focus on *lived experience* is crucial to this view, even in a study of the emergence of a collective representation. (For a forceful statement of such a position, see Kleinman and Kleinman 1989.) We can now make headway by merging these groups of concerns with an accountability to history and political economy. One important "bridge concept" might be the cultural model—an idea formalized by cognitive anthropologists seeking to show how "cultural models frame experience, supplying interpretations of that experience and inferences about it, and goals for action" (Quinn and Holland 1987, p. 6).

But as the case of HIV-related disorders shows, cultural models and theories about them need constant correction by the nosological and social environment itself (Farmer and Good 1991).

2. This processual ethnography of changing understandings of AIDS in Do Kay is based on a large body of interviews, most of which are not cited here, although they all inform my understanding of the significance of the comments that are cited. This larger project was initiated in 1983. At least once during each of the subsequent six years, I interviewed the same twenty villagers regarding tuberculosis and AIDS; most of these conversations were tape-recorded. (In 1988, a research assistant took my place with seven of the informants.) During three of these years, a third disorder (*move san*) was also discussed. The taped exchanges were initiated by me and took place in a variety of settings, most often in the informants' houses. Of the twenty adults, two have died, and one has left Do Kay. The interviews were open-ended and usually focused on specific "illness stories." We always discussed the following topics for each of the three illnesses: its key features (including typical presentation, causes, course, understandings of pathogenesis when relevant), the appropriate therapeutic interventions, its relation to other sicknesses common in the area, and questions of risk and vulnerability.

In addition to these interviews, the research involved lengthy conversations with all villagers afflicted with tuberculosis and AIDS and the majority of those with *move san*. I also interviewed members of victims' families as well as other key actors in the events described here. These qualitative data were complemented by information from several structured surveys and an annual census, conducted by myself and other members of Proje Veye Sante. And, of course, I personally witnessed the changes described here, having spent an average of six months per year in Do Kay since May of 1983.

3. For discussion of the political changes during this period, see Farmer 1994.

4. See Centers for Disease Control and Prevention 1982a and Nachman and Dreyfuss 1986.

5. The anti-Haitian backlash may have been felt as keenly in New York, Miami, Boston, Montreal, and other North American cities in which large numbers of Haitians now reside. See Farmer 1990a, Farmer 1992, and Sabatier 1988 for a review of AIDS-related discrimination against Haitians.

6. Three of the five who had never heard the term were men who "never traveled to Port-au-Prince." Such homebodies are rare in the Central Plateau, whose inhabitants are highly involved in the marketing of produce.

7. In Haiti, market women are known for their up-to-date information. Their "frequent trips to neighboring cities and to Port-au-Prince make [them] aware of everything—not just the rise and fall of prices, but also national events, not only the genuine ones, but the false rumors that spread through the marketplaces" (Bastien [1951] 1985, p. 128). My translation.

8.   It should be noted, however, that Ti Malou was widely believed to have *move san*, a common disorder that is treated by herbal medications and not transfusion (Farmer 1988a).

9.   For more on *move san*, see Farmer 1988a.

10. Weidman 1978. For more information about the blood paradigm, see also Farmer 1988a and Laguerre 1987.

11. Such commentaries are not without a basis in truth. Ferguson (1987) and Hagen (1982) document the role of *duvaliériste* Luckner Cambronne in a trade in Haitian blood, which was used for medical experiments and for its antibody-rich serum. Thus, the antigenic challenges of daily life in Haiti could become a source of wealth—though not for the blood donors, who were paid a pittance.

12. See Gaines and Farmer 1986 for a discussion of rhetorics of complaint and their relevance to illness representations. It has long been noted that Haitians have complicated, multifactorial ideas about illness causation. A large body of ethnographic literature shows that rural Haitians often entertain explanatory frameworks that make room for "naturalistic" causation as well as lines of causality dominated by human agency. Particularly relevant is Coreil's (1980) study of an anthrax epidemic in rural Haiti.

13. For discussion of health care practitioners in rural Haiti, see Coreil 1983 and Laguerre 1987.

14. As Sabatier notes, "Syphilis was referred to by the Spanish as 'the sickness of Hispaniola,' believing it to have come from what is now Haiti when Columbus returned from his voyage to the Americas" (1988, p. 42).

15. The advent of AIDS to this village is more fully described in Farmer 1992.

16. The term "expedition" is also used to describe this process, which requires the services of a *houngan*, or voodoo priest. In translating the term "*voye yon mò sida*," I have used the less accurate "send a *sida* death" rather than the more cumbersome "send a dead person who has died from *sida*."

17. Métraux [1959] 1972, p. 274.

18. This story is told more fully in Farmer and Kleinman 1989.

19. Things do not appear to have changed altogether. Ethnographic research conducted decades ago led Métraux to observe that "in everyday life the threat of charms, sorcery and spells makes it but one more care to be listed with drought and the price of coffee and bananas. Magic is at least an evil against which man is not entirely powerless" ([1959] 1972, p. 269). Hurbon offers a similar insight when he notes that "spells are part of the daily struggle in a world already littered with traps" (1987, p. 260). My translation.

20. See Garro 1988.

21. Good 1977, p. 54.

22. Métraux [1959] 1972, p. 274.

23. Taussig 1980, p. 7.

24.   See Moore 1987.

25.   This expression is borrowed from Bateson and Goldsby 1988. A similar image has been used by Lindenbaum in her classic study of sorcery and the advent of kuru, another novel infectious disease, in rural Papua New Guinea: "A geography of fear tracks unequal relations" (1979, p. 146).

CHAPTER 7

1.   World Health Organization 1996.

2.   "TB Returns with a Vengeance" 1996.

3.   Ott 1996, p. 157.

4.   Bloom and Murray 1992.

5.   Ryan 1993, p. 8.

6.   Dubos and Dubos 1992, pp. xiv–xv, n. 1.

7.   Rosenkrantz is quoted from her introduction to Dubos and Dubos 1992, p. xxi.

8.   Feldberg 1995, p. 1.

9.   Dubos and Dubos 1992, p. 22.

10.   See Farmer, Robin, Ramilus, and Kim 1991; Spence, Hotchkiss, Williams, and Davies 1993.

11.   For an in-depth exploration of the effects of *fujishock* on the health of Peru's urban poor, see Kim, Shakow, Bayona, et al. 1999.

12.   Current standards would favor initiating empiric treatment with four drugs to avoid the development of resistant strains of *M. tuberculosis*.

13.   World Health Organization 1996.

14.   McBride 1991.

15.   Frieden, Fujiwara, Washko, and Hamburg 1995.

16.   Brudney and Dobkin 1991a.

17.   Frieden, Fujiwara, Washko, and Hamburg 1995, p. 229.

18.   Mahmoudi and Iseman 1993.

19.   Cited in Feldberg 1995, p. 214.

20.   "Whether as a result of changing definitions of disease, new methods of record-keeping, or actual changes in mortality, the number of recorded deaths dropped by almost one-third between 1850 and 1890" (ibid., p. 13).

21.   Ibid., pp. 11–12; emphasis added.

22.   Ibid.

23.   Ibid., p. 23. Feldberg further notes that many Southern antebellum physicians "believed that the physician could make no greater error than to treat 'negroes' as though they were 'white men in black skins'" (ibid., pp. 24–25). See McBride 1991 for a more thorough review of this subject.

24.   Cited in Feldberg 1995, p. 14.

25. Ibid., p. 26. Not all Southern physicians shared the locally dominant explanatory models, however. Feldberg notes that in 1873 one doctor from Richmond, Virginia, trenchantly observed that "the most marked difference between the diseases of the two races is in the far greater prevalence and mortality of tubercular diseases amongst the blacks."

26. For a review, see Rieder 1989.

27. Cited in Feldberg 1995, p. 439.

28. Henry Wiley, cited in Feldberg 1995, p. 30.

29. Dubos and Dubos 1992, p. 210.

30. Cited in Feldberg 1995, p. 101.

31. Cited in ibid., p. 105.

32. Ibid., p. 4.

33. Cited in ibid., p. 4.

34. Rosenkrantz is quoted from her excellent introduction to Dubos and Dubos 1992, p. xxii.

35. Huber cited by Rosenkrantz, in ibid., pp. xxv–xxvi.

36. Cited in McBride 1991, p. 58.

37. Cited in Feldberg 1995, p. 48.

38. Kraut 1994.

39. Cited in McBride 1991, p. 46.

40. On the relationship between xenophobia and tuberculosis, see Kraut 1994.

41. Cited in McBride 1991, p. 61.

42. Ibid., p. 151.

43. Ibid., p. 126.

44. Cited in ibid., p. 129. Preferential attention to polio continued, as Feldberg notes: "In 1949, as polio cases rose to the 'epidemic' rate of 30/100,000, the tuberculous case rate exceeded 90/100,000; in 1951 alone, there were 119,000 new cases of tuberculosis. Tuberculous mortality also exceeded that for polio almost threefold" (1995, p. 2).

45. McBride 1991, p. 151.

46. Michael and Michael 1994.

47. Snider, Salinas, and Kelly 1989, p. 647.

48. Chaulet 1996, p. 7. My translation.

49. Iseman 1985.

50. Farmer, Robin, Ramilus, and Kim 1991.

51. Curry 1968.

52. Frieden, Fujiwara, Washko, and Hamburg 1995.

53. Telzak, Sepkowitz, Alpert, et al. 1995.

54. Cole and Telenti 1995, p. 701s.

55. Reichman 1997, p. 7.

56. Feldberg 1995, p. 38.

57. Krause cited in ibid., p. 107.

58.   The term "public health nihilism" was coined by Ron Bayer of Columbia University; it is discussed in Farmer and Nardell 1998.
59.   Dubos and Dubos 1992, p. 225.
60.   Ibid., p. 207.

CHAPTER 8

1.   Third East African/British Medical Research Council Study 1980; Cohn, Catlin, Peterson, Judson, and Sbarbaro 1990; Hong Kong Chest Service/British Medical Research Council 1982; Snider, Graczyk, Bek, and Rogowski 1984; Singapore Tuberculosis Service/British Medical Research Council 1988.
2.   See "If More Widely Used" 1997, p. 14.
3.   World Health Organization 1997c.
4.   Murray and Lopez 1996.
5.   See Farmer 1997d for a review of immodest claims of causality about the persistence or reemergence of tuberculosis.
6.   Menzies, Rocher, and Vissandjee 1993, p. 33. See also Addington 1979; Fox 1983; Kopanoff, Snider, and Johnson 1988; Yeats 1986; and Haynes 1979.
7.   World Health Organization 1991.
8.   Snider 1989, p. S336.
9.   Wiese 1971, p. 38. Regarding the European introduction of tuberculosis to Haiti, Kiple concurs: "Tuberculosis and bacterial pneumonia apparently were fairly new to the region when the first Europeans arrived—and in fact those Europeans probably brought the diseases to many" (1984, p. 13). The Africans in the Caribbean were not, however, as susceptible as their Indian predecessors; some note that the Africans were also less susceptible than their oppressors. As Kiple writes, "the Spanish quickly noticed how durable [the African slaves] were in the face of illnesses that were felling Indians" (1984, p. 12). Kiple argues that the slaves constituted "an immunological élite as survivors of one of the most formidable disease environments in the world." If this is true, the appalling death rates of the plantations must have been almost wholly due to "work" conditions.
10.   Service d'Hygiène 1933, p. 12.
11.   Moreau de Saint-Méry 1984, p. 1068. A review of the literature from colonial times and extensive fieldwork in contemporary Haiti led Wiese to assert that "the disease took its place in their medical beliefs and practices, many of which have remained essentially unchanged down to the present" (1971, p. 100).
12.   Tardo-Dino 1985, p. 198.
13.   Cauna 1984.
14.   Foubert 1987, p. 3.
15.   Bordes 1979, pp. 16–17; my translation. Bordes fails to note that many of these health workers were not allowed to "bleed or to bandage" white patients; see Moreau de Saint-Méry 1984, p. 559.

16.   In a devastating review, Jean-Louis states that only 5 percent of rural Haitians have access to potable water. He then compares this figure to that of neighboring islands: 60 percent in the Dominican Republic; 62 percent in Panama; 86 percent in Jamaica; 99 percent in Trinidad and Tobago; "almost the entire population" in Cuba (1989, p. 14).

17.   Feilden, Allman, Montague, and Rohde 1981, p. 1.

18.   Dr. Henec Titus, at a conference entitled "Santé, Médecine et Democratie," held on 10 November 1988 in Port-au-Prince, offered the following data: as of late August 1988, 202,700 infants had been born in Haiti during that year; 30,360 were stillborn. Furthermore, 38,000 children aged 1 to 4 years had also perished. Dr. Titus continued: "If we combine these two figures, that would give more than 50,000 deaths per 200,000 births, yielding a mortality of 250 percent. In 1965, during the Decade of Nutrition, I conducted a study on infant mortality, which at that time was estimated at 203 percent. This means that, despite certain progress in the environment, despite the important development of vaccination . . . we have not really improved our situation on this score" (p. 2 of the proceedings of this conference, *Forum Libre* 1). My translation.

19.   "Haitian Child Dies Every 5 Minutes" 1987. See the reviews by Beghin, Fougère, and King 1970 and by Feilden, Allman, Montague, and Rohde 1981.

20.   Wiese 1971, p. 40.

21.   Leyburn 1966, p. 275.

22.   United Nations 1949, pp. 70–72.

23.   Pan American Health Organization 1967, p. 290.

24.   See Feilden, Allman, Montague, and Rohde 1981 for a review of these data.

25.   Desormeaux, Johnson, Coberly, et al. 1996.

26.   Pape and Johnson 1988.

27.   Long, Scalcini, Manfreda, et al. 1991.

28.   Scalcini, Carré, Jean-Baptiste, et al. 1990. Until recently, multidrug-resistant strains have not been reported, but this is probably because they have not been sought out. We readily identified eight cases in our small group of patients in the Central Plateau; see Farmer, Bayona, Becerra, et al. 1997.

29.   Shears 1988.

30.   Wiese 1974.

31.   Farmer and Nardell 1998.

32.   Proje Veye Sante and the region it serves are described more thoroughly in Farmer 1992.

33.   Note that apparent inconsistencies between this essay and Farmer, Robin, Ramilus, and Kim 1991 are the result of an increase in the number of villages served by Proje Veye Sante.

34.   Rifampin has since replaced streptomycin in the initial treatment of adults with tuberculosis. The clinic also stocks second-line drugs for culture-proven cases of MDRTB.

35.   One person who initially lived in Sector 1 later moved out of the catchment area and was no longer served by a community health worker. This patient, rumored to have died some months after leaving the area, is not considered in any of the data analysis of either group.

36.   See Kleinman, Eisenberg, and Good 1978 for a concise review of this methodology. See Kleinman 1995b, pp. 5–15, for his assessment of the methodology's limitations.

37.   The preponderance of women waned over subsequent years, suggesting a backlog of untreated women facing significant barriers to care.

38.   The presence of acid-fast bacilli in a sputum sample usually signals the presence of active pulmonary tuberculosis. Although it is an imperfect test for tuberculosis—as all patients with extrapulmonary disease and many with pulmonary disease will have falsely negative smears—sputum microscopy is the standard test in most settings in the developing world, including Haiti.

39.   Farmer 1990c.

40.   Murray, Styblo, and Rouillon 1990.

41.   Styblo 1989.

42.   Murray, Styblo, and Rouillon 1990.

43.   Brudney and Dobkin 1991a; see also Brudney and Dobkin 1991b.

44.   Menzies, Rocher, and Vissandjee 1993, p. 36.

45.   Reichman 1997, p.11.

46.   Chaulet 1987, p. 21.

47.   Horton 1995.

48.   Sumartojo 1993, p. 1318. Dr. Sumartojo prefers the term "adherence."

49.   World Health Organization 1991.

50.   Weil 1994.

CHAPTER 9

1.   Dubos and Dubos 1992, p. xxxvii.

2.   Snider and Roper 1992.

3.   Mann, Tarantola, and Netter 1992.

4.   In large part because of increasing co-incidence of HIV and TB infections, especially in the poorest parts of the world, Schulzer and co-workers, using mathematical models, predict a 60 percent increase in smear-positive tuberculosis among young adults by the end of the millennium (Schulzer, Fitzgerald, Enarson, Grzybowski 1992). It is this upsurge that led editorialists writing in *Lancet* to ask, "Is Africa Lost?" (Stanford, Grange, and Pozniak 1991).

5.   A third mechanism, exogenous reinfection with a resistant strain, has recently been described among those with HIV infection; see Small, Shafer, Hopewell, et al. 1993. Exogenous reinfection may even occur in immunocompe-

tent patients but appears to be rare (Peter Small, personal communication to the author).

6.   Farmer, Bayona, Becerra, et al. 1997.

7.   Frieden and co-workers recently reported that "the tide is turning" as a result of improved tuberculosis-control strategies; see Frieden, Fujiwara, Washko, and Hamburg 1995.

8.   For an excellent overview of the effects of these changes in TB policy, see Brudney and Dobkin 1991b.

9.   Garrett 1995a, p. 523.

10.   See Goble, Iseman, Madsen, et al. 1993.

11.   Iseman 1993, p. 785.

12.   For additional information about the incidence of tuberculosis in Haiti, see Chapter 8.

13.   Scalcini, Carré, Jean-Baptiste, et al. 1990, p. 510.

14.   The case of Robert David led us to search more aggressively for other cases of MDRTB. We discovered six other patients who were also sick with this disease. The resistance patterns in these cases were different from those of the strain that infected Robert David. Two additional cases were referred to us by other clinics.

15.   Iseman 1993, p. 784.

16.   Scalcini, Carré, Jean-Baptiste, et al. 1990, p. 509.

17.   See Weil 1994 for more on the global supply of antituberculous drugs. The situation is even worse in Russia, where the collapse of the Soviet-era TB-control infrastructure has led to increasingly erratic tuberculosis treatment. Acquired MDRTB strains have become epidemic, in part through institutional amplification inside prisons and detention centers; see Englund 1998.

18.   Farmer and Kim 1998.

19.   Iseman 1985; Maloney, Pearson, Gordon, Del Castillo, Boyle, and Jarvis 1995.

20.   Centers for Disease Control and Prevention 1990b.

21.   McKenna, McCray, and Onorato 1995.

22.   Chaulet 1996, p. 8. My translation.

23.   For an ethnographically rich exploration of official silences about the scale of epidemic disease, see Briggs and Briggs 1997.

24.   Weis, Slocum, Blais, et al. 1994; Frieden, Fujiwara, Washko, and Hamburg 1995.

25.   Patients with cavitary tuberculosis are believed to be highly infectious because each cavity may contain billions of organisms.

26.   Rullán, Herrera, Cano, et al. 1996, p. 125.

27.   At this writing, I have just returned from a fact-finding mission in Siberia, where outbreaks of tuberculosis in prisons have veered out of control. Attempts to treat all prisoners diagnosed with TB with an empiric regimen of first-line drugs have led to an amplification of resistance—which was already at daunting levels—and low cure rates. In the Tomsk prison system, for example, a 1998

cohort study of 212 prisoners with active tuberculosis reveals that most have been previously treated and that most have drug-resistant disease.

28.	Snider, Kelly, Cauthen, Thompson, and Kilburn 1985.

29.	DiPerri, Cade, Castelli, et al. 1993.

30.	Beck-Sague, Dooley, Hutton, et al. 1992; Pearson, Jereb, Frieden, et al. 1992.

31.	Rullán, Herrera, Cano, et al. 1996.

32.	Kritski, Ozorio-Marques, Rabahi, et al. 1996.

33.	Weis, Slocum, Blais, et al. 1994, p. 1182.

34.	Brudney and Dobkin 1991a, p. 749.

35.	Weis, Slocum, Blais, et al. 1994, p. 1183.

36.	Weise 1974, p. 359.

37.	Rubel and Garro 1992, p. 627.

38.	de Villiers 1991, p. 72.

39.	Nightingale, Hannibal, Geiger, Hartmann, Lawrence, and Spurlock 1990, p. 2098.

40.	Packard 1989, p. xvi.

41.	Mata 1985, p. 57.

42.	Ibid., p. 59.

43.	Ibid., pp. 62, 60, 61, 58.

44.	Ibid., pp. 62, 63.

45.	Barnhoorn and Adriaanse 1992, p. 296.

46.	Ibid., pp. 299, 302.

47.	Ibid., pp. 291 (emphasis added), 301, 302.

48.	Rubel and Garro 1992, p. 630, referring to a paper by R. Lieban (1976); emphasis added.

49.	Valeza and McDougall cited in Sumartojo 1993, p. 1314.

50.	Rubel and Garro 1992, p. 630.

51.	Friemodt-Möller 1968, p. 22. In most studies, improving the quality of services inevitably results in drastically improved outcomes. In discussion of tuberculous meningitis in urban India, where access to care was significantly better, one large study found that "default was not a very serious problem, despite the fact that about half the patients come from outside Madras City. Patients attended punctually on 90% of occasions. Furthermore, in 95% of the remaining unpunctual occasions, drugs were missed for less than a week which, as there was no proper retrieval action, is very commendable. All those who attended late had valid reasons for their unpunctuality" (Ramachandran and Prabhakar 1992, p. 171). See also Grange and Festenstein 1993.

52.	Chaulet puts this sharply in an editorial castigating health care professionals for *their* noncompliance: "It is only after these general measures have been applied that we can turn our attention to improving compliance" (1987, p. 20).

53.	McKeown 1979. Note, however, that McKeown's position lends itself to the Luddite position I criticize in this book.

54.   For sharply divergent interpretations of tuberculosis control, see the disturbing essay by Steven Nachman, an anthropologist who worked briefly among Haitians detained by the U.S. Immigration and Naturalization Service (Nachman 1993). Nachman offers compelling ethnography without making immodest claims of causality. For a review stressing the importance of patients' perspectives, see Conrad 1985. Too few of the papers reviewed underline the enormous difference between failure to adhere to an isoniazid prophylaxis regimen and failure to adhere to treatment for active disease.

55.   Collando cited in Rubel and Garro 1992, p. 627.

56.   Rubel and Garro 1992.

57.   Sumartojo 1993.

58.   Onoge 1975, p. 221. Medical anthropologists are not the only ones who lend importance to factors that cannot be considered central in the shaping of tuberculosis pandemics. While René Dubos was at times tough-minded in his assessments, calling TB "the first penalty that capitalistic society had to pay for the ruthless exploitation of labor," he saw the disease as a reflection of the human failure to adapt harmoniously to the environment. This failure was most obvious in the "anonymous gloom of the industrial cities" of the nineteenth century that had replaced the more sensible pastoral lifestyle of the days before the Industrial Revolution: "The most destitute villager in his native land had learned to adorn the dullness and drudgery of existence with bright ribbons and jolly tunes, and with the pageantry of his church." See Dubos and Dubos 1992, pp. 207, 202. René Dubos tended, at times, to adopt a Luddite stance, even after the development of effective antituberculous chemotherapy. As regarded smallpox, he once wrote that "eradication programs will eventually become a curiosity item on library shelves, just as have all social utopias" (cited in Oldstone 1998, p. 41).

59.   For a helpful review, see Porter and McAdam 1994.

60.   Addington 1979, p. 741.

61.   Sumartojo 1993, p. 1312.

62.   Rosenkrantz is quoted from her excellent introduction to Dubos and Dubos 1992, p. xxi.

63.   See McMichael 1995.

64.   Margono, Garely, Mroueh, and Minkoff 1993. Although biological universals are important—cell-mediated immunity wanes during pregnancy—TB is strikingly patterned even among pregnant women. Poor, urban women of color are disproportionately affected among U.S. women. See also Snider 1992. It is important to note, however, that the majority of U.S. cases have in recent years been among men.

65.   See, for example, Patel 1987.

66.   Farmer 1991.

67.   See, for example, the review by Small and Moss 1993.

68.   Sumartojo 1993, p. 1318.

69.   Rosenkrantz is quoted from her introduction to Dubos and Dubos 1992, p. xxxiv.

CHAPTER 10

1.   Of course, estimates of world prevalence and incidence of HIV infection are the subject of much debate. If we rely, however, on the Joint United Nations Program on HIV/AIDS, this estimate of 30 million is conservative. UNAIDS and the WHO have estimated that 5.8 million people were infected with HIV in the course of 1997. "The more we know about the AIDS epidemic, the worse it appears to be," commented Peter Piot, in releasing these figures. "We are now realizing that rates of HIV transmission have been grossly underestimated—particularly in sub-Saharan Africa, where the bulk of infections have been concentrated to date. South Africa now estimates that one in 10 adults are living with HIV—up by more than one-third since 1996. And in Namibia, AIDS now kills nearly twice as many people as malaria, the next most common killer." See "HIV Claims" 1997, pp. 14, 29.

2.   "Successes Offer Hope" 1996. Several articles and editorials along these lines appeared in the press. For example, see Warsh 1997; noting the gloom of previous world AIDS conferences, Warsh writes: "From the vantage point of 1997, however, the 15-year search for a treatment has turned out to be—suddenly, amazingly—successful."

3.   See Charnow 1996, Stephenson 1996, and Fauci 1996.

4.   Barnett 1996.

5.   Sanford 1996, p 1.

6.   Leland 1996.

7.   O'Brien, Hartigan, Martin, et al. 1996.

8.   See, for example, Ho 1995.

9.   Historian Sheldon Watts puts it well: "The last half-century has seen the triumphal emergence of medicine as a fully scientific discipline of proven effectiveness in curing and preventing life-threatening diseases. Yet it has *also* seen the emergence of a widening gap in the provisioning (and non-provisioning) of effective health services for the privileged few and the underprivileged many" (1998, p. 269).

10.   Mann, Tarantola, and Netter 1996.

11.   Centers for Disease Control and Prevention 1995.

12.   See Bastian, Bennett, Adams, et al. 1993; Lemp, Hirozawa, Cohen, et al. 1992; Easterbrook, Keruly, Creagh-Kirk, et al. 1991; and Hogg, Strathdee, Craib, et al. 1994.

13.   Centers for Disease Control and Prevention 1994b.

14.   Soto-Ramírez, Renjifo, McLane, et al. 1996.

15. See Farmer, Connors, and Simmons 1996, pt. 2, for a critical review of these hypotheses.

16. Chaisson, Keruly, and Moore 1995, p. 755.

17. Bloom and Murray 1992

18. World Health Organization 1996.

19. Wise 1993, p. 13.

20. Group Interassociatif TRT-5/Traitements et Recherche Thérapeutique 1996.

21. Waldholz 1996, p. 1.

22. Ibid.

23. See Sontag and Richardson 1997, pp. 1, 31.

24. Leland 1996, p. 68.

25. For reviews, see Mushlin and Appel 1977; Wardman, Knox, Muers, and Page 1988. Fortunately, some physicians active in planning HIV care are aware of their inability to predict future compliance. "I don't think we have a right or a scientific background to exclude anyone as a general rule," said Dr. Charles Carpenter, chairman of the National Institutes of Health panel that is writing guidelines for the use of AIDS drugs. "I have been astonished by how many people, including those who are using IV drugs, have been able to stick to the regimen. I don't think we can tell a good or bad candidate in advance" (Sontag and Richardson 1997, p. 31). Recently, a strong appeal for access to highly active antiretroviral therapy for the U.S. poor has come from San Francisco, where Bangsberg and colleagues argue that "clinicians treating an indigent, largely minority population like the homeless should take a determined approach to making effective therapy possible" (Bangsberg, Tulsky, Hecht, and Moss 1997, p. 63).

26. Sanford 1996, p. A12.

27. See Richardson 1997, p. 25.

28. Waldholz 1996.

29. Leland 1996.

30. "For Mississippi AIDS Patients" 1997.

31. Brandt 1988, p. 168.

32. Reichman 1997.

33. Ibid., p. 4.

34. Iseman 1985, p. 735.

35. Hopewell, Sanchez-Hernandez, Baron, and Ganter 1984.

36. Hopewell, Ganter, Baron, and Sanchez-Hernandez 1985.

37. World Health Organization Global Tuberculosis Programme 1997.

38. Weil 1994, p. 124. This opposition has not been subtle. In a May 1998 interview with *TB Monitor* (see "Money Isn't the Issue" 1998), the deputy director of WHO's Global Tuberculosis Programme "singled out for criticism those who advocate treatment for MDRTB patients." I am identified as "chief among critics" of arguments against treating patients with MDRTB.

39. Blower, Small, and Hopewell 1996, p. 500.

40. McKenna, McCray, and Onorato 1995.

41. Economist Intelligence Unit 1997.

42. The "bargain" may have backfired, notes the *New York Times:* the jets, purchased from Belarus, came without a warranty or service contract. See "Peru's Cut-Rate Fighter Jets" 1997.

43. Nancy Tomes has recently written about a "socialism of the microbe," whose proponents argued that the health problems of the poor and the immigrant should be central to the grand project of social revolution; see Tomes 1998, chap. 9.

44. Budd [1874] 1931, pp. 174–75.

45. Hirsh and Klaidman 1997, p. 42.

46. Hasan 1996, p. 1055.

47. Rousseau [1755] 1994, pp. 81, 85. "Rousseau is often considered a rebel against inequality," notes Louis Dumont, "but in reality his ideas remained very moderate and were to a large extent traditional" (Dumont 1970, p. 12).

48. Documentation on the impact of growing inequality is wanting. For more on the health effects of some recent large-scale economic policies, see Kim, Millen, and Gershman 1999. On the simultaneous growth of poverty and wealth in the United States, see Krugman 1990. The U.S. Congressional Budget Office offers the following data: between 1977 and 1992, the poorest 10 percent of the population lost 20.3 percent of its post-tax income, while the top 10 percent gained 40.9 percent, and the top 5 percent gained 59.7 percent. The top 1 percent gained 135.7 percent. See Piven and Cloward 1996, pp. 74–75.

49. Wilkinson 1996, p. 212.

50. Ibid., p. 216.

51. McMichael 1995, p. 634.

52. Kleinman 1995b, p. 69.

53. Bourdieu 1993, p. 944. My translation.

References

Abbott, E.
    1988.   *Haiti: The Duvaliers and Their Legacy.* New York: McGraw-Hill.
Addington, W. W.
    1979.   "Patient Compliance: The Most Serious Remaining Problem in the Control of Tuberculosis in the United States." *Chest* 76 (6, Suppl.): 741–43.
Ad Hoc Committee to Defend Health Care.
    1997.   "For Our Patients, Not for Profits: A Call to Action." *Journal of the American Medical Association* 278 (21): 1733–34.
Adler, N. E., T. Boyce, M. A. Chesney, et al.
    1994.   "Socioeconomic Status and Health: The Challenge of the Gradient." *American Psychologist* 49 (1): 15–24.
Aïach, P., R. Carr-Hill, S. Curtis, and R. Illsley.
    1987.   *Les Inégalités Sociales de Santé en France et en Grande-Bretagne.* Paris: INSERM.
Alexander, A.
    1997.   "Does WHO Policy Create More MDR-TB?" *TB Monitor International,* May, pp. 1–3.

Alexander, P.
1988.   *Prostitutes Prevent AIDS: A Manual for Health Educators.* San Francisco: CAL-PEP.

———.

1995.   "Sex Workers Fight Against AIDS: An International Perspective." In *Women Resisting AIDS: Feminist Strategies of Empowerment,* edited by B. E. Schneider and N. E. Stoller, pp. 99–123. Philadelphia: Temple University Press.

Allman, J.
1980.   "Sexual Unions in Rural Haiti." *International Journal of Sociology of the Family* 10:15–39.

Allman, T. D.
1989.   "After Baby Doc." *Vanity Fair* 52 (1): 74–116.

Altman, D.
1986.   *AIDS in the Mind of America.* Garden City, N.Y.: Anchor Books.

Altman, L. K.
1983.   "Debate Grows on U.S. Listing of Haitians in AIDS Category." *New York Times,* 31 July, p. 1.

Ambinder, R. F., C. Newman, G. S. Hawyard, R. Biggar, et al.
1987.   "Lack of Association of Cytomegalovirus with Endemic African Kaposi's Sarcoma." *Journal of Infectious Diseases* 156 (1): 193–97.

Anastos, K., and C. Marte.
1989.   "Women: The Missing Persons in the AIDS Epidemic." *Health PAC Bulletin* 19 (4): 6–13.

André, S., O. Schatz, J. R. Bogner, et al.
1997.   "Detection of Antibodies Against Viral Capsid Proteins of Human Herpesvirus 8 in AIDS-Associated Kaposi's Sarcoma." *Journal of Molecular Medicine* 75 (2): 145–52.

Angell, M.
1997a.   "Editorial: The Ethics of Clinical Research in the Third World." *New England Journal of Medicine* 337 (12): 847–49.

———.

1997b.   "Tuskegee Revisited." *Wall Street Journal,* 28 October, p. A22.

Antonovsky, A.
1967.   "Social Class, Life Expectancy, and Overall Mortality." *Milbank Memorial Fund Quarterly* 45:31–73.

Aral, S., and K. Holmes.
1991.   "Sexually Transmitted Diseases in the AIDS Era." *Scientific American* 264 (2): 62–69.

Asad, T., ed.
1975.   *Anthropology and the Colonial Encounter.* London: Ithaca Press.

Ayanian, J. Z.

1993.   "Editorial: Heart Disease in Black and White." *New England Journal of Medicine* 329 (9): 656–58.

———.

1994.   "Editorial: Race, Class, and the Quality of Medical Care." *Journal of the American Medical Association* 271 (15): 1207–8.

Ayanian, J. Z., S. Udvarhelyi, C. A. Gatsonis, C. L. Pashos, and A. M. Epstein.

1993.   "Racial Differences in the Use of Revascularization Procedures After Coronary Angiography." *Journal of the American Medical Association* 269 (20): 2642–46.

Bangsberg, D., J. P. Tulsky, F. M. Hecht, and A. R. Moss.

1997.   "Protease Inhibitors in the Homeless." *Journal of the American Medical Association* 278 (1): 63–65.

Barnett, A.

1996.   "Protease Inhibitors Fly Through FDA." *Lancet* 347:678.

Barnhoorn, F., and H. Adriaanse.

1992.   "In Search of Factors Responsible for Noncompliance Among Tuberculosis Patients in Wardha District, India." *Social Science and Medicine* 34 (3): 291–306.

Barros, J.

1984.   *Haïti de 1804 à Nos Jours.* 2 vols. Paris: Éditions l'Harmattan.

Bartholemew, C., C. Saxinger, J. Clark, et al.

1987.   "Transmission of HTLV-1 and HIV Among Homosexual Men in Trinidad." *Journal of the American Medical Association* 257 (19): 2604–8.

Bastian, L., C. Bennett, J. Adams, et al.

1993.   "Differences Between Men and Women with HIV-Related *Pneumocystis Carinii* Pneumonia: Experience from 3,070 Cases in New York City in 1987." *Journal of Acquired Immune Deficiency Syndromes* 6 (6): 617–23.

Bastien, R.

1961.   "Haitian Rural Family Organization." *Social and Economic Studies* 10 (4): 478–510.

———.

[1951] 1985. *Le Paysan Haïtien et sa Famille: Vallée de Marbial.* Paris: Karthala.

Batchelor, W.

1984.   "AIDS: A Public Health and Psychological Emergency." *American Psychologist* 39 (11): 1279–84.

Bateson, M. C., and R. Goldsby.

1988.   *Thinking AIDS: The Social Response to the Biological Threat.* Reading, Mass.: Addison-Wesley.

Bayer, R.

1990.   "The Ethics of Research on HIV/AIDS in Community-Based Settings." *AIDS* 4 (12): 1287–88.

Beach, R., and P. Laura.
   1983.   "Nutrition and the Acquired Immune Deficiency Syndrome." *Annals of Internal Medicine* 99 (4): 565–66.
Beck-Sague, C., S. W. Dooley, M. D. Hutton, et al.
   1992.   "Hospital Outbreak of Multidrug-Resistant *Mycobacterium tuberculosis* Infections: Factors in Transmission to Staff and HIV-Infected Patients." *Journal of the American Medical Association* 268 (10): 1280–86.
Beghin, I., W. Fougère, and K. King.
   1970.   *L'Alimentation et la Nutrition en Haiti.* Paris: Presses Universitaires de France.
Behets, F. M. T., J. Desormeaux, D. Joseph, et al.
   1995.   "Control of Sexually Transmitted Diseases in Haiti: Results and Implications of a Baseline Study Among Pregnant Women Living in Cité Soleil Shantytowns." *Journal of Infectious Diseases* 172 (3): 764–71.
Benoist, J., and A. Desclaux, eds.
   1995.   *Sida et Anthropologie: Bilan et Perspectives.* Paris: Karthala.
Berkelman, R. L., and J. M. Hughes.
   1993.   "The Conquest of Infectious Diseases: Who Are We Kidding?" *Annals of Internal Medicine* 119 (5): 426–28.
Bifani, P. J., B. B. Plikaytis, V. Kapur, K. Stockbauer, X. Pan, M. L. Lutfey, S. L. Moghazeh, W. Eisner, T. M. Daniel, M. H. Kaplan, J. T. Crawford, J. M. Musser, B. N. Krieswirth.
   1996.   "Origina and Interstate Spread of a New York City Multidrug-resistant Mycobacterium Tuberculosis Clone Family." *Journal of the American Medical Association* 275 (6): 452–57.
Bloom, B. R.
   1992.   "Tuberculosis: Back to a Frightening Future." *Nature* 358:538–39.
Bloom, B., and C. J. L. Murray.
   1992.   "Tuberculosis: Commentary on a Resurgent Killer." *Science* 257:1055–63.
Blower, S. M., P. M. Small, and P. C. Hopewell.
   1996.   "Control Strategies for Tuberculosis Epidemics: New Models for Old Problems." *Science* 273:497–500.
Bolton, R., M. Lewis, and G. Orozco.
   1991.   "AIDS Literature for Anthropologists: A Working Bibliography." *Journal of Sex Research* 28 (2): 307–46.
Boodhoo, K.
   1984.   "The Economic Dimension of U.S. Caribbean Policy." In *The Caribbean Challenge: U.S. Policy in a Volatile Region,* edited by H. Erisman, pp. 72–91. Boulder, Colo.: Westview Press.
Bordes, A.
   1979.   *Évolution des Sciences de la Santé et de l'Hygiène Publique en Haïti.* Vol. 1. Port-au-Prince: Centre d'Hygiène Familiale.

Bourdieu, P.
1990.   *In Other Words: Essays Towards a Reflexive Sociology.* Cambridge: Polity.
———, ed.
1993.   *La Misère du Monde.* Paris: Seuil.
Bourgois, P.
1995.   *In Search of Respect: Selling Crack in El Barrio.* Cambridge: Cambridge University Press.
Bourque, S., and K. Warren.
1989.   "Democracy Without Peace: The Cultural Politics of Terror in Peru." *Latin American Research Review* 24 (1): 7–35.
Brandt, A.
1987.   *No Magic Bullet: A Social History of Venereal Disease in the United States Since 1880.* New York: Oxford University Press.
———.
1988.   "AIDS: From Social History to Social Policy." In *AIDS: The Burdens of History,* edited by E. Fee and D. M. Fox, pp. 147–71. Berkeley: University of California Press.
———.
1997.   "Behavior, Disease, and Health in the Twentieth-Century United States: The Moral Valence of Individual Risk." In *Morality and Health,* edited by A. M. Brandt and P. Rozin, pp. 53–77. New York: Routledge.
Briggs, C. L., and C. M. Briggs.
1997.   "'The Indians Accept Death as a Normal, Natural Event': Institutional Authority, Cultural Reasoning, and Discourses of Genocide in a Venezuelan Cholera Epidemic." *Social Identities* 3 (3): 439–69.
Brown, P.
1983.   "Introduction: Anthropology and Disease Control." *Medical Anthropology* 7 (3): 1–8.
Brudney, K., and J. Dobkin.
1991a.   "Resurgent Tuberculosis in New York City: Human Immunodeficiency Virus, Homelessness, and the Decline of Tuberculosis Control Programs." *American Review of Respiratory Disease* 144:745–49.
———.
1991b.   "A Tale of Two Cities: Tuberculosis Control in Nicaragua and New York City." *Seminars in Respiratory Infections* 6:261–72.
Brutus, J. R.
1989a.   "Problèmes d'éthique Liés au Dépistage du Virus HIV-1." Paper presented at the Congrès des Médecins Francophones d'Amérique, 12–16 June, Fort-de-France, Martinique.
———.
1989b.   "Séroprévalence de HIV Parmi les Femmes Enceintes à Cité Soleil, Haïti." Paper presented at the Fifth International Conference on AIDS, 5–7 June, Montreal, Canada.

Budd, W.

[1874] 1931. *Typhoid Fever: Its Nature, Mode of Spreading, and Prevention*. New York: George Brady Press.

Bunker, J. P., D. S. Gomby, and B. H. Kehrer, eds.

1989.   *Pathways to Health: The Role of Social Factors*. Menlo Park, Calif.: The Henry J. Kaiser Family Foundation.

Carovano, K.

1991.   "More Than Mothers and Whores: Redefining the AIDS Prevention Needs of Women." *International Journal of Health Services* 21 (1): 131–42.

Carpenter, F.

1930.   *Lands of the Caribbean*. Garden City, N.Y.: Doubleday, Doran and Co.

Castro, K. G., and D. E. Snider.

1995.   "Editorial: The Good News and the Bad News About Multidrug-Resistant Tuberculosis." *Clinical Infectious Diseases* 21:1265–66.

Cauna, J.

1984.   "L'état Sanitaire des Esclaves sur une Grande Sucrérie (Habitation Fleuriau de Bellevue, 1777–1788)." *Revue de la Société Haïtienne d'Histoire et de Géographie* 42 (145): 18–78.

Centers for Disease Control and Prevention.

1981.   "Pneumocystis Pneumonia—Los Angeles." *Morbidity and Mortality Weekly Report* 30 (21): 250–52.

———.

1982a.   "Opportunistic Infections and Kaposi's Sarcoma Among Haitians in the United States." *Morbidity and Mortality Weekly Report* 31 (14): 353–54, 360–61.

———.

1982b.   "Update on Kaposi's Sarcoma and Opportunistic Infections in Previously Well Persons—United States." *Morbidity and Mortality Weekly Report* 31 (22): 294, 300–301.

———.

1990a.   "AIDS in Women—United States." *Morbidity and Mortality Weekly Report* 39 (47): 845–46.

———.

1990b.   "Outbreak of Multi-Drug Resistant Tuberculosis—Texas, California, and Pennsylvania." *Morbidity and Mortality Weekly Report* 39 (22): 369–72.

———.

1992.   "Meeting the Challenge of Multidrug-Resistant Tuberculosis: Summary of a Conference." *Morbidity and Mortality Weekly Report* 41 (RR-11): 51–57.

———.

1993a.   "Diphtheria Outbreak—Russian Federation, 1990–1993." *Morbidity and Mortality Weekly Report* 42 (43): 840–47.

———.

1993b.   "Sexually Transmitted Disease Guidelines." *Morbidity and Mortality Weekly Report* 42 (RR-14).

———.

1994a.   *Addressing Emerging Infectious Disease Threats: A Prevention Strategy for the United States.* Atlanta: U.S. Department of Health and Human Services.

———.

1994b.   "AIDS Among Racial/Ethnic Minorities—United States, 1993." *Morbidity and Mortality Weekly Report* 43 (35): 644–47, 653–55.

———.

1995.   "Update: AIDS Among Women—United States, 1994." *Morbidity and Mortality Weekly Report* 44 (5): 81–85.

———.

1996.   "Update: Mortality Due to HIV Infection Among Persons Aged 25–44 Years—United States, 1994." *Morbidity and Mortality Weekly Report* 45 (6): 121–24.

———.

1997.   *HIV/AIDS Surveillance Report* 9 (2): 1–43.

Chaisson, R. E., J. C. Keruly, and R. D. Moore.

1995.   "Race, Sex, Drug Use, and Progression of Human Immunodeficiency Virus Disease." *New England Journal of Medicine* 333 (12): 751–56.

Chambers, V.

1995.   "Betrayal Feminism." In *Listen Up: Voices from the Next Feminist Generation,* edited by B. Findlen, pp. 21–28. Seattle: Seal Press.

Charnow, J.

1996.   "Mood Upbeat at International AIDS Conference." *Infectious Disease News* 9 (8): 10.

Chaulet, P.

1987.   "Compliance with Anti-Tuberculosis Chemotherapy in Developing Countries." *Tubercle* 68 (Suppl.): 19–24.

———.

1996.   "Les Nouveaux Tuberculeux." *Le Journal de la Tuberculose et du Sida* 6 (4): 6–8.

Chaze, W.

1983.   "In Haiti, A View of Life at the Bottom." *U.S. News and World Report,* 31 October, pp. 41–42.

Clatts, M. C.

1994.   "All the King's Horses and All the King's Men: Some Personal Reflections on Ten Years of AIDS Ethnography." *Human Organization* 53 (1): 93–95.

———.

1995.   "Disembodied Acts: On the Perverse Use of Sexual Categories in the Study of High-Risk Behavior." In *Culture and Sexual Risk: Anthropological Perspectives,* edited by H. ten Brummelhuis and G. Herdt, pp. 241–56. New York: Gordon and Breach.

Cohen, J.

1996.   "The Marketplace of HIV/AID$." *Science* 272:1880–81.

Cohn, D. L., B. J. Catlin, K. L. Peterson, F. N. Judson, and J. A. Sbarbaro.

1990.   "A 62-Dose, 6-Month Therapy for Pulmonary and Extrapulmonary Tuberculosis: A Twice-Weekly, Directly Observed, and Cost-Effective Regimen." *Annals of Internal Medicine* 112 (6): 407–15.

Cole, S. T., and A. Telenti.

1995.   "Drug Resistance in *Mycobacterium tuberculosis.*" *European Respiratory Journal* 20 (Suppl.): 701–13s.

Collaborative Study Group of AIDS in Haitian-Americans.

1987.   "Risk Factors for AIDS Among Haitians Residing in the United States: Evidence of Heterosexual Transmission." *Journal of the American Medical Association* 257 (5): 635–39.

Collins, P. H.

1990.   *Black Feminist Thought: Knowledge, Consciousness, and the Politics of Empowerment.* New York: Routledge.

Comhaire-Sylvain, S.

1960.   "Les fiançailles dans la région de Kenscoff, Haïti." *Bulletin d'Ethnologie de la République Dhaïti,* 3:23–24–25.

Connors, M.

1995.   "The Politics of Marginalization: The Appropriation of AIDS Prevention Messages Among Injection Drug Users." *Culture, Medicine, and Psychiatry* 19 (4): 1–28.

Conrad, P.

1985.   "The Meaning of Medications: Another Look at Compliance." *Social Science and Medicine* 20 (1): 29–37.

Coreil, J.

1980.   "Traditional and Western Responses to an Anthrax Epidemic in Rural Haiti." *Medical Anthropology* 4 (4): 79–105.

———.

1983.   "Parallel Structures in Professional Folk Health Care: A Model Applied to Rural Haiti." *Culture, Medicine, and Psychiatry* 7 (2): 131–51.

Cueto, M.

1992.   "'Sanitation from Above': Yellow Fever and Foreign Intervention in Peru, 1919–1922." *Hispanic American Historical Review* 72 (1): 1–22.

Curry, F. J.

1968.   "Neighborhood Clinics for More Effective Outpatient Treatment of Tuberculosis." *New England Journal of Medicine* 279 (23): 1262–67.

d'Adesky, A. C.
  1991.   "Silence + Death = AIDS in Haiti." *The Advocate* 577:30–36.
Das, S.
  1995.   "AIDS in India: An Ethnography of HIV/AIDS Amongst Bombay's
           Commercial Sex Workers." Undergraduate honors thesis, Depart-
           ments of Anthropology and Sanskrit and Indian Studies, Harvard
           University, Cambridge, Mass.
de Bruyn, M.
  1992.   "Women and AIDS in Developing Countries." *Social Science and
           Medicine* 34 (3): 249–62.
De Cock, K. M., B. Soro, I. M. Coulibaly, and S. B. Lucas.
  1992.   "Tuberculosis and HIV Infection in Sub-Saharan Africa." *Journal of
           the American Medical Association* 268 (12): 1581–87.
Degregori, C.
  1986.   *Sendero Luminoso.* Lima: IEP.
Degregori, C., J. Coronel, P. del Pino, and O. Starn, eds.
  1996.   *Las Rondas Campesinas y la Derrota de Sendero Luminoso.* Lima: IEP.
Denison, R.
  1995.   "Call Us Survivors! Women Organized to Respond to Life-
           Threatening Diseases (WORLD)." In *Women Resisting AIDS:
           Feminist Strategies of Empowerment,* edited by B. E. Schneider
           and N. E. Stoller, pp. 195–207. Philadelphia: Temple
           University Press.
Deschamps, M. M., et al.
  1992.   "HIV Seroconversion Related to Heterosexual Activity in Discor-
           dant Haitian Couples." Poster presented at the Eighth International
           Conference on AIDS/Third STD World Congress, 19–24 July, Am-
           sterdam. Abstract C1087.
Deschamps, M. M., J. W. Pape, A. Hafner, and W. D. Johnson.
  1996.   "Heterosexual Transmission of HIV in Haiti." *Annals of Internal
           Medicine* 125 (4): 324–30.
Deschamps, M. M., J. W. Pape, P. Williams-Russo, S. Madhavan, J. Ho, and W.
Johnson.
  1993.   "A Prospective Study of HIV-Seropositive Asymptomatic Women of
           Childbearing Age in a Developing Country." *Journal of Acquired Im-
           mune Deficiency Syndromes* 6 (5): 446–51.
DesJarlais, D. C., and S. R. Friedman.
  1988.   "Needle Sharing Among IVDUs at Risk for AIDS." *American Journal
           of Public Health* 78 (11): 1498–99.
DesJarlais, D. C., S. R. Friedman, and T. Ward.
  1993.   "Harm Reduction: A Public Health Response to the AIDS Epidemic
           Among Injecting Drug Users." *Annual Review of Public Health*
           14:413–50.

DesJarlais, D. C., N. Padian, and N. Winklestein, Jr.
    1994.   "Targeted HIV-Prevention Programs." *New England Journal of Medicine* 331 (21): 1451–53.
Desormeaux, J., M. P. Johnson, J. S. Coberly, et al.
    1996.   "Widespread HIV Counseling and Testing Linked to a Community-Based Tuberculosis Control Program in a High-Risk Population." *Bulletin of the Pan American Health Organization* 30 (1): 1–8.
Desvarieux, M., and J. W. Pape.
    1991.   "HIV and AIDS in Haiti: Recent Developments." *AIDS Care* 3 (3): 271–79.
de Villiers, S.
    1991.   "Tuberculosis in Anthropological Perspective." *South African Journal of Ethnology* 14:69–72.
DiBacco, T.
    1998.   "Tuberculosis on the Rebound." *Washington Post*, 27 January, p. A9.
Diedrich, B., and A. Burt.
    1986.   *Papa Doc et les Tontons Macoutes.* Translated by Henri Drevet. Port-au-Prince: Imprimerie Henri Deschamps.
DiPerri, G., G. P. Cade, F. Castelli, et al.
    1993.   "Transmission of HIV-Associated Tuberculosis to Health Care Workers." *Infection Control and Hospital Epidemiology* 14:67–72.
Dozon, J., and L. Vidal, eds.
    1995.   *Les Sciences Sociales Face au Sida: Cas Africains autour de l'Exemple Ivoirien.* Paris: Orstom.
Dubos, R., and J. Dubos.
    1992.   *The White Plague: Tuberculosis, Man, and Society.* 2d ed. New Brunswick, N.J.: Rutgers University Press. First ed. published 1952.
Dumont, L.
    1970.   *Homo Hierarchicus: The Caste System and Its Implications.* Chicago: University of Chicago Press.
Dunn, F.
    1984.   "Social Determinants in Tropical Disease." In *Tropical and Geographic Medicine*, edited by K. Warren and A. Mahmoud, pp. 1086–96. New York: McGraw-Hill.
Dunn, F., and C. Janes.
    1986.   "Introduction: Medical Anthropology and Epidemiology." In *Anthropology and Epidemiology*, edited by C. Janes, R. Stall, and S. Gifford, pp. 3–34. Dordrecht: D. Reidel.
Dupuy, A.
    1997.   *Haiti in the New World Order: The Limits of the Democratic Revolution.* Boulder, Colo.: Westview Press.

Dutton, D. B., and S. Levin.
   1989.   "Socioeconomic Status and Health: Overview, Methodological
            Critique, and Reformulation." In *Pathways to Health: The Role of
            Social Factors,* edited by J. P. Bunker, D. S. Gomby, and B. H.
            Kehrer, pp. 29–69. Menlo Park, Calif.: The Henry J. Kaiser Family
            Foundation.
Easterbrook, P. J., J. C. Keruly, J. Creagh-Kirk, et al.
   1991.   "Racial and Ethnic Differences in Outcome in Zidovudine Treated
            Patients with Advanced HIV Disease." *Journal of the American Med-
            ical Association* 266 (19): 2713–18.
Eckardt, I.
   1994.   "Challenging Complexity: Conceptual Issues in an Approach to
            New Disease." *Annals of the New York Academy of Sciences*
            740:408–17.
Economist Intelligence Unit.
   1997.   "First Quarter 1997 Report." *The Economist,* p. 329.
"Editorial: The Ethics Industry."
   1997.   *Lancet* 360 (9082): 897.
Eisenberg, L.
   1984.   "Rudolf Ludwig Karl Virchow, Where Are You Now That We Need
            You?" *American Journal of Medicine* 77 (3): 524–32.
Eisenberg, L., and A. Kleinman.
   1981.   *The Relevance of Social Science to Medicine.* Dordrecht: D. Reidel.
Ellerbrock, T. V., S. Lieb, P. Harrington, et al.
   1992.   "Heterosexually Transmitted Human Immunodeficiency Virus In-
            fection Among Pregnant Women in a Rural Florida Community."
            New England Journal of Medicine 327 (24): 1704–9.
Englund, W.
   1998.   "Resistant TB Strains Spreading from Russia." *Baltimore Sun,* 14
            September, p. 1A.
Epstein, P. R.
   1992.   "Pestilence and Poverty: Historical Transitions and the Great Pan-
            demics." *American Journal of Preventive Medicine* 8:263–78.
Escobar, E.
   1992.   "Culture, Practice, and Politics: Anthropology and the Study of So-
            cial Movements." *Critique of Anthropology* 12 (4): 395–432.
Escobedo, L. G., W. H. Giles, and R. F. Anda.
   1997.   "Socioeconomic Status, Race, and Death from Coronary Heart Dis-
            ease." *American Journal of Preventive Medicine* 13 (2): 123–30.
Evans, R. G., M. L. Barer, and T. R. Marmor.
   1994.   *Why Are Some People Healthy and Others Not? The Determinants of
            Health of Populations.* Hawthorne, N.Y.: Aldine de Gruyter.

Fabian, J.
    1983.   *Time and the Other: How Anthropology Makes Its Object.* New York: Columbia University Press.
Farmer, P. E.
    1988a.   "Bad Blood, Spoiled Milk: Bodily Fluids as Moral Barometers in Rural Haiti." *American Ethnologist* 15 (1): 131–51.

    ———.
    1988b.   "Blood, Sweat, and Baseballs: Haiti in the West Atlantic System." *Dialectical Anthropology* 13:83–99.

    ———.
    1990a.   "AIDS and Accusation: Haiti, Haitians, and the Geography of Blame." In *AIDS and Culture: The Human Factor,* edited by D. Feldman, pp. 67–91. New York: Praeger.

    ———.
    1990b.   "The Exotic and the Mundane: Human Immunodeficiency Virus in the Caribbean." *Human Nature* 1:415–45.

    ———.
    1990c.   "Sending Sickness: Sorcery, Politics, and Changing Concepts of AIDS in Rural Haiti." *Medical Anthropology Quarterly* 4 (1): 6–27.

    ———.
    1991.   "New Disorder, Old Dilemmas: AIDS and Anthropology in Haiti." In *The Time of AIDS,* edited by G. Herdt and S. Lindenbaum. Los Angeles: Sage.

    ———.
    1992.   *AIDS and Accusation: Haiti and the Geography of Blame.* Berkeley: University of California Press.

    ———.
    1994.   *The Uses of Haiti.* Monroe, Maine: Common Courage Press.
    ———.
    1995a.   "Culture, Poverty, and the Dynamics of HIV Transmission in Rural Haiti." In *Culture and Sexual Risk: Anthropological Perspectives on AIDS,* edited by H. ten Brummelhuis and G. Herdt, pp. 3–28. New York: Gordon and Breach.

    ———.
    1995b.   "Medicine and Social Justice: Insights from Liberation Theology." *America* 173 (2): 14.

    ———.
    1996a.   "Haiti's Lost Years: Lessons for the Americas." *Current Issues in Public Health* 2:143–51.

    ———.
    1996b.   "On Suffering and Structural Violence: A View from Below." *Dædalus* 125 (1): 261–83.

———.

1996c. "Social Inequalities and Emerging Infectious Diseases." *Emerging Infectious Diseases* 2 (4): 259–69.

———.

1997a. "AIDS and Anthropologists: Ten Years Later." *Medical Anthropology Quarterly* 11 (4): 516–25.

———.

1997b. "Ethnography, Social Analysis, and the Prevention of Sexually Transmitted HIV Infections Among Poor Women in Haiti." In *The Anthropology of Infectious Disease*, edited by M. Inhorn and P. Brown, pp. 413–38. New York: Gordon and Breach.

———.

1997c. "Letter from Haiti." *AIDS Clinical Care* 9 (11): 83–85.

———.

1997d. "Social Scientists and the New Tuberculosis." *Social Science and Medicine* 44 (3): 347–58.

Farmer, P. E., J. Bayona, M. Becerra, et al.

1997. "Poverty, Inequality, and Drug Resistance: Meeting Community Needs in the Global Era." In *Proceedings of the International Union Against Tuberculosis and Lung Disease, North American Region Conference*, 27 February–2 March, Chicago, Ill., pp. 88–101.

Farmer, P. E., J. Bayona, S. Shin, L. Alvarez, M. Becerra, E. Nardell, C. Nunez, E. Sanchez, R. Timperi, and J. Y. Kim.

1998. "Preliminary Results of Community-Based MDRTB Treatment in Lima, Peru." Poster presented at the Conference on Global Lung Health and the 1998 Annual Meeting of the International Union Against Tuberculosis and Lung Disease, 23–26 November, Bangkok.

Farmer, P. E., M. Becerra, J. Bayona, et al.

1997. "The Emergence of MDRTB in Urban Peru: A Population-Based Study Using Conventional, Molecular, and Ethnographic Methods." Poster presented at the Conference on Global Lung Health and the 1997 Annual Meeting of the International Union Against Tuberculosis and Lung Disease, 1–4 October, Paris.

Farmer, P. E., M. Connors, and J. Simmons, eds.

1996. *Women, Poverty, and AIDS: Sex, Drugs, and Structural Violence.* Monroe, Maine: Common Courage Press.

Farmer, P. E., and B. J. Good.

1991. "Illness Representations in Medical Anthropology: A Critical Review and a Case Study of the Representation of AIDS in Haiti." In *Mental Representation in Health and Illness*, edited by J. A. Skelton and R. T. Croyle, pp. 132–62. New York: Springer-Verlag.

Farmer, P. E., and J. Y. Kim.

1991.   "Anthropology, Accountability, and the Prevention of AIDS." *Journal of Sex Research* 28 (2): 203–21.

————.

1996.   Introduction to Series in Health and Social Justice. In *Women, Poverty, and AIDS: Sex, Drugs, and Sructural Violence,* edited by P. E. Farmer, M. Connors, and J. Simmons, pp. xiii–xxi. Monroe, Maine: Common Courage Press.

————.

1998.   "Community-Based Approaches to the Control of Multidrug-Resistant Tuberculosis: Introducing 'DOTS-Plus.'" *British Medical Journal* 317:671–74.

Farmer, P. E., and A. Kleinman.

1989.   "AIDS as Human Suffering." *Dædalus* 118 (2): 135–60.

Farmer, P. E., and E. Nardell.

1998.   "Nihilism and Pragmatism in Tuberculosis Control." *American Journal of Public Health* 88 (7): 4–5.

Farmer, P. E., M. Raymonville, S. Robin, S. L. Ramilus, and J. Y. Kim.

1992.   "The Dynamics of HIV Transmission in Rural Haiti." Poster presented at the Eighth International Conference on AIDS/ Third STD World Congress, 19–24 July, Amsterdam. Abstract C4608.

Farmer, P. E., S. Robin, S. L. Ramilus, and J. Y. Kim.

1991.   "Tuberculosis, Poverty, and 'Compliance': Lessons from Rural Haiti." *Seminars in Respiratory Infections* 6:373–79.

Fass, S.

1988.   *Political Economy in Haiti: The Drama of Survival.* New Brunswick, N.J.: Transaction.

Fassin, D.

1996a.   "Exclusion, Underclass, Marginalidad." *Revue Française de Sociologie* 37:37–75.

————.

1996b.   *L'Espace Politique de la Santé: Essai de Généalogie.* Paris: Presses Universitaires de France.

Fauci, A.

1996.   "AIDS in 1996: Much Accomplished, Much to Do." *Journal of the American Medical Association* 276 (2): 155–56.

"Federal Poverty Level Not Realistic."

1994.   *Omaha World Herald,* 18 October, p. 9.

Feilden, R., J. Allman, J. Montague, and J. Rohde.

1981.   *Health, Population, and Nutrition in Haiti: A Report Prepared for the World Bank.* Boston: Management Sciences for Health.

Feinsilver, J.
   1993.   *Healing the Masses: Cuban Health Politics at Home and Abroad.* Berkeley: University of California Press.
Feldberg, G. D.
   1995.   *Disease and Class: Tuberculosis and the Shaping of Modern North American Society.* New Brunswick, N.J.: Rutgers University Press.
Ferguson, J.
   1987.   *Papa Doc, Baby Doc: Haiti and the Duvaliers.* Oxford: Basil Blackwell.
Ferguson, J. A., W. M. Tierney, G. R. Westmoreland, L. A. Mamlin, D. S. Segar, G. J. Eckert, X. H. Zhao, D. K. Martin, and M. Weinberger.
   1997.   "Examination of Racial Differences in Management of Cardiovascular Disease." *Journal of the American College of Cardiology* 30 (7): 1707–13.
Field, M. G.
   1995.   "The Health Crisis in the Former Soviet Union: A Report from the 'Post-War' Zone." *Social Science and Medicine* 41 (11): 1469–78.
Fife, E., and C. Mode.
   1992.   "AIDS Incidence and Income." *Journal of Acquired Immune Deficiency Syndromes* 5 (11): 1105–10.
Fineberg, H. V., and M. E. Wilson.
   1996.   "Social Vulnerability and Death by Infection." *New England Journal of Medicine* 334 (13): 859–60.
Finzi, D., M. Hermankova, T. Pierson, et al.
   1997.   "Identification of a Reservoir for HIV-1 in Patients on Highly Active Antiretroviral Therapy." *Science* 278:1295–1300.
Fitzgerald, D.
   1996.   *Final Report HAS: Project 2005.* Boston: Management Sciences for Health.
Fleming, P.
   1996.   "Update: Trends in AIDS Incidence—United States." *Morbidity and Mortality Weekly Report* 46:861–67.
"For Mississippi AIDS Patients, A Lifeline May Be Cut Off."
   1997.   *Boston Globe,* 2 June.
Foubert, B.
   1987.   "L'habitation Lemmens à Saint-Dominque au début de la Révolution." *Revue de la Société Haïtienne d'Histoire et de Géographie* 45 (154): 1–29.
Fox, R. G., and O. Starn, eds.
   1997.   *Between Resistance and Revolution: Cultural Politics and Social Protest.* New Brunswick, N.J.: Rutgers University Press.
Fox, W.
   1983.   "Compliance of Patients and Physicians: Experience and Lessons from Tuberculosis." *British Medical Journal* 287:33–35.

Franceschi, S., L. Dal Maso, A. Lo Re, D. Serraino, and C. La Vecchia.
1997.   "Trends of Kaposi's Sarcoma at AIDS Diagnosis in Europe and the
United States, 1987–94." *British Journal of Cancer* 76 (1): 114–17.

Francisque, E.
1986.   *La Structure Économique et Sociale d'Haïti.* Port-au-Prince: Imprimerie
Henri Deschamps.

French, H.
1997.   "AIDS Research in Africa: Juggling Risks and Hopes." *New York
Times,* 10 October, pp. 1, 14.

Frenk, J., and F. Chacon.
1991.   "Bases Conceptuales de la Nueva Salud Internacional." *Salud
Pública de México* 33:307–13.

Frieden, T., P. Fujiwara, R. Washko, and M. Hamburg.
1995.   "Tuberculosis in New York City—Turning the Tide." *New England
Journal of Medicine* 333 (4): 229–33.

Friedman, L. N., M. T. Williams, T. P. Singh, and T. R. Frieden.
1996.   "Tuberculosis, AIDS, and Death Among Substance Abusers on
Welfare in New York City." *New England Journal of Medicine*
334 (13): 828–33.

Friedman, S.
1993.   "AIDS as a Sociohistorical Phenomenon." *Advances in Medical Sociology* 3:19–36.

Friemodt-Möller, J.
1968.   "Domiciliary Drug Therapy of Pulmonary Tuberculosis in a Rural
Population in India." *Tubercle* 49 (Supp.): 22–23.

Fullilove, M. T., R. E. Fullilove, K. Haynes, et al.
1990.   "Black Women and AIDS Prevention: A View Towards Understanding the Gender Rules." *Journal of Sex Research* 27 (1): 47–64.

Fullilove, M., A. Lown, and R. E. Fullilove.
1992.   "Crack 'Hos and Skeezers: Traumatic Experiences of Women Crack
Users." *Journal of Sex Research* 29 (2): 275–87.

Fullilove, R. E.
1995.   "Community Disintegration and Public Health: A Case Study of
New York City." In *Assessing the Social and Behavioral Science Base for
HIV/AIDS Prevention and Intervention Workshop Summary,* pp.
93–116. Washington, D.C.: National Academy Press.

Fumento, M.
1993.   *The Myth of Heterosexual AIDS.* 2d ed. Washington, D.C.: Regnery
Gateway.

Gail, M., P. Rosenberg, and J. Goedert.
1990.   "Therapy May Explain Recent Deficits in AIDS Incidence." *Journal
of Acquired Immune Deficiency Syndromes* 3 (4): 296–306.

Gaines, A., and P. Farmer.
  1986.   "Visible Saints: Social Cynosures and Dysphoria in the Mediter-
          ranean Tradition." *Culture, Medicine, and Psychiatry* 11 (4): 295–330.
García, R.
  1991.   "Tourism and AIDS: A Dominican Republic Study." *AIDS and Soci-
          ety* 2 (3): 1–3.
Garrett, L.
  1995a. *The Coming Plague.* New York: Farrar, Straus and Giroux.
———.
  1995b. "Public Health and the Mass Media." *Current Issues in Public Health*
          1:147–50.
Garris, I., E. M. Rodríguez, E. A. De Moya, et al.
  1991.   "AIDS Heterosexual Predominance in the Dominican Republic."
          Journal of Acquired Immune Deficiency Syndromes 4 (12): 1173–78.
Garro, L.
  1988.   "Explaining High Blood Pressure: Variation in Knowledge About
          Knowledge." *American Ethnologist* 15 (1): 98–119.
Geertz, C.
  1988.   *Works and Lives: The Anthropologist as Author.* Stanford, Calif.: Stan-
          ford University Press.
Geiger, H. J.
  1992.   "Urban Health and the Social Contract: Poverty, Race, and Death."
          Henry Ford Hospital Medical Journal 40 (1–2): 29–34.
Gerstoft, J., J. Nielsen, E. Dickmeiss, T. Ronne, P. Platz, and L. Mathiesen.
  1985.   "The Acquired Immunodeficiency Syndrome (AIDS) in Denmark."
          Acta Medica Scandinavica 217:213–24.
Gifford, S.
  1986.   "The Meaning of Lumps: A Case Study of the Ambiguities of Risk."
          In *Anthropology and Epidemiology,* edited by C. Janes, R. Stall, and S.
          Gifford, pp. 213–46. Dordrecht: D. Reidel.
Giles, W. H., R. F. Anda, M. L. Caspar, L. G. Escobedo, and H. A. Taylor.
  1995.   "Race and Sex Differences in Rates of Invasive Cardiac Procedures
          in U.S. Hospitals: Data from the National Hospital Discharge Sur-
          vey." *Archives of Internal Medicine* 155:318–24.
Gilman, S.
  1988.   "AIDS and Syphilis: The Iconography of Disease." In *AIDS: Culture
          Analysis/Cultural Activism,* edited by D. Crimp, pp. 87–107. Cam-
          bridge, Mass.: MIT Press.
Girault, C.
  1984.   "Commerce in the Haitian Economy." In *Haiti—Today and Tomorrow:
          An Interdisciplinary Study,* edited by C. Foster and A. Valdman,
          pp. 173–79. Lanham, Md.: University Press of America.

Glick-Schiller, N.
1993.   "The Invisible Women: Caregiving and the Construction of AIDS Health Services." *Culture, Medicine, and Psychiatry* 17 (4): 487–512.

Glick-Schiller, N., and G. Fouron.
1990.   "'Everywhere We Go We Are in Danger': Ti Manno and the Emergence of a Haitian Transnational Identity." *American Ethnologist* 17 (2): 329–47.

Global AIDS Policy Coalition.
1995.   *Status and Trends of the HIV/AIDS Pandemic as of January 1, 1995.* Cambridge, Mass.: Harvard School of Public Health/François-Xavier Bagnoud Center for Health and Human Rights.

———.
1996.   *Status and Trends of the HIV/AIDS Pandemic as of January 1, 1996.* Cambridge, Mass.: Harvard School of Public Health/François-Xavier Bagnoud Center for Health and Human Rights.

Goble, M., M. Iseman, L. Madsen, et al.
1993.   "Treatment of 171 Patients with Pulmonary Tuberculosis Resistant to Isoniazid and Rifampin." *New England Journal of Medicine* 328 (8): 527–32.

Goeman, J., A. Méheus, and P. Piot.
1991.   "L'Epidemiologie des Maladies Sexuellement Transmissibles dans les Pays en Développement à l'Ere du Sida." *Annales de la Société Belge de la Médecine Tropicale* 71:81–113.

Goldberger, J., G. Wheeler, and E. Sydenstricker.
1920.   "A Study of the Relation of Family Income and Other Economic Factors to Pellagra Incidence in Seven Cotton-Mill Villages of South Carolina in 1916." *Public Health Reports* 35:2673–714.

Goma Epidemiology Group.
1995.   "Public Health Impact of Rwandan Refugee Crisis: What Happened in Goma, Zaïre, in July, 1994?" *Lancet* 345:339–44.

Good, B.
1977.   "The Heart of What's the Matter: The Semantics of Illness in Iran." *Culture, Medicine, and Psychiatry* 1 (1): 25–58.

Good, B., and M. J. D. Good.
1982.   "Toward a Meaning-Centered Analysis of Popular Illness Categories: 'Fright Illness' and 'Heart Distress' in Iran." In *Cultural Conceptions of Mental Health and Therapy,* edited by A. J. Marsella and G. M. White, pp. 141–66. Boston: Reidel.

Gorman, M.
1986.   "The AIDS Epidemic in San Francisco: Epidemiological and Anthropological Perspectives." In *Anthropology and Epidemiology,* edited by C. Janes, R. Stall, and S. Gifford, pp. 157–74. Dordrecht: D. Reidel.

Goudsmit, J.
  1983.   "Malnutrition and Concomitant Herpesvirus Infection as a Possible
           Cause of Immunodeficiency Syndrome in Haitian Infants." *New
           England Journal of Medicine* 309 (9): 554–55.
Gould, P.
  1993.   *The Slow Plague: A Geography of the AIDS Pandemic.* Cambridge,
           Mass.: Blackwell.
Grange, J., and F. Festenstein.
  1993.   "The Human Dimension of Tuberculosis Control." *Tubercle and
           Lung Disease* 74:219–22.
Greco, R. S.
  1983.   "Haiti and the Stigma of AIDS." *Lancet* 2 (8348): 515–56.
Green, E. C.
  1994.   *AIDS and STDs in Africa: Bridging the Gap Between Traditional Healing
           and Modern Medicine.* Boulder, Colo.: Westview Press.
Greene, G.
  1966.   *The Comedians.* London: Bodley Head.
Greenfield, W.
  1986.   "Night of the Living Dead II: Slow Virus Encephalopathies and AIDS:
           Do Necromantic Zombiists Transmit HTLV-III/LAV During Voodooistic
           tic Rituals?" *Journal of the American Medical Association* 256 (16): 2199–200.
Groopman, J.
  1983.   "Viruses and Human Neoplasia: Approaching Etiology." *American
           Journal of Medicine* 75 (3): 377–80.
Grosskurth, H., F. Mosha, J. Todd, et al.
  1995.   "Impact of Improved Treatment of Sexually Transmitted Diseases
           on HIV Infection in Rural Tanzania: Randomised Controlled Trial."
           Lancet 346:530–36.
Group Interassociatif TRT-5/Traitements et Recherche Thérapeutique.
  1996.   "Communiqué: Accès aux Antirétroviraux; l'Europe en Panne." 31
           October, Paris.
Grover, J. Z.
  1988.   "AIDS: Keywords." In *AIDS: Cultural Analysis/Cultural Activism*,
           edited by D. Crimp, pp. 17–30. Cambridge, Mass.: MIT Press.
Grunwald, J., L. Delatour, and K. Voltaire.
  1984.   "Offshore Assembly in Haiti." In *Haiti—Today and Tomorrow: An In-
           terdisciplinary Study,* edited by C. Foster and A. Valdman,
           pp. 231–52. Lanham, Md.: University Press of America.
Guérin, J., R. Malebranche, R. Elie, et al.
  1984.   "Acquired Immune Deficiency Syndrome: Specific Aspects of the
           Disease in Haiti." *Annals of the New York Academy of Sciences*
           437:254–61.

Guinan, M., P. Thomas, P. Pinsky, et al.
1984.   "Heterosexual and Homosexual Patients with the Acquired Immunodeficiency Syndrome." *Annals of Internal Medicine* 100 (2): 213–18.

Gwatkin, D. R., and P. Heuveline.
1997.   "Improving the Health of the World's Poor." *British Medical Journal* 315:497.

Gwinn, M., M. Pappaioanou, J. R. George, et al.
1991.   "Prevalence of HIV Infection in Childbearing Women in the United States: Surveillance Using Newborn Blood Samples." *Journal of the American Medical Association* 265 (13): 1704–8.

Haan, M., G. A. Kaplan, and T. Camacho.
1987.   "Poverty and Health: Prospective Evidence from the Alameda County Study." *American Journal of Epidemiology* 125 (6): 989–98.

Hagen, P.
1982.   *Blood: Gift or Merchandise?* New York: Alan R. Liss.

Haggett, P.
1994.   "Geographical Aspects of the Emergence of Infectious Diseases." *Geographic Annals* 76:91–104.

Hahn, R. A., E. Eaker, N. D. Barker, S. M. Teutsch, W. Sosniak, and N. Krieger.
1995.   "Poverty and Death in the United States—1973 to 1991." *Epidemiology* 6 (5): 490–97.

"Haitian Child Dies Every 5 Minutes."
1987.   *Miami Herald,* 25 April, p. 20A.

Halsey, N., et al.
1990.   "Transmission of HIV-1 Infections from Mothers to Infants in Haiti." *Journal of the American Medical Association* 264 (16): 2088–92.

Halsey, N., R. Boulos, J. Brutus, et al.
1987.   "HIV Antibody Prevalence in Pregnant Haitian Women." *Abstracts of the Third International Conference on AIDS,* June, Washington, D.C., p. 174.

Handwerker, W. P.
1997.   "Universal Human Rights and the Problem of Unbounded Cultural Meanings." *American Anthropologist* 99 (4): 799–809.

Harvard AIDS Institute.
1990.   "HAI Forum Panelists Debate the True Numbers of the AIDS Epidemic." *Harvard AIDS Institute Monthly Report,* May, pp. 2–6.

Hasan, M. M.
1996.   "Let's End the Non-Profit Charade." *New England Journal of Medicine* 334 (16): 1055–57.

Haynes, R. B.
1979. "A Critical Review of the 'Determinants' of Patient Compliance with Therapeutic Regimens." In *Compliance in Health Care*, edited by B. Haynes, D. W. Tayler, and D. Sackett, pp. 26–39. Baltimore: Johns Hopkins University Press.

Herzfeld, M.
1992. *The Social Production of Indifference: Exploring the Symbolic Roots of Western Bureaucracy.* Chicago: University of Chicago Press.

Hiatt, H.
1987. *Medical Lifeboat.* New York: Harper & Row.

Hirsh, M., and D. Klaidman.
1997. "Bad Practices." *Newsweek*, 11 August, pp. 42–43.

"HIV Claims Close to 16,000 New Victims Each Day."
1997. *Infectious Disease News* 10 (12): 14, 29.

Ho, D.
1995. "Time to Hit HIV, Early and Hard." *New England Journal of Medicine* 333 (7): 450–51.

Hogg, R. S., S. A. Strathdee, K. J. P. Craib, et al.
1994. "Lower Socioeconomic Status and Shorter Survival Following HIV Infection." *Lancet* 344 (8930): 1120–24.

Hollibaugh, A.
1995. "Lesbian Denial and Lesbian Leadership in the AIDS Epidemic: Bravery and Fear in the Construction of a Lesbian Geography of Risk." In *Women Resisting AIDS: Feminist Strategies of Empowerment*, edited by B. E. Schneider and N. E. Stoller, pp. 219–30. Philadelphia: Temple University Press.

Holmes, K., and S. Aral.
1991. "Behavioral Interventions in Developing Countries." In *Research Issues in Human Behavior and Sexually Transmitted Diseases in the AIDS Era*, edited by J. Wasserheit, S. Aral, and K. Holmes, pp. 318–44. Washington, D.C.: American Society for Microbiology.

Hong Kong Chest Service/British Medical Research Council.
1982. "Controlled Trial of 4 Three-Times Weekly Regimens and a Daily Regimen All Given for 6 Months for Pulmonary Tuberculosis. Second Report: The Results Up to 24 Months." *Tubercle* 63:89–98.

Hopewell, P. C., B. Ganter, R. B. Baron, and M. Sanchez-Hernandez.
1985. "Operational Evaluation of Treatment for Tuberculosis: Results of 8- and 12-Month Regimens in Peru." *American Review of Respiratory Disease* 132 (4): 737–41.

Hopewell, P. C., M. Sanchez-Hernandez, R. B. Baron, and B. Ganter.
1984. "Operational Evaluation of Treatment for Tuberculosis: Results of a 'Standard' 12-Month Regimen in Peru." *American Review of Respiratory Disease* 129 (3): 439–43.

Horton, R.
  1995.   "Towards the Elimination of Tuberculosis." *Lancet* 346:790.
Hospedales, J.
  1989.   "Heterosexual Spread of HIV Infection." *Reviews of Infectious Diseases* 11 (4): 663–64.
Hunt, N. R.
  1997.   "Condoms, Confessors, Conferences: Among AIDS Derivatives in Africa." *Journal of the International Institute* (University of Michigan) 4 (3): 1, 16–18.
Hunter, N. D.
  1995.   "Complications of Gender: Women, AIDS, and the Law." In *Women Resisting AIDS: Feminist Strategies of Empowerment,* edited by B. E. Schneider and N. E. Stoller, pp. 32–56. Philadelphia: Temple University Press.
Hurbon, L.
  1987.   *Le Barbare Imaginaire.* Port-au-Prince: Éditions Henri Deschamps. "If More Widely Used, DOTS Could Strike Powerful Blow Against TB."
———.
  1997.   *Infectious Disease News* 10 (10): 52–53.
"Infectious Diseases Continue to Be Dangerous Global Health Crisis."
  1996.   *Infectious Disease News* 9 (6): 1.
Inhorn, M.
  1995.   "Medical Anthropology and Epidemiology: Divergences or Convergences?" *Social Science and Medicine* 40 (3): 285–90.
Inhorn, M., and P. Brown.
  1990.   "The Anthropology of Infectious Disease." *Annual Reviews in Anthropology* 19:89–117.
———, eds.
  1997.   *The Anthropology of Infectious Diseases.* New York: Gordon and Breach.
International Monetary Fund.
  1984.   "Directions of Trade Statistics." In 1984 Yearbook. Washington, D.C.: International Monetary Fund.
Iseman, M.
  1985.   "Tailoring a Time-Bomb." *American Review of Respiratory Disease* 132:735–36.
———.
  1993.   "Treatment of Multidrug-Resistant Tuberculosis." *New England Journal of Medicine* 329 (11): 784–91.
Jaffe, H. W., W. W. Darrow, and D. F. Echenberg.
  1985.   "The Acquired Immunodeficiency Syndrome in a Cohort of Homosexual Men: A Six-Year Follow-Up Study." *Annals of Internal Medicine* 103 (2): 210–14.

Janes, C.
1986. "Migration and Hypertension: An Ethnography of Disease Risk in an Urban Samoan Community." In *Anthropology and Epidemiology*, edited by C. Janes, R. Stall, and S. Gifford, pp. 175–212. Dordrecht: D. Reidel.

Janes, C., R. Stall, and S. Gifford, eds.
1986. *Anthropology and Epidemiology*. Dordrecht: D. Reidel.

Jean, S., et al.
1997. "Clinical Manifestations of Human Immunodeficiency Virus Infection in Haitian Children." *Pediatric Infectious Disease Journal* 16 (6): 600–606.

Jean-Louis, R.
1989. "Diagnostic de l'état de Santé en Haïti." *Forum Libre (Santé, Médicine et Democratie en Haïti)* 1:11–20.

Jencks, C.
1992. *Rethinking Social Policy: Race, Poverty, and the Underclass*. Cambridge, Mass.: Harvard University Press.

Johnson, K. M., P. A. Webb, J. V. Lange, and F. A. Murphy.
1977. "Isolation and Partial Characterization of a New Virus Causing Acute Hemorrhagic Fever in Zaïre." *Lancet* 1 (8011): 569–71.

Johnson, W., and J. W. Pape.
1989. "AIDS in Haiti." In *AIDS: Pathogenesis and Treatment*, edited by J. Levy, pp. 65–78. New York: Marcel Dekker.

Kadlec, D.
1997. "How CEO Pay Got Away." *Newsweek*, 28 April, pp. 59–60.

Kajiyama, W., S. Kashwagi, H. Ikematsu, et al.
1986. "Intrafamilial Transmission of Adult T-Cell Leukemia Virus." *Journal of Infectious Diseases* 154 (5): 851–57.

Kaus, M.
1992. *The End of Equality*. New York: Basic Books.

Kawachi, I., B. P. Kennedy, K. Lochner, and D. Prothrow-Stith.
1997. "Social Capital, Income Inequality, and Mortality." *American Journal of Public Health* 87 (9): 1491–98.

Kendig, N.
1998. "Tuberculosis Control in Prisons." *International Journal of Tuberculosis and Lung Disease* 2 (9): 557–63.

Kennedy, B. P., I. Kawachi, and D. Prothrow-Stith.
1996. "Income Distribution and Mortality: Test of the Robin Hood Index in the United States." *British Medical Journal* 312:1004–8.

Kim, J. Y., J. Millen, and J. Gershman, eds.
1999. *Dying for Growth: Global Restructuring and the Health of the Poor*. Monroe, Maine: Common Courage Press.

Kim, J. Y., A. Shakow, J. Bayona, et al.

1999.   "Sickness Amidst Recovery: Public Debt and Private Suffering in a Peruvian Shantytown." In *Dying for Growth: Global Restructuring and the Health of the Poor,* edited by J. Y. Kim, J. Millen, J. Gershman, and A. Irwin. Monroe, Maine: Common Courage Press.

King, A. D., ed.

1997.   *Culture, Globalization, and the World-System: Contemporary Conditions for the Representation of Identity.* Minneapolis: University of Minnesota Press.

King, N.

1996.   "Routinization and Emergence." Manuscript in the author's possession.

Kinsella, J.

1989.   *Covering the Plague: AIDS and the American Media.* New Brunswick, N.J.: Rutgers University Press.

Kiple, K.

1984.   *The Caribbean Slave: A Biological History.* Cambridge: Cambridge University Press.

Kitagawa, E. M., and P. M. Hauser.

1973.   *Differential Mortality in the United States: A Study in Socioeconomic Epidemiology.* Cambridge, Mass.: Harvard University Press.

Kleinman, A.

1995a.   "Medicine, Anthropology of." In *Encyclopedia of Bioethics,* edited by W. T. Reich, pp. 1667–72. New York: Simon & Schuster Macmillan.

———.

1995b.   *Writing at the Margin: Discourse Between Anthropology and Medicine.* Berkeley: University of California Press.

Kleinman, A., V. Das, and M. Lock, eds.

1997.   *Social Suffering.* Berkeley: University of California Press.

Kleinman, A., L. Eisenberg, and B. Good.

1978.   "Culture, Illness, and Care: Clinical Lessons from Anthropologic and Cross-Cultural Research." *Annals of Internal Medicine* 88 (2): 251–58.

Kleinman, A., and J. Kleinman.

1989.   "Suffering and Its Professional Transformation: Toward an Ethnography of Experience." Paper presented at the First Conference of the Society for Psychological Anthropology, 6–8 October, San Diego, Calif.

———.

1996.   "The Appeal of Experience; The Dismay of Images: Cultural Appropriations of Suffering in Our Times." *Dædalus* 125 (1): 1–23.

———.
1997.   "Moral Transformations of Health and Suffering in Chinese Soci-
         ety." In *Morality and Health*, edited by A. M. Brandt and P. Rozin,
         pp. 101–18. New York: Routledge.

Klepp, K., P. M. Biswalo, and A. Talle, eds.
1995.   *Young People at Risk: Fighting AIDS in Northern Tanzania*. Oslo: Scan-
         dinavian University Press.

Kluegel, J. R., and E. R. Smith.
1986.   *Beliefs About Inequality: Americans' View of What Is and What Ought to
         Be*. New York: Aldine de Gruyter.

Koenig, E. L., G. Brach, and J. A. Levy.
1987.   "Response to K. W. Payne." *Journal of the American Medical Associa-
         tion* 258 (1): 46–47.

Koenig, E., J. Pittaluga, M. Bogart, et al.
1987.   "Prevalence of Antibodies to Human Immunodeficiency Virus in
         Dominicans and Haitians in the Dominican Republic." *Journal of the
         American Medical Association* 257 (5): 631–34.

Kopanoff, D. E., D. E. Snider, and M. Johnson.
1988.   "Recurrent Tuberculosis: Why Do Patients Develop Disease
         Again?" *American Journal of Public Health* 78 (1): 30–33.

Kosa, J.
1969.   "The Nature of Poverty." In *Poverty and Health: A Sociological Analy-
         sis*, edited by J. Kosa, A. Antonovsky, and I. Zola, pp. 1–34. Cam-
         bridge, Mass.: Harvard University Press.

Kosa, J., A. Antonovsky, and I. Zola, eds.
1969.   *Poverty and Health: A Sociological Analysis*. Cambridge, Mass.: Har-
         vard University Press.

Kraut, A.
1994.   *Silent Travelers: Germs, Genes, and the "Immigrant Menace."* New
         York: Basic Books.

Krieger, N., and E. Fee.
1994.   "Social Class: The Missing Link in U.S. Health Data." *International
         Journal of Health Services* 24 (1): 25–44.

Krieger, N., D. Rowley, A. Herman, B. Avery, and M. Phillips.
1993.   "Racism, Sexism, and Social Class: Implications for Studies of
         Health, Disease, and Well-Being." *American Journal of Preventive
         Medicine* 9 (Suppl.): 82–122.

Krieger, N., and S. Zierler.
1995.   "Accounting for Health of Women." *Current Issues in Public Health*
         1:251–56.

———.
1996.   "What Explains the Public's Health? A Call for Epidemiologic The-
         ory." *Epidemiology* 7 (1): 107–9.

Kritski, A. L., M. J. Ozorio-Marques, M. F. Rabahi, et al.
    1996.   "Transmission of Tuberculosis to Close Contacts of Patients with
             Multidrug-Resistant Tuberculosis." *American Journal of Respiratory &
             Critical Care Medicine* 153:331–35.
Krueger, L. E., R. W. Wood, P. H. Diehr, and C. L. Maxwell.
    1990.   "Poverty and HIV Seropositivity: The Poor Are More Likely to Be
             Infected." *AIDS* 4 (8): 811–14.
Krugman, P.
    1990.   *The Age of Diminished Expectations: U.S. Economic Policy in the 1990s.*
             Cambridge, Mass.: MIT Press.
Laga, M., M. Alary, N. Nzila, et al.
    1994.   "Condom Promotion, Sexually Transmitted Diseases Treatment,
             and Declining Incidence of HIV-1 Infection in Female Zaïrian Sex
             Workers." *Lancet* 344 (8917): 246–48.
Laga, M., A. Manoka, M. Kivuvu, et al.
    1993.   "Non-Ulcerative Sexually Transmitted Diseases as Risk Factors for
             HIV-1 Transmission in Women: Results from a Cohort Study." *AIDS*
             7 (1): 95–102.
Laguerre, M.
    1982.   *Urban Life in the Caribbean.* Cambridge, Mass.: Schenkman.

    ———.
    1987.   *Afro-Caribbean Folk Medicine.* Granby, Mass.: Bergin and Garvey.
Lange, W. R., and J. Jaffe.
    1987.   "AIDS in Haiti." *New England Journal of Medicine* 316 (22):
             1409–10.
Langley, L.
    1989.   *The United States and the Caribbean in the Twentieth Century.* 4th ed.
             Athens, Ga.: University of Georgia Press.
Langone, J.
    1985.   "AIDS: The Latest Scientific Facts." *Discover,* December, pp. 40–56.
Larson, A.
    1989.   "Social Context of Human Immunodeficiency Virus Transmission
             in Africa." *Reviews of Infectious Diseases* 11 (5): 716–31.
Latour, B.
    1988.   *The Pasteurization of France.* Translated by A. Sheridan and J. Law.
             Cambridge, Mass.: Harvard University Press.
Lawless, R.
    1992.   *Haiti's Bad Press.* Rochester, Vt.: Schenkman Books.
Lederberg, J., R. E. Shope, and S. C. Oaks.
    1992.   *Emerging Infections: Microbial Threats to Health in the United
             States.* Institute of Medicine. Washington, D.C.: National
             Academy Press.

Lee, J.

1995a.   "Beyond Bean Counting." In *Listen Up: Voices from the Next Feminist Generation*, edited by Barbara Findlen, pp. 205–11. Seattle: Seal Press.

———.

1995b.   "Sisterhood May Be Global, But Who Is in That Sisterhood?" In *Women Resisting AIDS: Feminist Strategies of Empowerment*, edited by B. E. Schneider and N. E. Stoller, pp. 205–11. Philadelphia: Temple University Press.

Leibowitch, J.

1985.   *A Strange Virus of Unknown Origin*. Translated by Richard Howard. New York: Ballantine Books.

Leland, J.

1996.   "The End of AIDS?" *Newsweek*, 2 December, pp. 64–73.

Lemp, G. F., A. Hirozawa, J. Cohen, et al.

1992.   "Survival for Women and Men with AIDS." *Journal of Infectious Diseases* 166 (1): 74–79.

Lemp, G. F., A. M. Hirozawa, D. Givertz, et al.

1994.   "Seroprevalence of HIV and Risk Behaviors Among Young Homosexual and Bisexual Men: The San Francisco/Berkeley Young Men's Survey." *Journal of the American Medical Association* 272 (6): 449–54.

Lerner, B. H.

1996.   "Does Stress Cause Disease? Revisiting the Tuberculosis Research of Thomas Holmes, 1949–1961." *Annals of Internal Medicine* 124 (7): 673–80.

———.

1997.   "From Careless Consumptives to Recalcitrant Patients: The Historical Construction of Noncompliance." *Social Science and Medicine* 45 (9): 1423–31.

Lerner, M.

1969.   "Social Differences in Physical Health." In *Poverty and Health: A Sociological Analysis*, edited by J. Kosa, A. Antonovsky, and I. Zola, pp. 69–112. Cambridge, Mass.: Harvard University Press.

Levine, N.

1964.   Editor's Preface to *Selections from Drake's "Malaria in the Interior Valley of North America."* Urbana: University of Illinois Press.

Levins, R.

1995.   "Preparing for Uncertainty." *Ecosystem Health* 1:47–57.

Lewis, D. K.

1995.   "African-American Women at Risk: Notes on the Sociocultural Context of HIV Infection." In *Women Resisting AIDS: Feminist Strategies of Empowerment*, edited by B. E. Schneider and N. E. Stoller, pp. 57–73. Philadelphia: Temple University Press.

Lewis, O.
   1969.   "The Culture of Poverty." In *On Understanding Poverty: Perspectives from the Social Sciences*, edited by D. P. Moynihan, pp. 187–200. New York: Basic Books.

Leyburn, J.
   1966.   *The Haitian People*. New Haven, Conn.: Yale University Press.

Liautaud, B., et al.
   1992.   "Preliminary Data on STDs in Haiti." Poster presented at the Eighth *International Conference on AIDS/Third STD World Congress*, 19–24 July, Amsterdam. Abstract C4302.

Liautaud, B., C. Laroche, J. Duvivier, and C. Péan-Guichard.
   1983.   "Le Sarcome de Kaposi en Haïti: Foyer Méconnu ou Récemment Apparu?" *Annals of Dermatological Venereology* 110:213–19.

Liautaud, B., J. W. Pape, and M. Pamphile.
   1988.   "Le Sida dans les Caraïbes." *Médecine et Maladies Infectieuses* 18 (Suppl.): 687–97.

Lieban, R.
   1976.   "Traditional Medical Beliefs and the Choice of Practitioners in a Philippine City." *Social Science and Medicine* 10 (6): 289–96.

Lief, L.
   1990.   "Where Democracy Isn't About to Break Out." *U.S. News and World Report*, 12 February, pp. 34–36.

Lindenbaum, S.
   1979.   *Kuru Sorcery: Disease and Danger in the New Guinea Highlands*. Palo Alto, Calif.: Mayfield.

Locher, U.
   1984.   "Migration in Haiti." In *Haiti—Today and Tomorrow: An Interdisciplinary Study*, edited by C. Foster and A. Valdman, pp. 325–36. Lanham, Md.: University Press of America.

Lockett, G.
   1995.   "CAL-PEP: The Struggle to Survive." In *Women Resisting AIDS: Feminist Strategies of Empowerment*, edited by B. E. Schneider and N. E. Stoller, pp. 32–56. Philadelphia: Temple University Press.

Long, R., B. Maycher, M. Scalcini, and J. Manfreda.
   1991.   "The Chest Roentgenogram in Pulmonary Tuberculosis Patients Seropositive for Human Immunodeficiency Virus Type 1." *Chest* 99 (1): 123–27.

Long, R., M. Scalcini, J. Manfreda, et al.
   1991.   "Impact of Human Immunodeficiency Virus Type 1 on Tuberculosis in Rural Haiti." *American Review of Respiratory Disease* 143:69–73.

Lowenthal, I.
   1984.   "Labor, Sexuality, and the Conjugal Contract in Rural Haiti." In *Haiti—Today and Tomorrow: An Interdisciplinary Study*, edited by C.

Foster and A. Valdman, pp. 15–33. Lanham, Md.: University Press of America.

Lurie, P., P. Hintzen, and R. A. Lowe.

1995.   "Socioeconomic Obstacles to HIV Prevention and Treatment in Developing Countries: The Roles of the International Monetary Fund and the World Bank." *AIDS* 9 (6): 539–46.

Lurie, P., and S. M. Wolfe.

1997.   "Unethical Trials of Interventions to Reduce Perinatal Transmission of the Human Immunodeficiency Virus in Developing Countries." *New England Journal of Medicine* 337 (12): 853–56.

Lykes, M. B.

1996.   "Meaning Making in a Context of Genocide and Silencing." In *Myths About the Powerless: Contesting Social Inequalities,* edited by M. B. Lykes, A. Banuazizi, R. Liem, and M. Morris, pp. 159–78. Philadelphia: Temple University Press.

Lykes, M. B., A. Banuazizi, R. Liem, and M. Morris, eds.

1996.   *Myths About the Powerless: Contesting Social Inequalities.* Philadelphia: Temple University Press.

Lynch, J. W., G. A. Kaplan, and J. T. Salonen.

1997.   "Why Do Poor People Behave Poorly? Variation in Adult Health Behaviours and Psychosocial Characteristics by Stages of the Socio-economic Lifecourse." *Social Science and Medicine* 44 (6): 809–19.

MacKenzie, W., N. Hoxie, M. Proctor, et al.

1994.   "A Massive Outbreak in Milwaukee of *Cryptosporidium* Infection Transmitted Through the Water Supply." *New England Journal of Medicine* 331 (3): 161–67.

Mahmoudi, A., and M. D. Iseman.

1993.   "Pitfalls in the Care of Patients with Tuberculosis: Common Errors and Their Association with the Acquisition of Drug Resistance." *Journal of the American Medical Association* 270 (1): 65–68.

Maloney, S. A., M. L. Pearson, M. T. Gordon, R. Del Castillo, J. F. Boyle, and W. R. Jarvis.

1995.   "Efficacy of Control Measures in Preventing Nosocomial Transmission of Multidrug-Resistant Tuberculosis to Patients and Health Care Workers." *Annals of Internal Medicine* 122 (2): 90–95.

Mann, J.

1991.   "Global AIDS: Critical Issues for Prevention in the 1990s." *International Journal of Health Services* 21 (3): 553–59.

Mann, J., D. Tarantola, and T. Netter, eds.

1992.   *AIDS in the World.* Cambridge, Mass.: Harvard University Press.

———.

1996.   *AIDS in the World.* 2d ed. Cambridge, Mass.: Harvard University Press.

Marcus, G., and M. Fischer.

1986.   *Anthropology as Cultural Critique: An Experimental Moment in the Human Sciences.* Chicago: University of Chicago Press.

Margono, F., A. Garely, J. Mroueh, and H. Minkoff.

1993.   "Tuberculosis Among Pregnant Women—New York City, 1985–1992." *Morbidity and Mortality Weekly Report* 42 (31): 605–12.

Marmot, M. G.

1994.   "Social Differentials in Health Within and Between Populations." *Dædalus* 123 (4): 197–216.

Marmot, M. G., and G. D. Smith.

1989.   "Why Are the Japanese Living Longer?" *British Medical Journal* 299:1547–51.

Martinez, H.

1980.   *Migraciones Internas en Peru.* Lima: IEP.

Mata, J. I.

1985.   "Integrating the Client's Perspective in Planning a Tuberculosis Education and Treatment Program in Honduras." *Medical Anthropology* 9 (1): 57–64.

Mathai, R., P. V. Prasad, M. Jacob, et al.

1990.   "HIV Seropositivity Among Patients with Sexually Transmitted Diseases in Vellore." *Indian Journal of Medical Research* 91:239–41.

McBarnett, L.

1988.   "Women and Poverty: The Effects on Reproductive Status." In *Too Little, Too Late: Death with the Health Needs of Women in Poverty,* edited by C. Perales and L. Young, pp. 55–81. Binghamton, N.Y.: Harrington Park Press.

McBride, D.

1991.   *From TB to AIDS: Epidemics Among Urban Blacks Since 1900.* Albany: SUNY Press.

McCarthy, S., R. McPhearson, and A. Guarino.

1992.   "Toxigenic *Vibrio Cholera* O1 and Cargo Ships Entering the Gulf of Mexico." *Lancet* 339:624.

McClintock, C.

1984.   "Why Peasants Rebel: The Case of Peru's Sendero Luminoso." *World Politics* 27 (1): 48–84.

McCord, C., and H. Freeman.

1990.   "Excess Mortality in Harlem." *New England Journal of Medicine* 322 (3): 173–77.

McKenna, M. T., E. McCray, and I. Onorato.

1995.   "The Epidemiology of Tuberculosis Among Foreign-Born Persons in the United States, 1986 to 1993." *New England Journal of Medicine* 332 (16): 1071–76.

McKeown, T.

1979. *The Role of Medicine: Dream, Mirage, or Nemesis?* 2d ed. Princeton, N.J.: Princeton University Press.

McMichael, A.

1995. "The Health of Persons, Populations, and Planets: Epidemiology Comes Full Circle." *Epidemiology* 6 (6): 633–36.

Mellon, R. L., B. Liautaud, J. W. Pape, W. D. Johnson, Jr.

1995. "Association of HIV and STDs in Haiti: Implications for Blood Banks and HIV Vaccine Trials." *Journal of Acquired Immune Deficiency Syndrome and Human Retrovirology* 8 (2): 214.

Mellors, J. W., and M. Barry.

1984. "Malnutrition or AIDS in Haiti?" *New England Journal of Medicine* 310 (17): 1119–20.

Menzies, R., I. Rocher, and B. Vissandjee.

1993. "Factors Associated with Compliance in Treatment of Tuberculosis." *Tubercle and Lung Disease* 74:32–37.

Merino, N., R. Sanchez, A. Muñoz, G. Prada, C. García, and B. F. Polk.

1990. "HIV 1, Sexual Practices, and Contact with Foreigners in Homosexual Men in Colombia, South America." *Journal of Acquired Immune Deficiency Syndromes* 3 (4): 330–34.

Métellus, J.

1987. *Haïti: Une Nation Pathétique.* Paris: Denoël.

Métraux, A.

[1959] 1972. *Haitian Voodoo.* Translated by Hugo Charteris. New York: Schocken.

Michael, J. M., and M. A. Michael.

1994. "Health Status of the Australian Aboriginal People and the Native Americans—A Summary Comparison." *Asia-Pacific Journal of Public Health* 7 (2): 132–36.

Miller, J.

1993. "'Your Life Is on the Line Every Night You're on the Streets': Victimization and Resistance Among Street Prostitutes." *Humanity and Society* 17:422–46.

Miller, S. J.

1996. "Equality, Morality, and the Health of Democracy." In *Myths About the Powerless: Contesting Social Inequalities,* edited by M. B. Lykes, A. Banuazizi, R. Liem, and M. Morris, pp. 17–33. Philadelphia: Temple University Press.

Mintz, S. W.

1964. "The Employment of Capital by Market Women in Haiti." In *Capital, Saving, and Credit in Peasant Societies,* edited by R. Firth and B. Yamey, pp. 56–78. Chicago: Aldine.

————.

1977.   "The So-Called World System: Local Initiative and Local Response." *Dialectical Anthropology* 2:253–70.

Mitchell, J. L., J. Tucker, P. D. Loftmann, and S. B. Williams.

1992.   "HIV and Women: Current Controversies and Clinical Relevance." *Journal of Women's Health* 1 (1): 35–39.

"Money Isn't the Issue; It's (Still) Political Will."

1998.   *TB Monitor* 5 (5): 53.

Moore, A., and R. LeBaron.

1986.   "The Case for a Haitian Origin of the AIDS Epidemic." In *The Social Dimensions of AIDS: Method and Theory*, edited by D. Feldman and T. Johnson, pp. 77–93. New York: Praeger.

Moore, M., I. M. Onorato, E. McCray, and K. G. Castro.

1997.   "Trends in Drug-Resistant Tuberculosis in the United States, 1993–1996." *Journal of the American Medical Association* 278 (10): 833–37.

Moore, S. F.

1987.   "Explaining the Present: Theoretical Dilemmas in Processual Ethnography." *American Ethnologist* 14 (4): 123–32.

Moral, P.

1961.   *Le Paysan Haïtien.* Port-au-Prince: Les Éditions Fardins.

Moreau de Saint-Méry, M. L. E.

1984.   *Description Topographique, Physique, Civile, Politique et Historique de la Partie Française de l'Isle Saint-Domingue* (1797–1798). 3 vols. Edited by B. Maurel and E. Taillemite. Paris: Société de l'Histoire des Colonies Françaises and Librarie Larose.

Morris, M.

1996.   "Culture, Structure, and the Underclass." In *Myths About the Powerless: Contesting Social Inequalities*, edited by M. B. Lykes, A. Banuazizi, R. Liem, and M. Morris, pp. 34–49. Philadelphia: Temple University Press.

Morris, M., and J. B. Williamson.

1982.   "Stereotyping and Social Class: A Focus on Poverty." In *In the Eye of the Beholder: Contemporary Issues in Stereotyping*, edited by A. G. Miller, pp. 411–65. New York: Praeger.

Morse, S.

1995.   "Factors in the Emergence of Infectious Diseases." *Emerging Infectious Diseases* 1 (1): 7–15.

Moses, P., and J. Moses.

1983.   "Haiti and the Acquired Immune Deficiency Syndrome." *Annals of Internal Medicine* 99 (4): 565.

Muecke, M. A.

1992.   "Mother Sold Food, Daughter Sells Her Body: The Cultural Continuity of Prostitution." *Social Science and Medicine* 35 (7): 891–901.

Muir, D., and M. Belsey.
    1980.   "Pelvic Inflammatory Disease and Its Consequences in the Developing
             World." *American Journal of Obstetrics and Gynecology* 138:913–28.
Murphy, E., P. Figeroa, W. Gibbs, et al.
    1989.   "Sexual Transmission of Human T-Lymphotropic Virus Type I
             (HTLV-I)." *Annals of Internal Medicine* 111 (7): 555–60.
Murray, C.
    1991.   "Social, Economic, and Operational Research on Tuberculosis: Re-
             cent Studies and Some Priority Questions." *Bulletin of the Interna-
             tional Union Against Tuberculosis and Lung Disease* 66 (4): 149–56.
Murray, C. J., and A. D. Lopez, eds.
    1996.   *The Global Burden of Disease.* Cambridge, Mass.: Harvard University
             Press.
Murray, C. J., K. Styblo, and A. Rouillon.
    1990.   "Tuberculosis in Developing Countries: Burden, Intervention, and
             Cost." *Bulletin of the International Union Against Tuberculosis and
             Lung Disease* 65 (1): 6–24.
Murray, G.
    1976.   "Women in Perdition: Ritual Fertility Control in Haiti." In *Culture,
             Natality, and Family Planning,* edited by J. Marshall and S. Polgar,
             pp. 59–78. Chapel Hill: Carolina Population Center, University of
             North Carolina.
Murray, S.
    1986.   "A Note on Haitian Tolerance of Homosexuality." In *Male Homosex-
             uality in Central and South America,* edited by S. Murray, pp. 92–100.
             Gai Saber Monograph 5.
Murray, S., and K. Payne.
    1988.   "Medical Policy Without Scientific Evidence: The Promiscuity Para-
             digm and AIDS." *California Sociologist* 11:13–54.
Mushlin, A. I., and F. A. Appel.
    1977.   "Diagnosing Potential Noncompliance." *Archives of Internal Medi-
             cine* 137:318–21.
Nachman, S.
    1993.   "Wasted Lives: Tuberculosis and Other Health Risks of Being Hai-
             tian in a U.S. Detention Camp." *Medical Anthropology Quarterly* 7
             (3): 227–59.
Nachman, S., and G. Dreyfuss.
    1986.   "Haitians and AIDS in South Florida." *Medical Anthropology Quar-
             terly* 17 (2): 32–33.
Nader, L.
    1997.   "The Phantom Factor: Impact of the Cold War on Anthropology." In
             *The Cold War and the University: Toward an Intellectual History of the Post-
             war Years,* edited by Andre Schiffrin, pp. 107–46. New York: New Press.

Naik, T. N., S. Sarkar, H. L. Singh, et al.
  1991.   "Intravenous Drug Users—A New High-Risk Group for HIV Infection in India." *AIDS* 5 (1): 117–18.
Nardell, E. A., and P. W. Brickner.
  1996.   "Tuberculosis in New York City—Focal Transmission of an Often Fatal Disease." *Journal of the American Medical Association* 276 (15): 1259–60.
Nardell, E. A., J. Salter, D. Boutotte, et al.
  1991.   "HIV Seroprevalence in an Asymptomatic, PPD-Positive Predominantly Non-White, Foreign-Born, Inner-City TB Clinic Population." *American Review of Respiratory Diseases* 143:A278.
Nataraj, S.
  1990.   "Indian Prostitutes Highlight AIDS Dilemmas." *Development Forum* (November–December): 1, 16.
Nations, M.
  1986.   "Epidemiological Research on Infectious Disease: Quantitative Rigor or Rigormortis? Insights from Ethnomedicine." In *Anthropology and Epidemiology*, edited by C. Janes, R. Stall, and S. Gifford, pp. 97–124. Dordrecht: D. Reidel.
Navarro, V.
  1990.   "Race or Class Versus Race and Class: Mortality Differentials in the United States." *Lancet* 336:1238–40.
Neptune-Anglade, M.
  1986.   *"L'Autre Moitié du Développement: A Propos du Travail des Femmes en Haïti."* Pétion-Ville, Haïti: Éditions des Alizés.
Nicholls, D.
  1985.   *Haiti in Caribbean Context: Ethnicity, Economy, and Revolt.* New York: St. Martin's Press.
Nightingale, E. O., K. Hannibal, H. J. Geiger, L. Hartmann, R. Lawrence, and J. Spurlock.
  1990.   "Apartheid Medicine: Health and Human Rights in South Africa." *Journal of the American Medical Association* 164 (16): 2097.
Nyamathi, A., C. Bennett, B. Leake, et al.
  1993.   "AIDS-Related Knowledge, Perceptions, and Behaviors Among Impoverished Minority Women." *American Journal of Public Health* 83 (1): 65–71.
O'Brien, W., P. Hartigan, D. Martin, et al.
  1996.   "Changes in Plasma HIV-1 RNA and CD4+ Lymphocyte Counts and the Risk of Progression to AIDS." *New England Journal of Medicine* 334 (7): 426–31.
Oldstone, M.
  1998.   *Viruses, Plagues, and History.* New York: Oxford University Press.

Oliver, M., and T. Shapiro.
  1995.   *Black Wealth/White Wealth: A New Perspective on Racial Inequality.*
           London: Routledge.
Olliaro, P., J. Cattani, and D. Wirth.
  1996.   "Malaria, the Submerged Disease." *Journal of the American Medical
           Association* 275 (3): 230–33.
Onoge, O.
  1975.   "Capitalism and Public Health: A Neglected Theme in the Medical
           Anthropology of Africa." In *Topias and Utopias in Health,* edited by S.
           Ingman and A. Thomas, pp. 219–32. The Hague: Mouton.
Oppenheimer, G.
  1988.   "In the Eye of the Storm: The Epidemiological Construction of
           AIDS." In *AIDS: The Burdens of History,* edited by E. Fee and D. Fox,
           pp. 267–300. Berkeley: University of California Press.
Ortner, S.
  1984.   "Theory in Anthropology Since the Sixties." *Comparative Studies of
           Society and History* 26:126–66.
Osborn, J.
  1989.   "Public Health and the Politics of AIDS Prevention." *Dædalus* 118
           (3): 123–44.
———.
  1990.   "Policy Implications of the AIDS Deficit." *Journal of Acquired Im-
           mune Deficiency Syndromes* 3 (4): 293–95.
Osmond, D. H., K. Page, J. Wiley, et al.
  1994.   "HIV Infection in Homosexual and Bisexual Men 18 to 29 Years of
           Age: The San Francisco Young Men's Health Study." *American Jour-
           nal of Public Health* 84 (12): 1933–37.
Ott, K.
  1996.   *Fevered Lives: Tuberculosis in American Culture Since 1870.* Cam-
           bridge, Mass.: Harvard University Press.
Paavonen, J., L. Koutsky, and N. Kiviat.
  1990.   "Cervical Neoplasia and Other STD-Related Genital and Anal Neo-
           plasias." In *Sexually Transmitted Diseases,* edited by K. K. Holmes
           et al., pp. 561–62. New York: McGraw-Hill.
Packard, R.
  1989.   *White Plague, Black Labor: Tuberculosis and the Political Economy of
           Health and Disease in South Africa.* Berkeley: University of California
           Press.
Packard, R., and P. Epstein.
  1991.   "Epidemiologists, Social Scientists, and the Structure of Medical
           Research on AIDS in Africa." *Social Science and Medicine*
           33 (7): 771–94.

Palmer, D. S.
    1986.   "Rebellion in Rural Peru: The Origins and Evolution of Sendero Lu-
             minoso." *Comparative Politics* 18 (2): 127–46.
Pan American Health Organization.
    1967.   *Reported Cases of Notifiable Diseases in the Americas.* Scientific Publica-
             tion No. 149. Washington, D.C.
Panem, S.
    1988.   *The AIDS Bureaucracy.* Cambridge, Mass.: Harvard Univer-
             sity Press.
Pape, J. W., and W. Johnson.
    1988.   "Epidemiology of AIDS in the Caribbean." *Baillière's Clinical Tropical
             Medicine and Communicable Diseases* 3 (1): 31–42.

———.

    1989.   "HIV-1 Infection and AIDS in Haiti." In *The Epidemiology of AIDS:
             Expression, Occurrence, and Control of Human Immunodeficiency Virus
             Type 1 Infection,* edited by R. A. Kaslow and D. P. Francis,
             pp. 221–30. New York: Oxford University Press.

———.

    1993.   "AIDS in Haiti: 1982–1992." *Clinical Infectious Diseases* 17 (Suppl. 2):
             S341–45.
Pape, J. W., B. Liautaud, F. Thomas, J. R. Mathurin, M. M. St Amand, M. Boncy,
V. Péan, M. Pamphile, A. C. Laroche, and W. D. Johnson, Jr.
    1983.   "Characteristics of the Acquired Immunodeficiency Syn-
             drome (AIDS) in Haiti." *New England Journal of Medicine* 309 (16):
             945–50.

———.

    1984.   "Acquired Immunodeficiency Syndrome in Haiti (Abstract)." *Clini-
             cal Research* 32 (2): 379A.

———.

    1986.   "Risk Factors Associated with AIDS in Haiti." *American Journal of
             Medical Sciences* 291 (1): 4–7.
Pape, J. W., B. Liautaud, F. Thomas, J. R. Mathurin, M. M. St Amand, M. Boncy,
V. Péan, M. Pamphile, A. C. Laroche, J. Dehovitz, et al.
    1985.   "The Acquired Immunodeficiency Syndrome in Haiti." *Annals of In-
             ternal Medicine* 103 (5): 674–78.
Pappas, G., S. Queen, W. Hadden, and G. Fisher.
    1993.   "The Increasing Disparity in Mortality Between Socioeconomic
             Groups in the United States, 1960 and 1986." *New England Journal of
             Medicine* 329 (2): 103–9.
Patel, M.
    1987.   "Problems in the Evaluation of Alternative Medicine." *Social Science
             and Medicine* 25 (6): 669–78.

Patterson, O.
  1987.   "The Emerging West Atlantic System: Migration, Culture, and
           Underdevelopment in the U.S. and Circum-Caribbean Region." In
           Population in an Interacting World, edited by W. Alonzo, pp. 227–60.
           Cambridge, Mass.: Harvard University Press.
Patz, J., P. Epstein, T. Burke, and J. Balbus.
  1996.   "Global Climate Change and Emerging Infectious Diseases." *Jour-
           nal of the American Medical Association* 275 (3): 217–33.
Payne, K. W.
  1987.   "Response to Koenig et al." *Journal of the American Medical Associa-
           tion* 258 (1): 46–47.
Pearson, M. L., J. A. Jereb, T. R. Frieden, et al.
  1992.   "Nosocomial Transmission of Multidrug-Resistant *Mycobacterium
           tuberculosis:* A Risk to Patients and Health Care Workers." *Annals of
           Internal Medicine* 117 (3): 191–96.
Perez, J.
  1992.   "Situation and Trend Analysis of AIDS Epidemic in the Domini-
           can Republic." Programa Control Enfermedades Transmission
           Sexual y SIDA (PROCETS), Dominican Republic. Poster pre-
           sented at the Eighth International Conference on AIDS/Third
           STD World Congress, 19–24 July, Amsterdam. Abstract
           C254.
"Peru: Politics and Violence, Sendero's Strategy from Close Up."
  1989.   *Latin America Weekly Report,* 12 October, pp. 4–5.
"Peru's Cut-Rate Fighter Jets Were Too Good to Be True."
  1997.   *New York Times,* 30 May, p. 1.
Peterman, T. A., R. L. Stoneburner, J. R. Allen, et al.
  1988.   "Risk of Human Immunodeficiency Virus Transmission from Het-
           erosexual Adults with Transfusion-Associated Infections." *Journal of
           the American Medical Association* 259 (1): 55–58.
Piven, F. F., and R. A. Cloward.
  1996.   "Welfare Reform and the New Class War." In *Myths About the
           Powerless: Contesting Social Inequalities,* edited by M. B. Lykes, A.
           Banuazizi, R. Liem, and M. Morris, pp. 72–86. Philadelphia: Temple
           University Press.
Pivnick, A.
  1993.   "HIV Infection and the Meaning of Condoms." *Culture, Medicine,
           and Psychiatry* 17 (4): 431–53.
Pivnick, A., A. Jacobson, K. Eric, et al.
  1991.   "Reproductive Decisions Among HIV-Infected, Drug-Using
           Women: The Importance of Mother-Child Coresidence." *Medical
           Anthropology Quarterly* 5 (2): 153–69.

Plotnick, R. D.
  1992.   "Changes in Property, Income Inequality, and the Standard of Living During the Reagan Era." *Journal of Sociology and Social Welfare* 19 (1): 29–44.
Plummer, F. A.
  1998.   "Heterosexual Transmission of Human Immunodeficiency Virus Type 1 (HIV): Interactions of Conventional Sexually Transmitted Diseases, Hormonal Contraception, and HIV-1." *AIDS Research and Human Retroviruses* 14 (Suppl. 1): S5–10.
Poinsignon, Y., Z. Marjanovic, and D. Farge.
  1996.   "Maladies Infectieuses Nouvelles et Résurgentes Liées à la Pauvreté." *La Revue du Practicien* 46:1827–38.
Polakow, V.
  1995a.   *Lives on the Edge.* Chicago: University of Chicago Press.

———.
  1995b.   "Lives of Welfare Mothers: On a Tightrope Without a Net." *The Nation,* 1 May, pp. 590–92.
Population Crisis Committee.
  1992.   *The International Human Suffering Index.* Washington, D.C.: Population Crisis Committee.
Porter, J., and K. McAdam.
  1994.   "The Re-Emergence of Tuberculosis." *Annual Review of Public Health* 15:303–23.
Portes, A., and J. Walton.
  1982.   *Labor, Class, and the International System.* New York: Academic Press.
Preston, R.
  1994.   *The Hot Zone: A Terrifying True Story.* New York: Random House.
Price, L.
  1987.   "Ecuadorian Illness Stories: Cultural Knowledge in Natural Discourse." In *Cultural Models in Language and Thought,* edited by D. Holland and N. Quinn, pp. 313–42. Cambridge: Cambridge University Press.
Quinn, N., and D. Holland.
  1987.   "Culture and Cognition." In *Cultural Models in Language and Thought,* edited by D. Holland and N. Quinn, pp. 3–40. Cambridge: Cambridge University Press.
Ramachandran, P., and R. Prabhakar.
  1992.   "Defaults, Defaulter Action, and Retrieval of Patients During Studies of Tuberculous Meningitis in Children." *Tubercle and Lung Disease* 73:170–73.
Reeves, W., W. Rawls, and L. Brinton.
  1989.   "Epidemiology of Genital Papillomaviruses and Cervical Cancer." *Reviews of Infectious Diseases* 11 (3): 426–39.

Reichman, L. B.
1997.   "Tuberculosis Elimination—What's to Stop Us?" *International Journal of Tuberculosis and Lung Disease* 1 (1): 3–11.
Richardson, L.
1997.   "Whites Have More Access to Effective New AIDS Drugs, Survey Shows." *New York Times*, 27 July, p. 25.
Rieder, H. L.
1989.   "Tuberculosis Among American Indians of the Contiguous United States." *Public Health Report* 104 (6): 653–57.
Roizman, B., ed.
1995.   *Infectious Diseases in an Age of Change: The Impact of Human Ecology and Behavior on Disease Transmission.* Washington, D.C.: National Academy Press.
Roseberry, W.
1988.   "Political Economy." *Annual Review of Anthropology* 17:161–85.
———.
1992.   "Multiculturalism and the Challenge of Anthropology." *Social Research* 59 (4): 841–58.
Rosen, G.
1947.   "What Is Social Medicine?" *Bulletin of the History of Medicine* 21:674–733.
Rothenberg, R., M. Woelfel, R. Stoneburner, J. Milberg, R. Parker, and B. Truman.
1987.   "Survival with the Acquired Immunodeficiency Syndrome: Experience with 5833 Cases in New York City." *New England Journal of Medicine* 317 (21): 1297–302.
Rousseau, J.
[1755] 1994. *Discourse on the Origin of Inequality.* Oxford: Oxford University Press.
Rubel, A., and L. Garro.
1992.   "Social and Cultural Factors in the Successful Control of Tuberculosis." *Public Health Reports* 107:626–36.
Rullán, J. V., D. Herrera, R. Cano, et al.
1996.   "Nosocomial Transmission of Multidrug-Resistant *Mycobacterium tuberculosis* in Spain." *Emerging Infectious Diseases* 2 (2): 125–29.
Ryan, F.
1993.   *The Forgotten Plague: How the Battle Against Tuberculosis Was Won—and Lost.* Boston: Little, Brown.
Ryan, W.
1971.   *Blaming the Victim.* New York: Vintage.
———.
1981.   *Equality.* New York: Pantheon.
Saba, J., and A. Ammann.
1997.   "A Cultural Divide on AIDS Research." *New York Times*, 20 September, p. A25.

Sabatier, R.
  1988.   *Blaming Others: Prejudice, Race, and Worldwide AIDS.* Philadelphia:
           New Society Publishers.
Saltus, R.
  1997.   "Journal Departures Reflect AIDS Dispute." *Boston Globe,* 16 Octo-
           ber, p. A11.
Sampson, J., and J. Neaton.
  1994.   "On Being Poor with HIV." *Lancet* 344:1100–101.
Sanford, D.
  1996.   "Back to a Future: One Man's AIDS Tale Shows How Quickly Epi-
           demic Has Turned." *Wall Street Journal,* 8 November, pp. 1, A12.
Satcher, D.
  1995.   "Emerging Infections: Getting Ahead of the Curve." *Emerging Infec-
           tious Diseases* 1 (1): 1–6.
Scalcini, M., G. Carré, M. Jean-Baptiste, et al.
  1990.   "Antituberculous Drug Resistance in Central Haiti." *American Re-
           view of Respiratory Disease* 142 (3, Suppl.): 508–11.
Scheper-Hughes, N.
  1992.   *Death Without Weeping: The Violence of Everyday Life in Brazil.* Berke-
           ley: University of California Press.
————.
  1993.   "AIDS, Public Health, and Human Rights in Cuba." *Lancet* 342
           (8877): 965–67.
Schneider, B. E., and N. E. Stoller, eds.
  1995.   *Women Resisting AIDS: Feminist Strategies of Empowerment.* Philadel-
           phia: Temple University Press.
Schoenbaum, E. E., and M. P. Webber.
  1993.   "The Underrecognition of HIV Infection in Women in an Inner-
           City Emergency Room." *American Journal of Public Health* 83 (3):
           363–68.
Schoepf, B. G.
  1988.   "Women, AIDS, and the Economic Crisis in Central Africa." *Cana-
           dian Journal of African Studies* 22 (3): 625–44.
————.
  1993.   "Gender, Development, and AIDS: A Political Economy and Cul-
           ture Framework." In *Women and International Development Annual,*
           edited by R. Galin, A. Ferguson, and J. Harper, pp. 53–85. Boulder,
           Colo.: Westview Press.
Schulzer, M., J. M. Fitzgerald, D. A. Enarson, S. Grzybowski.
  1992.   "An Estimate of the Future Size of the Tuberculosis Problem in Sub-
           Saharan Africa Resulting from HIV Infection." *Tuberculosis and Lung
           Disease* 73 (1): 52–58.

Selik, R. M., S. Y. Chu, and J. W. Buehler.
  1993.   "HIV Infection as Leading Cause of Death Among Young Adults in
           U.S. Cities and States." *Journal of the American Medical Association*
           296 (23): 2991–94.
Sen, A.
  1992.   *Inequality Reexamined.* Cambridge, Mass.: Harvard University Press.
Serres, M.
  1980.   *Le Passage du Nord-Ouest.* Paris: Éditions de Minuit.
Service d'Hygiène.
  1933.   *Notes Bio-bibliographiques: Médecins et Naturalistes de l'Ancienne
           Colonie Française de Saint-Domingue.* Port-au-Prince: Imprimerie
           de l'État.
Shears, P.
  1988.   *Tuberculosis Control Programmes in Developing Countries.* OXFAM
           Practical Health Guide No. 4. 2d ed. Oxford: OXFAM.
Shilts, R.
  1987.   *And the Band Played On: Politics, People, and the AIDS Epidemic.* New
           York: St. Martin's Press.
"Significant Drop Seen in AIDS Cases in 1996."
  1997.   *Infectious Disease News* 10 (10): 10, 17.
Simonsen, J., P. Plummer, E. Ngugi, et al.
  1990.   "HIV Infection Among Lower Socio-economic Strata Prostitutes in
           Nairobi." *AIDS* 4 (2): 139–44.
Simpson, G.
  1942.   "Sexual and Family Institutions in Northern Haiti." *American An-
           thropologist* 44:655–74.
Singapore Tuberculosis Service/British Medical Research Council.
  1988.   "Five-Year Follow-Up of a Clinical Trial of Three 6-Month Regi-
           mens of Chemotherapy Given Intermittently in the Continuation
           Phase in the Treatment of Pulmonary Tuberculosis." *American Re-
           view of Respiratory Disease* 137:1147–50.
Singer, M.
  1994.   "AIDS and the Health Crisis of the U.S. Urban Poor: The Perspec-
           tive of Critical Medical Anthropology." *Social Science and Medicine*
           39 (7): 931–48.
Slutsker, L., J.-B. Brunet, J. Karon, et al.
  1992.   "Trends in the United States and Europe." In *AIDS in the World,*
           edited by J. Mann, D. Tarantola, and T. Netter, pp. 173–94. Cam-
           bridge, Mass.: Harvard University Press.
Small, P., and A. Moss.
  1993.   "Molecular Epidemiology and the New Tuberculosis." *Infectious
           Agents and Disease* 2:132–38.

Small, P., R. Shafer, P. Hopewell, et al.
 1993.   "Exogenous Reinfection with Multidrug-Resistant *Mycobacterium tuberculosis* in Patients with Advanced HIV Infection." *New England Journal of Medicine* 328 (16): 1137–44.

Smith, D. K., D. L. Warren, D. Vlahov, P. Schuman, M. D. Stein, B. L. Greenberg, and S. D. Holmberg.
 1997.   "Design and Baseline Participant Characteristics of the Human Immunodeficiency Virus Epidemiology Research (HER) Study: A Prospective Cohort Study of Human Immunodeficiency Virus Infection in U.S. Women." *American Journal of Epidemiology* 146 (6): 459–69.

Snider, D.
 1989.   "Research Toward Global Control and Prevention of Tuberculosis with an Emphasis on Vaccine Development." *Review of Infectious Diseases* II (S): 335–38.

———.
 1992.   "The Impact of Tuberculosis on Women, Children, and Minorities in the United States." *World Congress of Tuberculosis.* Bethesda, Md. Abstract C1.

Snider, D. E., J. Graczyk, E. Bek, and J. Rogowski.
 1984.   "Supervised Six-Months Treatment of Newly Diagnosed Pulmonary Tuberculosis Using Isoniazid, Rifampin, and Pyrazinamide With and Without Streptomycin." *American Review of Respiratory Disease* 130:1091–94.

Snider, D. E., G. D. Kelly, G. M. Cauthen, N. J. Thompson, and J. O. Kilburn.
 1985.   "Infection and Disease Among Contacts of Tuberculosis Cases with Drug-Resistant and Drug-Susceptible Bacilli." *American Review of Respiratory Disease* 132:125–32.

Snider, D., and W. Roper.
 1992.   "The New Tuberculosis." *New England Journal of Medicine* 326 (10): 703–5.

Snider, D. E., Jr., L. Salinas, and G. D. Kelly.
 1989.   "Tuberculosis: An Increasing Problem Among Minorities in the United States." *Public Health Report* 104 (6): 646–53.

Solórzano, A.
 1992.   "Sowing the Seeds of Neo-Imperialism: The Rockefeller Foundation's Yellow Fever Campaign in Mexico." *International Journal of Health Services* 22 (3): 529–54.

Sontag, D., and L. Richardson.
 1997.   "Doctors Withhold H.I.V. Pill Regimen from Some." *New York Times,* 2 March, pp. 1, 31.

Soto-Ramírez, L., B. Renjifo, M. McLane, et al.
 1996.   "HIV-1 Langerhans' Cell Tropism Associated with Heterosexual Transmission of HIV." *Science* 271 (5253): 1291–93.

Spence, D., J. Hotchkiss, C. Williams, and P. Davies.

1993.   "Tuberculosis and Poverty." *British Medical Journal* 307:759–61.

Standaert, B., and A. Méheus.

1985.   "Le Cancer du Col Utérin en Afrique." *Médecine en l'Afrique Noire* 32:406–15.

Stanford, J. L., J. M. Grange, and A. Pozniak.

1991.   "Is Africa Lost?" *Lancet* 338:557–58.

Starn, O.

1991.   *"Con Los Llanques Todo Barro"—Reflexiones Sobre Rondas Campesinas, Protesta Rural y Nuevos Movimientos Sociales.* Lima: IEP.

———.

1992.   "Missing the Revolution: Anthropologists and the War in Peru." In *Rereading Cultural Anthropology*, edited by G. Marcus, pp. 99–112. Durham, N.C.: Duke University Press.

The Status and Trends of the Global HIV/AIDS Pandemic Report.

1996.   Eleventh International Conference on AIDS, Vancouver, 7–12 July.

Stein, Z.

1994.   "What Was New at Yokohama—Women's Voices at the 1994 International HIV/AIDS Conference." *American Journal of Public Health* 84 (12): 1887–88.

Stephenson, J.

1996.   "New Anti-HIV Drugs and Treatment Strategies Buoy AIDS Researchers." *Journal of the American Medical Association* 275 (8): 579–80.

St. Louis, M., G. Conway, C. Hayman, et al.

1991.   "Human Immunodeficiency Virus in Disadvantaged Adolescents." *Journal of the American Medical Association* 266 (17): 2387–91.

Stolberg, S. G.

1997.   "The Better Half Got the Worse End." *New York Times*, 20 July, sect. 4, pp. 1, 4.

Strobel, J., Y. François, et al.

1989.   "Le Syndrome d'Immunosuppression Acquise en Guadeloupe." *Médecine Tropicale* 49 (1): 17–20.

Styblo, K.

1989.   "Overview and Epidemiological Assessment of the Current Global Tuberculosis Situation: With an Emphasis on Tuberculosis Control in Developing Countries." *Zeitschrift für Erkrankungen der Atmungsorgane* 173 (1): 6–17.

"Successes Offer Hope on AIDS."

1996.   *Boston Globe*, 7 July, p. 17.

Sumartojo, E.

1993.   "When Tuberculosis Treatment Fails: A Social Behavioral Account of Patient Adherence." *American Review of Respiratory Disease* 147:1311–20.

Syme, S. L., and L. F. Berkman.
　　1976.　"Social Class, Susceptibility, and Sickness." *American Journal of Epidemiology* 104 (1): 1–8.

Tardo-Dino, F.
　　1985.　*Le Collier de Servitude: La Condition Sanitaire des Esclaves aux Antilles Françaises du XVIIe au XIXe Siècle.* Paris: Éditions Caribéennes.

Taussig, M.
　　1980.　"Reification and the Consciousness of the Patient." *Social Science and Medicine* 148 (1): 3–13.

"TB Returns with a Vengeance."
　　1996.　*Washington Post,* 3 August, p. A19.

Telzak, E. E., K. Sepkowitz, P. Alpert, et al.
　　1995.　"Multidrug-Resistant Tuberculosis in Patients Without HIV Infection." *New England Journal of Medicine* 333 (14): 907–11.

"Ten Years of Commitment, A Lifetime of Solidarity."
　　1997.　*PIH Bulletin* 4 (1): 1.

Thiede, M., and S. Traub.
　　1997.　"Mutual Influences of Health and Poverty: Evidence from German Panel Data." *Social Science and Medicine* 45 (6): 867–77.

Third East African/British Medical Research Council Study.
　　1980.　"Controlled Clinical Trial of Four Short-Course Regimens of Chemotherapy for Two Durations in the Treatment of Pulmonary Tuberculosis: Second Report." *Tubercle* 61:59–69.

Tomes, N.
　　1998.　*The Gospel of Germs: Men, Women, and the Microbe in American Life.* Cambridge, Mass.: Harvard University Press.

Treichler, P. A.
　　1988.　"AIDS, Gender, and Biomedical Discourse: Current Contests for Meaning." In *AIDS: The Burdens of History,* edited by E. Fee and D. Fox, pp. 190–266. Berkeley: University of California Press.

Trouillot, M. R.
　　1986.　*Les Racines Historiques de l'État Duvaliérien.* Port-au-Prince: Imprimerie Henri Deschamps.

———.
　　1990.　*Haiti, State Against Nation: The Origins and Legacy of Duvalierism.* New York: Monthly Review Press.

Turner, J.
　　1987.　"Analytical Theorizing." In *Social Theory Today,* edited by A. Giddens and J. Turner, pp. 156–94. Stanford, Calif.: Stanford University Press.

Turshen, M.
　　1984.　*The Political Ecology of Disease in Tanzania.* New Brunswick, N.J.: Rutgers University Press.

United Nations.
   1949.   *Mission to Haiti: Report of the United Nations Mission of Technical As-*
            sistance to the Republic of Haiti. Lake Success, N.Y.: United Nations.
United Nations Development Program.
   1992.   *Young Women: Silence, Susceptibility, and the HIV Epidemic.* New
            York: UNDP.
Valentine, C. A.
   1968.   *Culture and Poverty: Critique and Counter-Proposals.* Chicago: Univer-
            sity of Chicago Press.
Varmus, H., and D. Satcher.
   1997.   "Complexities of Conducting Research in Developing Countries."
            New England Journal of Medicine 337 (14): 1003–5.
Viera, J.
   1985.   "The Haitian Link." In *Understanding AIDS: A Comprehensive Guide,*
            edited by V. Gong, pp. 90–99. New Brunswick, N.J.: Rutgers Uni-
            versity Press.
Vieux, S.
   1989.   *Le Plaçage: Droit Coutumier et Famille en Haïti.* Paris: Éditions
            Publisud.
Virchow, R.
   1848.   *Die Medizinische Reform,* no. 1, p. 182. Berlin: Druck und Verlag von
            G. Reimer.
Wagner, R.
   1975.   *The Invention of Culture.* Englewood Cliffs, N.J.: Prentice-Hall.
Waldholz, M.
   1996.   "Precious Pills: New AIDS Treatment Raises Tough Question of
            Who Will Get It." *Wall Street Journal,* 3 July, p. 1.
Wallace, R.
   1988.   "A Synergism of Plagues: 'Planned Shrinkage,' Contagious Housing
            Destruction and AIDS in the Bronx." *Environmental Research* 47:1–33.
   ———.
   1990.   "Urban Desertification, Public Health, and Public Order: 'Planned
            Shrinkage,' Violent Death, Substance Abuse, and AIDS in the
            Bronx." *Social Science and Medicine* 31 (7): 801–13.
Wallace, R., M. Fullilove, R. Fullilove, et al.
   1994.   "Will AIDS Be Contained Within U.S. Minority Populations?" *Social
            Science and Medicine* 39 (8): 1051–62.
Wallace, R., Y. S. Huang, P. Gould, and D. Wallace.
   1997.   "The Hierarchical Diffusion of AIDS and Violent Crime Among U.S.
            Metropolitan Regions: Inner-City Decay, Stochastic Resonance, and
            Reversal of the Mortality Transition." *Social Science and Medicine* 44
            (7): 935–47.

Wallace, R., and D. Wallace.
  1995.   "U.S. Apartheid and the Spread of AIDS to the Suburbs: A Multi-
          City Analysis of the Political Economy of Spatial Epidemic Thresh-
          old." *Social Science and Medicine* 41 (3): 333–45.
Wallerstein, I.
  1987.   "World-Systems Analysis." In *Social Theory Today,* edited by A. Giddens
          and J. Turner, pp. 309–24. Stanford, Calif.: Stanford University Press.
———.
  1994.   "Response to Eric Wolf." *Current Anthropology* 35 (1): 9–12.
———.
  1995.   *After Liberalism.* New York: The New Press.
Ward, M. C.
  1993.   "Poor and Positive: Two Contrasting Views from Inside the
          HIV/AIDS Epidemic." *Practicing Anthropology* 15 (4): 59–61.
Wardman, A. G., A. J. Knox, M. F. Muers, and R. L. Page.
  1988.   "Profiles of Non-Compliance with Antituberculous Therapy."
          British Journal of Diseases of the Chest 82:285–89.
Warner, D. C.
  1991.   "Health Issues at the US-Mexican Border." *Journal of the American
          Medical Association* 265 (2): 242–47.
Warsh, D.
  1997.   "AIDS: What Went Right?" *Boston Globe,* 13 July, sect. F, pp. 1, 3.
Wasser, S. C., M. Gwinn, and P. Fleming.
  1993.   "Urban-Nonurban Distribution of HIV Infection in Childbearing
          Women in the United States." *Journal of Acquired Immune Deficiency
          Syndromes* 6 (9): 1035–42.
Wasserheit, J., S. Aral, and K. K. Holmes, eds.
  1991.   *Research Issues in Human Behavior and Sexually Transmitted Diseases in
          the AIDS Era.* Washington, D.C.: American Society for Microbiology.
Waterston, A.
  1993.   *Street Addicts in the Political Economy.* Philadelphia: Temple Univer-
          sity Press.
Watts, S.
  1998.   *Epidemics and History: Disease, Power, and Imperialism.* New Haven:
          Yale University Press.
Weidman, H.
  1978.   *Miami Health Ecology Project Report: A Statement on Ethnicity and
          Health.* Miami: University of Miami.
Weil, D.
  1994.   "Drug Supply—Meeting a Global Need." In *Tuberculosis: Back to the
          Future,* edited by J. Porter and K. McAdam, pp. 124–49. Chichester:
          John Wiley.

Weis, S. E., P. C. Slocum, F. X. Blais, et al.
    1994. "The Effect of Directly Observed.Therapy on Rates of Drug Resistance and Relapse in Tuberculosis." *New England Journal of Medicine* 330 (17): 1179–84.

Wiese, H. J. C.
    1971. "The Interaction of Western and Indigenous Medicine in Haiti in Regard to Tuberculosis." Ph.D. diss., Department of Anthropology, University of North Carolina at Chapel Hill.

———.
    1974. "Tuberculosis in Rural Haiti." *Social Science and Medicine* 8 (6): 359–62.

Wilentz, A.
    1989. *The Rainy Season: Haiti After Duvalier.* New York: Simon and Schuster.

Wilkinson, R. G.
    1992. "National Mortality Rates: The Impact of Inequality?" *American Journal of Public Health* 82 (8): 1082–84.

———.
    1994. "The Epidemiological Transition: From Material Scarcity to Social Disadvantage." *Dædalus* 123 (4): 61–77.

———.
    1996. *Unhealthy Societies: The Afflictions of Inequality.* London: Routledge.

Wilson, C.
    1995. *Hidden in the Blood: A Personal Investigation of AIDS in the Yucatán.* New York: Columbia University Press.

Wilson, M.
    1995. "Travel and the Emergence of Infectious Diseases." *Emerging Infectious Diseases* 1 (2): 39–46.

Wilson, R., and M. Pounds.
    1993. "AIDS in African-American Communities and the Public Health Response: An Overview." *Transforming Anthropology* 4:9–16.

Winant, H.
    1994. *Racial Conditions: Politics, Theory, Comparisons.* Minneapolis: University of Minnesota Press.

Wise, P. H.
    1993. "Confronting Racial Disparities in Infant Mortality: Reconciling Science and Politics." *American Journal of Preventive Medicine* 9 (6): 7–16.

Wolf, E. R.
    1982. *Europe and the People Without History.* Berkeley: University of California Press.

———.
    1994. "Perilous Ideas: Race, Culture, People." *Current Anthropology* 35 (1): 1–9.

Wong, J. K., M. Hezareh, H. F. Günthard, et al.
 1997.   "Recovery of Replication-Competent HIV Despite Prolonged Sup-
          pression of Plasma Viremia." *Science* 278:1291–95.
Woodson, D.
 1997.   "*Lamanjay*, Food Security, Sécurité Alimentaire." *Culture and Agri-
          culture* 19 (3): 108–22.
World Bank.
 1997.   "Confronting the Spread of AIDS." News release 98/1513,
          3 November. Available online at
          http://rocks.worldbank.org/html/extdr/extme/1513.htm.
World Health Organization.
 1978.   "Ebola Hæmorrhagic Fever in Zaïre, 1976. Report of an International
          Commission." *Bulletin of the World Health Organization* 56:271–93.
 ———.
 1991.   *Guidelines for Tuberculosis Treatment in Adults and Children in National
          Tuberculosis Programmes.* Geneva: World Health Organization.
 ———.
 1992a.   "Cholera in the Americas." *Weekly Epidemiological Record* 67:33–39.
 ———.
 1992b.   *Global Health Situation and Projections.* Geneva: World Health
          Organization.
 ———.
 1995a.   *Bridging the Gaps: The World Health Report.* Geneva: World Health
          Organization.
 ———.
 1995b.   *Facing the Challenges of HIV/AIDS/STDs: A Gender-Based Response.*
          Geneva: World Health Organization.
 ———.
 1996.   *Groups at Risk: WHO Report on the Tuberculosis Epidemic.* Geneva:
          World Health Organization.
 ———.
 1997a.   *Anti-Tuberculosis Drug Resistance in the World.* Geneva: World Health
          Organization.
 ———.
 1997b.   "New Report Confirms Global Spread of Drug-Resistant Tuberculo-
          sis." WHO Press Release 74, 22 October.
 ———.
 1997c.   *WHO Report on the Tuberculosis Epidemic.* Geneva: World Health
          Organization.
 ———.
 1998.   *Report on the Global HIV/AIDS Epidemic.* Geneva: World Health
          Organization.

World Health Organization Global Tuberculosis Programme.
   1997.   *TB Treatment Observer*, 24 March, no. 2. (Available at
             http://www.who.int/gtb/publications/treatobserver/issue2.)
Wyatt, G. E.
   1995.   "Transaction Sex and HIV Risks: A Woman's Choice?" Paper pre-
             sented at the conference HIV Infection in Women: Setting a New
             Agenda, 22–24 February, Washington, D.C. Abstract WA1-1.
Yeats, J. R.
   1986.   "Attendance Compliance for Short Course Tuberculosis
             Chemotherapy at Clinics in Estcourt and Surroundings." *South
             African Medical Journal* 30:265–66.
Zierler, S.
   1997.   "Hitting Hard: HIV and Violence." In *Gender Politics of HIV*, edited
             by N. Goldstein and J. Manlowe, pp. 207–21. New York: New York
             University Press.
Zimmerman, T.
   1997.   "Fighting TB: A Second Chance to Do It Right." *U.S. News and
             World Report*, 31 March, p. 45.
Zinsser, H.
   1934.   *Rats, Lice, and History: The Biography of a Bacillus.* Boston:
             Little, Brown.
Zyporyn, T.
   1988.   *Disease in the Popular American Press: The Case of Diphtheria, Typhoid
             Fever, and Syphilis, 1870–1920.* New York: Greenwood Press.

Index